Dr Penny Stanway

Breast is Best

PAN BOOKS

First published 2005 by Pan Books
an imprint of Pan Macmillan Ltd
20 New Wharf Road, London N1 9RR
Basingstoke and Oxford
Associated companies throughout the world
www.panmacmillan.com

Originally published 1978 by Pan Books
as *Breast Is Best* by Drs Andrew and Penny Stanway

ISBN 0 330 43630 9

1 3 5 7 9 8 6 4 2

A CIP catalogue record for this book is available from
the British Library.

Typeset by SetSystems Ltd, Saffron Walden, Essex
Printed and bound in Great Britain by
Mackays of Chatham plc, Chatham, Kent

To Susannah, Amy and Ben

Contents

Acknowledgements

I would like to thank the many women and their helpers from around the world whose shared experiences have enriched this book, and my husband Andrew for his wise comments and his unfailing support.

Preface

Does it matter in the twenty-first century whether babies are breastfed?

It most certainly does. Breastfeeding offers a great many advantages to babies and to their parents, both in developed countries and in developing ones.

Breast Is Best explains these advantages and provides practical guidance on how to breastfeed successfully. The information is based on many women's experiences of breastfeeding; on my own experiences of breastfeeding three babies for a total of over seven years, and of helping thousands of other women to breastfeed; and on a substantial volume of scientific literature from around the world.

This edition is fully revised and updated. Since the first edition twenty-seven years ago, many people have asked why I don't include full scientific and other references. My reasoning is that there are so many, it's more helpful to most people if the available space provides practical information about breastfeeding. Anyone who needs to access the original research papers can do so with the help of a specialist library.

I refer to a baby or a child as 'he' throughout, in the hope that this is more reader-friendly (or, at least, less annoying!) than saying 'he or she', or even 's/he', each time.

ONE

Breastfeeding today

Breastfeeding offers a unique way of being with, responding to and mothering your baby and is endorsed by many official bodies, including the World Health Organization (WHO), the American Academy of Pediatrics and the UK Department of Health. Indeed, in 2001, WHO recommended exclusive breastfeeding (which means giving no other milk or other food or drink) for six months, plus continued breastfeeding for up to two years or beyond. The reason that these endorsements and recommendations are necessary is that women today have a choice over how to feed their babies – they can either breastfeed or give their baby formula.

Once there was no choice – a woman either breastfed or her baby died, unless someone else breastfed for her, but the advent of cows' milk formula feeds in the first half of the twentieth century offered an easy alternative for the first time. This apparent advance has had two worrying results. One is that many babies today have a higher risk of many immediate, short-term and long-term health problems because they are formula-fed. The other is that fewer people are familiar with the womanly art of breastfeeding.

Changes in lifestyle over the last few decades have exerted an important influence too, with the number of babies born each year shrinking, the number born to over-thirties growing, more babies being born to single mums and more women planning to work full-time after their babies are born. Choosing how to feed her baby can have particular implications for an older mum, for a woman who will probably have only one or two babies, and for a woman who is unpartnered or intends going back to work.

When making her feeding choice, a woman might consider the benefits of breastfeeding (or, more aptly, the disadvantages of formula-feeding) to her baby's health, development and contentment, and to her own health, well-being, convenience, purse and relationship with the baby. She might think about how her chosen method of feeding will affect her partner and other children. She'll factor in her previous experiences of feeding, her observations of how other women feed, and her perception of other people's enthusiasm or lack of it for breastfeeding. Lastly, she'll have her own beliefs about how breastfeeding could affect her love life, weight, figure, sleep, self-confidence and freedom, and what it means at a deeper level in terms of loving, giving and receiving.

For you, making the choice may or may not be simple, but it's clearly a vitally important and multifaceted affair. It also offers the potential for better understanding of yourself and of your baby's needs. And with good information and support, nearly all women can breastfeed successfully for as long as they, or their babies, want.

HOW POPULAR IS BREASTFEEDING?

Breastfeeding rates vary widely from one country to another. The following figures represent the proportions of all babies that start off breastfed and those that are still being breastfed at six months.

- Australia: 87 per cent and 48 per cent.
- Italy: 85 per cent and 19 per cent.
- The Netherlands: 75 per cent and 37 per cent.
- Canada: 72 per cent and 31 per cent.
- UK: 71 per cent and 29 per cent.
- US: 70 per cent and 32 per cent.

In Norway, to its great credit, 99 per cent of babies start off breastfed, while Sweden and Denmark at 98 per cent and Ghana with 97 per cent aren't far behind; New Zealand, Poland and Portugal, at 93 per cent, also do very well.

There have been big changes in breastfeeding rates over the years, with gradual improvements in many developed countries over the past ten to fifteen years.

In the US, for example, the most recent figures (above, for 2001) are a great improvement on comparable sets of figures for babies who started off breastfed, and were breastfeeding at six months, in 1990 (51 and 17 per cent) and 1998 (64 and 28 per cent).

In Australia, 87 per cent of babies started off breastfeeding in 1995 and 47 per cent were being breastfed at six months. In contrast, estimates suggest that in the 1970s only 40–45 per cent of babies were being breastfed on discharge from hospital.

In the UK, surveys commissioned by the Department of Health provide an interesting comparison of the numbers of women breastfeeding at different ages from 1975 to 2000. The most recent report, *Infant Feeding 2000*, is published by The Stationery Office, and the following table refers to babies in England and Wales.

	1975	*1980*	*1985*	*1990*	*1995*	*2000*
	%	%	%	%	%	%
Birth	51	67	65	64	68	71
1 week	42	58	56	54	58	57
2 weeks	35	54	53	51	54	54
6 weeks	24	42	40	39	44	43
4 months	13	27	26	25	28	29
6 months	9	23	21	21	22	22
9 months	0	12	11	12	14	14

Overall this shows considerable improvement. Further breakdown of the figures shows that the percentage of mothers who start breastfeeding grew in every part of the UK from 1995 to 2000, but only in Scotland did an increasing percentage carry on breastfeeding. This improvement in Scotland may reflect greater awareness of the benefits of breastfeeding, plus higher levels of enthusiasm and skill among health workers.

However, although the figures in the UK as a whole for the number of women starting to breastfeed are improving over the years, they are still nowhere near the Department of Health's goal for women to breastfeed exclusively, meaning to give no other milk or solid food, for six months. *And they certainly don't meet the World Health Organization recommendation of exclusive breastfeeding for six months and continued breastfeeding for up to two years or beyond.*

WHY NOT BOTTLE-FEED?

Giving babies formula deprives them of the special and unique milk nature intended for them.

Humans have been around for about five million years, yet have reared milk-producing animals only for the last 10,000 or so. Only in the last seventy years has the use of cows' milk as a source of infant food become widespread.

Giving formula based on cows' milk to babies at so crucial a time in their life is an intervention without parallel in our history, and it's so massive and uncontrolled a change that it's been called the greatest uncontrolled trial ever to have been done on humans. For the stark fact is that huge numbers of studies suggest it can be hazardous both to short-term and long-term health.

The first doubts about infant formula arose fairly quickly, when scientists pointed out that compared with breast milk it lacked vitamin B_6, vitamin E and linoleic acid (a fatty acid) and had too much protein, sodium and phosphorus. As the years went by they found breast milk contained high levels of antibodies capable of protecting against disease. They then pointed out that formula doesn't contain the live cells, enzymes and hormones of breast milk, said that protein from milk formula could encourage allergy by leaking from a baby's gut into the blood, and clarified the fact that each mother's milk is designed to meet the needs of her own baby.

Formula manufacturers have repeatedly changed their recipes

to try to keep pace with the ongoing discoveries. There has even been talk of vaccinating cows to give them immunity against human diseases, so that cows'-milk-based formula could protect human babies. But it's simply impossible ever to replicate breast milk.

Given the health benefits of breastfeeding, but the comparatively low rates of doing it, let's look at what can be done to help.

SCHOOL EDUCATION

Nowadays, with most modern families being so small, a girl may reach motherhood without ever seeing a baby at the breast. Yet a girl who sees a baby being breastfed is much more likely to become a breastfeeder later.

So teachers are doing something very valuable if they ask a woman to talk to a biology or parentcraft class about breastfeeding, and, baby permitting, to breastfeed in front of them. It's even better if the father of the breastfeeding baby can come in too. The children also benefit from the opportunity to discuss breastfeeding. The subject can be introduced at any age, and teachers can be creative in the way their class learns. If it's left until the teenage years, many girls and boys in mixed classes are too embarrassed to learn anything much.

The Norwich Joint Breastfeeding Initiative has created breastfeeding education packs for teachers to use with children of different ages (see Appendix).

PROFESSIONAL BACK-UP

While your baby probably won't need to be taught how to feed (because searching for and getting milk from the breast are instinctive behaviours), many women need help and encouragement if they are to succeed with breastfeeding.

Professional helpers have an enormously influential role. For example, studies show that a paediatrician who is enthusiastic about breastfeeding can make all the difference to the numbers of women who breastfeed. They can also encourage other health professionals (and perhaps also cleaners, clerks and others who come into contact with mothers) to work together to make sure their hospital is 'Baby Friendly' (see page 102). Health professionals can also encourage breastfeeding by ensuring that women have good antenatal education, continuous care during childbirth, and early close contact with their newborns. They can make sure mothers in hospital are allowed to have their babies by them all the time (called 'rooming-in') and are offered expert help in positioning their baby at the breast and helping the baby latch on (take the nipple and areola into his mouth). They can encourage unrestricted feeding. And they can also promote women's confidence in themselves as breastfeeders and help them overcome any problems. All these are learnable skills.

Thankfully, breastfeeding education for doctors, midwives and other professional helpers has improved, but it's vital for all helpers to maintain their standards through ongoing in-service training.

FRIENDS, RELATIVES AND NEIGHBOURS

Some older people are more familiar with bottle-feeding than breastfeeding and, while not actively discouraging breastfeeding, may try to persuade a woman that bottle-fed babies are as contented and healthy as breastfed ones. If you have decided to breastfeed, it might help to arm yourself, and ideally your partner too, with information and a positive attitude in case you come into contact with anyone who is unsupportive about your decision. Any country that wants to improve its breastfeeding rates should remember to educate everyone about breastfeeding, not just mothers-to-be and professional helpers.

WORK

Today's young woman is brought up to think of herself as a wage-earner and career woman. When she leaves her parents' home, she'll almost certainly need her income to buy or rent a place of her own, and it may be difficult for her and her partner to surrender this when they have a baby.

Pregnant women tend to think of themselves more in relation to their career and partner than in relation to their unborn baby – the birth is often as far ahead as they see.

But when her baby arrives, a woman comes face to face with the reality of the choice between caring for it, going out to work, or somehow combining the two.

It's often claimed that many mothers don't breastfeed because they return to work so soon. However, in developed countries such as the UK, only a few women return to work while their children are very young, and working mothers breastfeed for as long as those who don't work.

It would be good to have a more realistic and informed debate about the lifestyle choices women face after having a baby, and this is probably best done before pregnancy.

GOVERNMENTS AND NON-GOVERNMENTAL ORGANIZATIONS

Companies selling infant formula and other drinks and foods for babies stand to gain vast amounts of money by pushing their products. But the International Code of Marketing of Breast Milk Substitutes, adopted by the World Health Assembly in 1981, aims to protect breastfeeding by controlling the way these companies market their products. They must not promote formula or feeding bottles and teats. Nor must they promote bottled water, juice, tea, glucose solution or cereal for babies under six months, or promote these products or follow-on milks for babies over six months as a replacement for that part of the diet best met by breast milk. They must also not market any infant food in a way that undermines breastfeeding.

In practice, this means they shouldn't advertise to mothers or health workers, imply their products are equivalent to breast milk, or provide free samples or supplies. Company representatives should make no contact with pregnant women or mothers of young children. There should be no promotion of products through health-care facilities – no posters, leaflets, videos, lectures, or sponsorship of events, for example. There should be no point-of-sale advertising in shops and no discount coupons, premiums, special sales, loss-leaders and tie-in sales. And companies shouldn't give gifts to mothers or health workers. The reason is that all these can provably undermine a mother's knowledge about and confidence in breastfeeding.

Even with the Code in place in many countries, the money put into marketing formula is still hugely more than the amount governments spend on promoting breastfeeding. In the UK in 2001, for example, the government spent £1.60 per baby promoting breastfeeding, while formula companies spent £18.

What we need is for all governments to protect, promote and support breastfeeding meaningfully and wholeheartedly.

We should also applaud non-governmental organizations such as the International Baby Food Action Network for their vitally important work of helping monitor companies' promotional tactics.

MOTHERS' STATUS

Fewer babies are being born in devleoped countries nowadays, and our society doesn't seem to value mothers as it once did, so mothering is seldom seen as a rewarding career in itself. Also, it's widely accepted that childminders, nursery nurses, au pairs, mother's helps and nannies are interchangeable with mothers. Not only have many millions accepted the concept that breast milk isn't essential, but they also seem to think mothers aren't all that important either.

What we need is encouragement for women who have children and breastfeed to think well of themselves for doing a job that is unique for each child, and an invaluable contribution to society.

THE MEDIA

Local and national newspapers and magazines have an important role to play in promoting breastfeeding.

They can do this by featuring the stories and views of breastfeeding women, and by giving space to groups campaigning for public acceptance of breastfeeding, and facilities to make it easier.

PEER SUPPORT

Breastfeeding counsellors or leaders in organizations such as La Leche League, the Australian Breastfeeding Association and, in the UK, the National Childbirth Trust have breastfed for long periods themselves and have also learned from practical experience with many women as well as from books and courses. They are deeply committed to positive attitudes and practices in a way professionals may find hard to equal. They have time to focus on breastfeeding. And they can provide a degree of one-to-one support that few professionals – because of other commitments – can match.

> Choosing to breastfeed is one of the most important choices you'll ever make, and those around you can do a great deal to help you make the choice and breastfeed successfully. Now let's take a look at breast milk – the perfect food.

TWO

Breast milk – the perfect food

Over scores of thousands of years each species of mammal has developed a milk unique to its young. Whale milk, for example, has a very high fat content, making it richer than double cream, because an infant whale needs to form a thick layer of blubber very quickly to protect it from the cold. Rabbit milk has a very high protein content, because protein provides the basic building blocks for growth, and a young rabbit grows particularly fast, doubling its birthweight in about six days. (In contrast, this takes a human baby about 140 days.) Animals whose milk contains large amounts of fat and protein (seals and deer, for example, as well as whales and rabbits) feed their young much less frequently than animals such as dogs, whose milk has less fat and protein. Those whose milk contains very little protein and fat (such as monkeys) carry their young around and feed them almost continuously. Human milk contains relatively little protein but moderate amounts of fat; it also contains more carbohydrate (mainly milk sugar, which is called lactose) than any other milk.

Over the years there have been a few reports of non-human mammals caring for the young of other species and feeding them, or of the occasional baby being fed on another animal's milk. Romulus and Remus, for example, were supposedly reared by a wolf, and people in various countries over the years have used goat, donkey, buffalo, sheep, llama, reindeer, horse and camel milk for their babies. But the first time any mammal used another mammal's milk to any great extent was when we started giving our babies cows' milk early in the twentieth century. So the widespread use of cows' milk is a new phenomenon, and today nearly all infant formulas are made by modifying cows' milk.

Why did we choose cows' milk as a substitute for breast milk? After all, it's by no means the nearest in composition – a donkey's, for example, is much closer. It came about because the great move towards artificial feeding started in the West, where cows were already being reared for meat and dairy produce, so their milk was convenient and cheap. Cows are also easily herded and milked and produce large volumes of milk.

DIFFERENCES BETWEEN BREAST MILK AND COWS' MILK

Ordinary cows' milk – pasteurized or raw, full-cream, semi-skimmed, skimmed, liquid or dry – is unsuitable for babies under six months because it's so different from breast milk. For example, it contains more protein and less sugar. This led doctors and scientists to modify it to resemble breast milk more closely. They did this originally by diluting it with water and adding sugar. This basic modification was used for years, with mothers either adapting ordinary cows' milk by diluting it with water, adding sugar, and then boiling it, or buying dried, evaporated or condensed milk and adding water and sugar. Modern dried milk formula needs only water added. However, over the years more differences between cows' milk and human milk have come to light and companies have made repeated modifications in their never-ending quest to replicate breast milk.

WHAT BREAST MILK CONTAINS

Breast milk, or 'white blood' as it's called in parts of India, is a fascinating fluid that's as much a food as a drink.

Water

Water makes up the main bulk, with the other constituents dissolved or suspended in it, making it white, creamy, translucent or yellow, depending on their proportions. Breast milk is the perfect food for babies because the proportion of water is just right, even if it looks rather watery. A thirsty baby given enough breast milk automatically gets the right amount of water to satisfy his thirst, so a breastfed baby who drinks enough breast milk never needs to drink water, though in very hot weather a breastfeeding *mother* needs to drink more so neither she nor her baby becomes dehydrated. In contrast, a thirsty bottle-fed baby who drinks a lot more formula than usual may risk getting too much of certain substances, especially if bottle-feeds are made up too strong. This can be particularly dangerous for a baby already dehydrated from diarrhoea, vomiting or a fever. Such a baby needs more drinks of water, not more formula, and certainly not more extra-strength formula.

Proteins

About 1.2 per cent of breast milk is protein. This comprises whey proteins – including lactalbumin, lactoglobulin (immunoglobulins or antibodies), lactoferrin, folate- and vitamin B_{12}-binding proteins, enzymes, hormones and growth factors – and curd protein, or casein. Unmodified cows' milk is 3.3 per cent protein.

When milk enters a baby's stomach it becomes curds (made of casein) and whey. Cows' milk contains six times as much casein as whey protein (necessary because a calf grows fast, doubling its birthweight in fifty days), whereas breast milk contains one and a half times as much whey protein as casein. Cows' milk curds are so bulky, tough and rubbery that babies would get indigestion if they were to drink unmodified milk. The main reason why companies dilute cows' milk when making formula is that adding water dilutes the tough indigestible casein. Boiling, homogenization and the addition of various chemicals also make it less tough and indigestible. Some formulas are whey dominant, with a whey:casein ratio similar to that of breast milk; others are casein dominant, with a whey:casein ratio close to that of cows' milk.

In contrast, breast-milk protein in the stomach forms finely separated curds that pass into the small intestine after about one and a half hours. This means a breastfed baby's stomach empties quickly, which is why breastfeds get hungry more quickly and need more frequent feeds. However, cows' milk curds stay in the stomach for about four hours. So four-hourly feeds for a bottle-fed baby are reasonable.

A bottle-fed baby assimilates (makes use of) only about half the nutritional protein in infant formula, whilst a breastfed uses 95 per cent of the nutritional protein in breast milk. The protein a bottle-fed baby doesn't assimilate is partly passed out in the stools (making them bulkier than those of a breastfed baby) and partly broken down and excreted in the urine. Because breast milk produces so little waste, breastfed babies need less milk than formula-fed babies.

Amino acids – All milk contains some free amino acids, as well as those in the form of proteins, but the proportions differ between human and cows' milk. Breast milk, for instance, contains more cystine, cows' milk contains more methionine; this is important, as preterm babies are incapable of using methionine until they become more mature. Cows' milk also contains less taurine than breast milk, which is why it's now added to infant formula.

Nucleotides – These are present in human milk but only in minimal amounts in cows' milk; the main nucleotide in cows' milk, orotic acid, isn't found in human milk at all. Nucelotides are building blocks for proteins and encourage the growth of 'friendly' bowel bacteria. Most babies can make their own nucleotides, but preterms and some full-terms can't make enough. Although scientists aren't aware that any babies have had deficiency problems, formula manufacturers add nucleotides to some products.

Fats

These are the predominant source of energy in both cows' milk and breast milk. They mostly occur as globules of triglyceride fats but are also present in other fatty substances, such as cholesterol, free fatty acids and phospholipids (in lecithin, for example). Fatty acids are the building blocks of fats and are classed as saturated, monounsaturated and polyunsaturated, depending on their structure. Those in breast milk are mainly unsaturated, those in cows' milk mainly saturated. The proportions of fatty acid types in breast and cows' milk reflect the types of fats eaten by the woman or the cows, though some fatty acids are made by breast or udder cells. The amount of fat in milk varies from one woman to another. The fat content of any one woman's milk varies during a feed, with two to three times as much at the end as at the beginning (from the first breast); it also changes over the months after childbirth.

Essential fatty acids – Our bodies can manufacture certain fatty acids that are vital to health but are unable to make certain polyunsaturated fatty acids (PUFAs), which is why they are called essential fatty acids and we must have them in our food.

Fats in general, PUFAs in particular, are necessary for many aspects of growth, especially the development of healthy, PUFA-rich coverings in certain nerve fibres in the brain and spinal cord and in the peripheral nerves.

Breast milk contains a higher percentage of PUFAs (including the essential fatty acid linoleic acid) than does cows' milk. Cows' milk formula contains enough of this to prevent deficiency symptoms of poor growth and thick scaly skin, but some formula manufacturers replace some of the saturated fat of cows' milk with vegetable oil in order to increase the PUFA content of a formula. There are two groups of PUFAs, omega-6s and omega-3s, and the amounts and proportions of these differ between breast milk and infant formula.

— Certain PUFAs are found only in breast milk. These are the ones with a 'long-chain' structure, such as DHA (docosahexanoic acid, an omega-3) and AA (arachidonic acid, an omega-6). These are also referred to as LCPs – long-chain polyunsaturated fatty acids. These fatty acids are important for brain, eye and nerve development. Indeed, about one-quarter of a baby's brain is made of DHA and AA! Interestingly, researchers have discovered that breastfed babies of women whose milk is relatively high in DHA sleep better than do those of women with lower levels.

Cows' milk formula also contains highly variable amounts, if any, of alpha-linolenic acid. Even if a formula contains enough alpha-linolenic and linoleic acids – the 'parent' PUFAs of the omega-6s and omega-3s from which healthy full-term babies make DHA, AA and other long-chain PUFAs – some bottle-fed babies, whether full-term or preterm, can't make these fast enough. Neither full-term nor preterm bottle-fed babies necessarily get enough DHA for optimal eyesight development from the usual types of formula. And preterm formula-fed babies may not get enough AA for optimal growth or mental development. Breastfed babies, in contrast, get all the DHA and AA they need from breast milk.

World Health Organization experts advised in 1978 that AA and DHA are desirable components of milk formula, but nothing was done. Recently, however, other scientists have recommended adding them to preterm formula, preferably in the same proportions as in breast milk, and questioned whether full-term formula-fed babies might benefit from a similar change. However, making the PUFA-profile of formula similar to that of breast milk is expensive. Nonetheless, some formulas – including most of those especially made for preterm babies and, in the UK, one made for full-term babies – are now enriched with these fatty acids.

Researchers wonder whether the amounts and ratio of saturated and monounsaturated fats and PUFAs in breast milk help protect a baby against heart disease and other arterial disease in later life. Evidence is lacking, but we do know there's more of another fat, cholesterol, in breast milk than in cows' milk, which may accustom babies to handling it. This could stand them in good stead in future and might even reduce the risk of heart disease later on.

Gut enzymes called lipases split fats into simpler fatty substances. The digestion of cows' milk fat by lipase releases palmitic acid, a fatty acid that combines with calcium before leaving the body in the bowel motions, so removing calcium. In human milk, palmitic acid is built into fat particles in such a way that when fat is digested, the palmitic acid is absorbed into the blood with part of the broken-down fat particle. This means calcium isn't lost, which is important because babies need plentiful calcium to build strong bones and teeth.

Human milk contains some lipase of its own, unlike cows' milk which relies solely on the baby's gut lipase for its digestion. The fat in breast milk starts being digested by milk lipase even before it reaches the gut. This means valuable fatty acids are available sooner from breast milk than from formula.

The digestion of both breast and cows' milk fats in a baby's stomach produces fatty acids as well as other, simpler, fats which help protect babies from infection.

If a breastfed baby brings up any milk, the smell isn't particularly unpleasant, whereas a bottle-fed baby's vomit has a much sourer smell which quickly permeates clothing. The difference is due to the presence in formula of a fatty acid called butyric acid, which smells nasty when partially digested.

Carbohydrates

Both breast and cows' milks contain lactose (milk sugar) but breast milk has more (7 g per 100 g of milk compared with 4.8 g). Up to 95 per cent of breast-milk carbohydrate is lactose, which is why it tastes so sweet. Given the choice between breast milk and formula, babies prefer breast milk, probably partly because it's sweeter. Some of the lactose is split into the simple sugars galactose and glucose in the gut. The rest, which travels through undigested, improves calcium absorption and encourages a healthy balance of micro-organisms in the large bowel. Galactose is an important constituent of the myelin coating of nerves, and besides getting it from breast milk a baby can make it from glucose in the liver.

Both breast milk and formula contain glucose, though some other sugars found in breast milk are completely absent, or present in much lower quantities, in formula.

Breast milk contains around twenty-five oligosaccharides, while formula contains only a very small amount of some of these sugars and none of others. Oligosaccharides seem to encourage a healthy population of micro-organisms in the gut, and protect against harmful bacteria by preventing them sticking to the gut lining. Also, when there's breast milk in the mouth and throat during and after a feed, its oligosaccharides help prevent bacteria such as pneumococci and *Haemophilus influenzae* (which can cause respiratory infections) sticking to the throat. They also help prevent urine infections.

Minerals

Cows' milk contains almost four times as many minerals as breast milk, which is one reason it has to be modified into infant formula or it might overload a baby's kidneys.

Infant formula has a much lower mineral content but in no formula is this as low as in breast milk.

Sodium – The amount in breast milk is ideal for babies. The level in infant formula is lower than in fresh cows' milk but higher than in breast milk. Sodium is closely linked with water in the body and an imbalance can be serious and even fatal. This is why formula-fed babies need particular care if they become dehydrated and why formula must never be made up too strong.

Calcium and magnesium – The levels are higher in cows' milk than in breast milk, but have been reduced in modern formulas. There's a little less calcium in breast milk than in modern formulas, but babies absorb breast-milk calcium more efficiently than that from formula, possibly because the high lactose level of breast milk promotes its transfer from gut to blood.

Phosphorus – There's less phosphorus in breast milk than in infant formula. Also, the amount in breast milk changes as a baby grows older, while that in formula remains constant.

Iron – This is present in larger amounts (twice as much) in breast milk than in cows' milk, though the levels in formula are higher than in breast milk because it is fortifed with iron. A fully breastfed full-term baby of a healthy mother almost never becomes anaemic in the first six months, partly because breastfed babies absorb about half the iron in breast milk, whereas bottle-fed babies absorb only one-tenth of that in formula. Vitamins C and E, lactose and copper, present in higher amounts in breast milk, encourage more efficient absorption of iron, and breast milk's relatively low concentration of proteins, calcium and phosphorus helps too.

Fluoride – See page 58.

Trace elements – These minerals include copper, zinc, manganese, chromium, cobalt, molybdenum, selenium, iodine, silicon and boron. Many are essential for babies as they form parts of enzymes. There's generally enough of most of them in breast milk and in infant formula, but breast milk may be low in selenium, which is an antioxidant (see **Vitamin A**, page 22), if a woman doesn't eat enough selenium-containing food. It's also possible that some formulas could be improved by having more selenium.

Vitamins

Breast milk contains more vitamins A, C and E than does cows' milk, but less vitamin K. In women who are well nourished in pregnancy and who eat a well-balanced diet while breastfeeding, evidence suggests that their fully breastfed babies don't normally need any vitamin supplements in the first six months.

Vitamin A – Both breast milk and cows' milk contain vitamin A and carotenoids. Carotenoids are yellowish substances that the body can make into vitamin A and also use as antioxidants to protect cells from damage by free radicals (unstable oxygen particles) during illness and stress, for example. Breast milk provides substantial amounts of vitamin A. Beta-carotene forms 24 per cent of the carotenoids in breast milk and 85 per cent of those in cows' milk; other carotenoids in breast milk include lycopene and beta-cryptoxanthine, but many remain unidentified. The amount of carotenoids varies considerably from one woman to another; it also varies in any one woman according to how many babies she's had and what she's eaten throughout the day.

Vitamin C – This is concentrated in breast milk, so the baby of a healthy mother who eats a healthy diet needs no extra. Even the babies of women with a vitamin-C deficiency aren't themselves deficient in vitamin C – it is only the mother who needs supplements of vitamin C.

Vitamin D – This enables minerals such as calcium to enter and strengthen bones, helping prevent rickets (soft, bendy bones). Colostrum (the milk made in the week or so after delivery) contains more vitamin D than does mature milk, but vitamin-D-fortified formula has much more than either. The amount of this vitamin in a breastfeeding woman's diet has only a small influence on her baby's vitamin-D level. Sunshine on the skin is a far better source for a breastfeeding mother and her baby than is the mother's food or the baby's milk; skin produces vitamin D after exposure to daylight and the body stores it for use in the darker months.

However, there isn't always enough vitamin D available from breast milk or daylight to strengthen a baby's bones, which is why all preterm and some full-term breastfed babies benefit from a supplement. This is especially important if the mother is malnourished or eats a vegetarian diet containing a lot of chapattis (chapatti flour contains substances which prevent calcium being absorbed). A supplement may also be important for breastfed babies whose mothers go outside very little, or always cover their skin outside and so get little exposure to bright daylight. However, some can solve the problem simply by getting more daylight on their skin. Also, babies whose faces are exposed to bright outdoor daylight for just a quarter of an hour each day in the summer months (in the UK, the US and countries at similar latitudes) make enough of their own vitamin D.

Vitamin K – Breast milk contains less of this than cows' milk does. Some babies suffer from haemorrhagic disease of the newborn, due to a shortage of vitamin K. This makes the gut bleed and is more common in breastfed babies. Many doctors recommend vitamin K after birth, either by injection, by mouth, or by both, for all newborns, whether or not the mother breastfeeds. It's worth pointing out that a woman who breastfeeds frequently is likely to produce more milk – and therefore more vitamin K – more quickly than a woman who breastfeeds according to a schedule.

Anti-infective factors

Many factors besides antibodies help fight infection.

The proportion of nutrients in breast milk compared with that in formula prevents the growth in the baby's gut of certain potentially harmful organisms, including *E. coli* (a common cause of gastro-enteritis in formula-fed babies) and dysentery and typhoid bacteria; the high lactose, low phosphorus and low protein levels are particularly helpful.

Micro-organisms – A baby's gut contains a huge number of micro-organisms. These vary from one baby to another and account for the unpleasant smell of a formula-fed baby's bowel motions compared with the sweeter smell of those of a breastfed baby. Many researchers report that the organisms in the breastfed baby's bowel are predominantly lactobacilli. These produce acetic and lactic acids which together prevent the growth of many disease-producing organisms such as *E. coli*, dysentery bacilli and candida

– yeast-like organisms that cause thrush. However, the balance of micro-organisms may vary according to whether a baby was full-term, the type of delivery, and whether he has had antibiotics.

The bifidus factor (also called gynolactose) is a mixture of ten oligosaccharides and there's about forty times as much of it in human milk as in cows' milk. It promotes the growth of lactobacilli, encouraging a healthy balance of micro-organisms in the gut, and may interfere with flu viruses too.

Lactoferrin – Colostrum and mature milk are unusually rich in this important anti-infective, iron-binding whey protein. Lactoferrin constitutes up to 25 per cent of breast-milk protein and there's ten to twenty times more of it in breast milk than in cows' milk. Lactoferrin mops up a potentially harmful excess of iron. Also, test-tube experiments show that together with immunoglobulin A (see below), it inhibits the growth of many potentially harmful organisms, including *E. coli*, yeasts, *Staphylococcus aureus* and, perhaps, viruses, by robbing them of the iron they need. Lactoferrin also kills some micro-organisms, makes some bacteria more susceptible to damage by lysozyme (see opposite), and has some anti-parasitic, anti-tumour and anti-inflammatory power.

Lactoferrin, like antibodies and enzymes, loses its anti-infective activity when milk is boiled, so the small amount present in fresh cows' milk becomes useless when this is processed into formula.

Dutch scientists are breeding dairy cows descended from a bull called Herman whose genetic material contains a human gene for lactoferrin. They hope to use lactoferrin-rich milk from these cows to make formula milk.

Immunoglobulins – These are specialized proteins, called antibodies, that help protect against infection. Immunoglobulin A – or IgA – is the most abundant; others include IgD, IgE, IgG and IgM, and colostrum contains especially large amounts. Breast-milk antibodies coat the gut lining and prevent many infective organisms and other large protein molecules from entering the blood; they can also be absorbed into the blood. Breast-milk IgA helps combat bacterial, fungal and viral illnesses from which the mother has suffered (for example, tetanus, whooping cough, pneumonia, diphtheria, *E. coli* gastro-enteritis, typhoid, dysentery, flu, rubella, polio and various other viral illnesses). It may also protect against infections to which the mother has been immunized, though any such protection is unpredictable. And it can protect against certain food antigens (food proteins that can trigger ill health in sensitive babies).

A growing baby gradually begins to manufacture its own antibodies in response to infection or immunization, with a full-term baby's gut cells sometimes beginning to make IgA at around twelve days, though the concentration of IgA-producing cells in a baby's gut doesn't reach the adult level until he is two years old. The early period of gradually increasing antibody formation by a baby is called the 'immunity gap'. This can be filled only by breast milk. This is because although cows' milk also contains antibodies, heating during formula manufacture renders them inactive.

Interestingly, calves reared on heat-treated milk or dried milk powder get more enteritis than those drinking fresh untreated milk. The treatment is fresh cows' milk! A parallel was seen in a nursery of formula-fed babies in Belgrade, where an epidemic of *E. coli* gastro-enteritis couldn't be stopped even when the babies were fed with donated and boiled breast milk. Not until breast milk was given unboiled was it controlled.

Lysozyme and complement – These proteins interact with IgA to kill bacteria and viruses. Lysozyme is present in breast milk in amounts 300 times greater than in cows' milk and has been dubbed a 'natural antibiotic'. Breast milk lysozyme levels fall in the first few months, then rise until at six months there is more than there was in colostrum, and at one year there is even more.

Anti-staphylococcal factor and hydrogen peroxide – These are present in breast milk and cows' milk, and together with vitamin C, they kill bacteria such as *E. coli*.

Fibronectin is a protein that encourages white cells to mop up harmful bacteria, and reduces any inflammation. The large amounts of fibronectin in colostrum explain why breastfed babies have higher levels in their blood than do formula-fed babies.

Live cells – These are white cells similar to some of those in blood, and they make breast milk a living fluid. Fresh cows' milk also contains living cells, but these are killed when the milk is processed into formula. White cells from a single breastfeed can stick to the gut lining and remain there for sixty hours. White cells called lymphocytes make antibodies as well as an antiviral substance called interferon, and can be absorbed into the blood where they continue making antibodies. Researchers believe hormonal and other factors in breastfeeding women send IgA-producing lymphocytes (T-cells) from the lymph tissue in her gut to her breasts. This means that her milk's lymphocytes know about the potentially harmful organisms in her bowel and can protect her baby from them. What's more, they 'remember' past infections and protect against new attacks for many years.

Neutrophils, granulocytes and epithelial cells are other live cells found in breast milk. They are present in even larger amounts in colostrum.

Macrophages are large cells that can engulf foreign particles such as bacteria. They also produce lactoferrin, lysozyme and complement, may help transport antibodies, and are thought to protect against a dangerous disorder in preterm babies called necrotizing enterocolitis.

Mucins – These large proteins are probably responsible for half the antiviral activity of breast milk. They contain protein and carbohydrate that can stick to unwanted bacteria and viruses and carry them from the body in the bowel motions. They are especially active against the rotaviruses that are often responsible for diarrhoea. Older babies make mucins in their gut. The mucins in cows' milk are removed during formula manufacture. One reseacher has suggested that if mucins could be synthesized they would make a useful addition to formula.

Hormones

Breast milk contains many hormones, hormone-releasing factors and hormone-like factors, including insulin, prolactin, corticosteroids, relaxin, oestrogens, progesterone, gonadotrophins, gonadotrophin-releasing hormone, thyroid hormones, thyroid-releasing and thyroid-stimulating hormones, parathyroid hormone and erythropoietin. Some come from the mother's blood, others are made in the breast.

Some of these hormones may stimulate the breast to make milk proteins and enzymes. Others, including insulin, prolactin, thyroxine and thyroid-stimulating hormone, are thought to be important to the baby.

Erythropoietin is a hormone in milk that helps regulate red cell production, and it's possible, though unproven, that it helps protect preterm babies from anaemia.

Prostaglandins

These hormone-like substances are found in breast milk but not in formula. A baby who gets a good balance of omega-3 and omega-6 polyunsaturated fatty acids can make a healthy balance of prostaglandins himself.

The concentration of certain prostaglandins (E and F) in breast milk is one hundred times that in a woman's plasma (the liquid part of blood). One function may be to help a baby absorb zinc from breast milk, which would explain the protective effect of breast milk against the rare inherited ulcerating skin disease acrodermatitis enteropathica.

Growth factors

Breast milk contains many growth factors. Epidermal growth factor, for example, is a hormone-like polypeptide (protein fragment) that stimulates the multiplication and development of several cells, including those in the gut lining. There's a lot of this in colostrum and researchers consider it particularly valuable for very immature preterm babies. There is very much less in infant formula.

Enzymes

More than seventy enzymes have been identified in breast milk. Some are important for a baby's digestion or development, and most are present in highest concentration in colostrum. Lipase has already been mentioned. Lactoperoxidase inhibits bacterial growth. Others include lysozyme, xanthine oxidase, aldolase, alkaline and acid phosphatases, anti-trypsin, amylase, glutathione peroxidase and catalase. Enzymes are destroyed by heating, which is one reason why any breast milk you express or pump for your own baby should ideally not be heated above body temperature, particularly if the baby is preterm. Most enzymes in cows' milk are destroyed by heating during the manufacture of formula.

Food traces, drugs, perfumes and environmental contaminants

Breast milk may contain such things as alcohol; caffeine from coffee, tea and caffeinated soft drinks; and trace amounts of whole food-protein molecules. It may also contain certain drugs taken by a breastfeeding woman, and certain perfume ingredients, such as musk.

Some newspapers made a lot of fuss in 2004 when they discovered breast milk could contain environmental contaminants to which a mother had been exposed via food or air, such as dioxins. But the good news is that the levels of these substances in breast milk are decreasing. Anyway, the many advantages of breastfeeding are thought greatly to outweigh any possibility of harm; experts believe breast milk may make such substances less potentially harmful; formula can contain these substances too; and formula-feeding is well known to have many possible disadvantages to a baby's health.

COLOURED MILK

Milk varies in colour. For example, colostrum is yellower than mature milk, and the milk produced early in a feed – especially from the first breast – tends to be more translucent than the later milk. However, very occasionally other colours are seen.

Yellow milk – Taking a supplement of beta-carotene (used by the body to make vitamin A) can colour milk yellow. Probably eating a large number of satsumas on a daily basis could do so too, as this can temporarily colour skin yellowish orange.

Red, pink, brown, orange or otherwise blood-stained milk – Seeing blood in your milk can be a shock, but it's rarely anything to worry about. Check your breasts and, if you are concerned about anything, consult your doctor. A cracked or sore nipple is the most likely cause of blood in milk.

Some women have blood-staining in the first week after delivery with no sign of anything else wrong. This is rare, generally disappears within two to five days and doesn't harm the baby. You can continue breastfeeding. The most likely cause, according to one researcher, is a tendency for the blood vessels to leak red blood cells; milk normally contains a few anyway, but quite a lot are needed to colour it.

Blood in milk occasionally comes from a tumour. This is almost always non-cancerous and the discoloration stops once breastfeeding is well under way. Discuss with your doctor whether investigations are necessary.

Green milk – Milk can go green if a woman takes the iron-containing drug called ferritin.

Milk of assorted hues – If milk stagnates in a blocked duct or in a milk-retention cyst (a cyst that gradually develops behind the block in an untreated blocked duct), it can turn one of many colours, including deep yellow, brown, green and even blue-black.

This results from the presence of various substances, including cholesterol, cholesterol 5,6-epoxides, oestrogens, and fluorescent compounds – including lipofucsin complexes – from oxidized fats. A smoker's milk may be even darker.

HOW BREAST MILK CHANGES

The composition of breast milk varies according to the time since childbirth and the time of day; it also varies during a feed. A calf feeding from its mother also benefits from similar changes in its mother's milk. However, a formula-fed baby drinks milk of a highly consistent composition, because milk from many cows, at different stages of lacatation and at different times of day, is pooled to make milk formula. Breast milk, on the other hand, is supplied on a one-off basis direct from producer to consumer and varies in composition considerably in any one woman over time and from one woman to another. These variations are important to the individual baby.

Studies in France and England have found that a baby turns to a pad that has been placed next to his mother's breast in preference to a clean pad that has no milk on it and hasn't been in contact with the breast. And they show that it's the contact of the pad with the breast skin itself that's most important, because babies don't turn to pads soaked in their mother's expressed breast milk. Babies prefer the smell of their own mother's breast to that of other mothers'. And one study found that twenty-two out of thirty babies preferred the smell of their mother's breast when it hadn't been washed. What it is on the mother's breast that enables this unique recognition isn't known, but it could be natural hormone-like substances called pheromones.

Bottle-fed babies like the smell of a pad soaked in breast milk, whoever it's from, better than that of a pad soaked in their usual milk formula.

Colostrum – This is the first milk a woman produces, and it's made from about halfway through pregnancy until up to a week or so after childbirth. It is rich in protein (nine times as much as in mature milk), certain amino acids, minerals (including calcium, magnesium, zinc), vitamins A, E, B_6 and B_{12} and epidermal growth factor, and has less sugar than later milk. It also has less fat but is particularly rich in DHA. Most important, colostrum contains large amounts of antibodies, which give the newborn baby resistance to infection at a time when he would otherwise be particularly susceptible.

Formula-fed babies don't get cows' colostrum, yet cows' colostrum (known as beestings) is considered so vital for calves that farmers save it for them or even buy it if necessary.

Colostrum often leaks from the nipples in the second half of pregnancy and looks yellow because of its high levels of beta-carotene. It speeds the passage of meconium – the sticky, tar-like early bowel motions – through a baby's gut, reducing the absorption of bile pigments, naturally occurring substances that might encourage newborn jaundice.

A few days after birth, colostrum becomes more milky and is sometimes called transitional milk. This gradually changes further to become mature milk. The amount of colostrum is not fixed, so expressing it antenatally doesn't reduce the supply available to the baby. Letting a baby suck frequently and for as long as he wants in the first few days not only provides more of this valuable colostrum but also hastens the production of mature milk.

Mature milk – This contains one-fifth of the protein of colostrum but more fat and sugar, and is thinner and whiter. A baby grows fastest in the first six months, when breast milk's protein level is highest, but the protein content gradually falls during the first year.

The content of the milk varies according to the mother's diet, the frequency of feeds and the age of her baby. Early in a feed from the first breast the milk usually tends to be relatively low in fat and look relatively thin and white or bluish white, and it contains around ten calories per 25 ml (1 fl oz). Later in the feed from that breast the milk usually tends to have more fat (up to two or three times as much) and more protein (up to one and a half times as much), making it look thicker and creamy-white, and giving it a different 'mouth-feel' for the baby, as it's more viscous and coats the mouth more. It contains around thirty calories per ounce. The increase in fat content occurs gradually throughout a feed.

The differences in the content, appearance and mouth-feel of milk at the beginning and end of a feed are less dramatic in the second breast, because let-downs of milk from the milk glands (see page 125) during the feed from the first breast mean this let-down milk mixes with the milk already in the ducts and reservoirs. The milk in the ducts and reservoirs at the beginning of a feed is sometimes known as foremilk, and the milk present towards the end of a feed is sometimes called hindmilk.

The changing composition of milk during a feed means a baby who feeds at the first breast as long as he or she wants finishes that side with higher-fat milk. If he then wants to feed from the second breast, the milk will be relatively thinner at first, but not as thin as the first milk from the first breast.

Milk removed from the breast by the strong milking and sucking action of a well latched-on baby tends to be higher in fat than milk that's let down without being milked by a baby or by hand expression. Higher-fat milk stays in the stomach and gut longer, so it satisfies a baby for longer, meaning he's likely to need fewer feeds than a baby who may get the same volume but doesn't suck or milk so strongly.

The fat concentration in breast milk is lowest in the early hours of the morning.

After the first few weeks many breastfeeding women produce around 700–940 ml (about 25–33 UK fl oz) of milk a day.

Monthly changes when periods return – When a mother eventually starts to ovulate again, her milk will alter slightly before and after ovulation. Five to six days before ovulation (which usually occurs between the tenth and fourteenth days of the cycle – the twelfth day of the average cycle – counting from the first day of a period) the milk changes in composition for between thirty and forty hours; a similar change happens six to seven days after ovulation. In both cases there's temporarily less lactose, glucose and potassium, and more sodium and chloride. Some experienced breastfeeders believe babies notice these changes. Others report a temporary decrease in milk supply, or a less reliable let-down reflex, around the time of a period.

Towards the end of breastfeeding – As a baby breastfeeds less and less, the mother's milk dwindles and looks thicker, yellower and more like colostrum.

Preterm milk – Mothers of preterm babies produce 'preterm milk'. This has a different composition from mature milk, with around 30 per cent more protein and higher concentrations of many minerals (including sodium, calcium and iron) and of lipase. As the baby grows, the milk gradually changes to meet his changing needs.

Breast milk is different from formula, however much this is modified. No longer is it reasonable for anyone to claim formula is close to breast milk – now we know better. In the next chapter we'll see why these differences matter to babies.

THREE

Best for baby?

Experts around the world strongly recommend breastfeeding as the best way of feeding babies.

THE PERFECT FOOD

Chapter 2 detailed the unique composition that makes breast milk the perfect food for babies.

Breastfeeding also has many other advantages to a baby's health. Let's look at some of the enormous and mounting evidence from around the world that it's the very best way of feeding your baby.

LESS OBESITY

A formula-fed baby has a statistically greater chance of being fat, and some studies, though not all, suggest that adolescents who were breastfed are less likely to be overweight or obese.

Does this matter? Well, it could, because up to one in five fat babies are still fat at five years old, and about 14 per cent of very fat babies (weighing over the ninetieth percentile for their age) are still obese twenty to thirty years later. The concern is that very overweight adults are more prone to heart disease, high blood pressure, diabetes, varicose veins and gallstones and, as a result, have a reduced life expectancy.

- A Scottish study (2002) found that breastfed babies were less likely to become obese in childhood.
- A large US study (2001) found that babies who received more breast milk than formula, or who were breastfed for longer periods, had a lower risk of being overweight in adolescence.

LESS ILLNESS

Babies who are breastfed – and especially those who are exclusively breastfed – are less likely to become ill in their first year and less likely to be admitted to hospital. Even more important, breastfeeding can save lives.

- The United Nations Children's Fund (UNICEF) estimates that reversing the decline in breastfeeding could save 1.5 million lives a year worldwide.
- A US study (2004) suggested that breastfeeding cuts by up to 38 per cent the risk of a baby dying in the first year.
- Research in 2001 suggested that exclusively breastfeeding babies for at least three months, and continuing to breastfeed for the rest of the first year, could prevent 52,000 infant deaths a year in Latin America alone.

FEWER INFECTIONS

Breast milk helps protect a baby from infection by bacteria, viruses, yeasts and other organisms. But just how important is this today, with hygiene precautions for bottle-feeding so good and treatment for infections so advanced?

Developing countries

Feeding with formula is risky, even life-threatening, for two-thirds of the world's babies. This is because the lack of adequate hygiene, sanitation and facilities for sterilizing bottle-feeding equipment means there is an extremely high risk of infective diarrhoea (gastro-enteritis). Also, formula contains few anti-infective factors, and poverty frequently means the family simply can't afford sufficient milk powder.

The combination of diarrhoea, dehydration and malnutrition is known as bottle-baby disease and is a frequent killer.

- An analysis (2000) of studies in Brazil, The Gambia, Ghana, Pakistan, the Phillipines and Senegal concluded that babies who aren't breast-fed are six times more likely to die from an infection in their first two months of life.

Developed countries

Even here infections are less likely in breastfed babies. Critics say that illness protection from breastfeeding is minimal in developed countries. However, part of the smallish DARLING study (1995) of babies born to relatively affluent families in the US, and fully breastfed or formula-fed for the first year, found that even here the protection breastfeeding gives against illness is significant to public health.

Diarrhoea (infective diarrhoea/gastro-enteritis)

This is much more likely in formula-fed babies.

For example:

- A review (2002) of twenty studies from around the world found that gastrointestinal infection was more common in formula-fed babies.
- A Brazilian study (2000) found that exclusively breastfed babies were eight times less likely to have diarrhoea.
- In California, in the DARLING study (1995), exclusively breastfed babies had only half as many attacks of diarrhoea in the first year as formula-fed babies.
- A study in Mexico (1992) found that breastfed babies were five times less likely than formula-fed babies to develop diarrhoea from infection from protozoa called giardia.

Also:

- Doctors in Calcutta, India (1995) reported that babies and young children with diarrhoea were nearly seven times more likely to become dehydrated if formula-fed.

It's a common misconception among mothers and health workers that milk formula is sterile. But it isn't:

- A study in the UK (2004) analysed eighty-two samples of powdered infant formula and found that eight contained stomach bacteria.

One problem with formula is that the number of bacteria it contains doubles every half-hour it's left at room temperature. Even in the fridge, the number doubles every ten hours.

Respiratory infections

In developing countries breastfeeding helps protect babies from bronchiolitis (infection in the lungs' small airways) and pneumonia. The evidence from developed countries is mixed.

- An analysis (2003) of thirty-three studies found that formula-fed babies were more than three times at risk of needing hospital treatment for respiratory infections (and asthma) compared with breastfeds.
- An Australian study (2002) found that breastfeeding for at least six months, and continued breastfeeding for up to a year, reduced the risk of respiratory infection.
- A Saudi Arabian study (2001) found that the longer a child was breastfed, the fewer respiratory infections he had.
- A Brazilian study (1999) found that one in eighteen young children admitted to hospital for pneumonia were formula-fed.
- A large Canadian study (1995) reported fewer respiratory illnesses in breastfed babies.
- In Italy (1994) babies with pneumonia or bronchiolitis were much more likely to be formula-fed.
- Swedish research (1994) found that breastfed babies had fewer colds and other upper respiratory infections.

- A large US study (1993) reported that breastfeeding helped protect children aged under two years from pneumonia.
- A large study in Dundee, Scotland (1990) found that breastfeeding for thirteen weeks or more significantly reduced the risk of respiratory infection.

Middle ear infection (otitis media)

Many studies report less middle ear infection in breastfed babies. The duration of any protective effect depends on how how long breastfeeding continues. This is important because not only is middle ear infection painful but it can also lead to deafness. Also, bacteria from infected middle ears can slide along the Eustachian tubes to the throat, be swallowed and cause diarrhoea. They can also slide down the throat to the lungs, leading to lung infection.

There are three reasons why breastfed babies have a lower risk of middle ear infection. Firstly, breastfeeding mothers tend to hold their babies more upright than do bottle-feeding mothers, so milk is less likely to escape from the throat along the Eustachian tubes to the middle ear cavities, where it can encourage infection. Secondly, anti-infective and anti-inflammatory factors in breast milk reduce the risk of infection developing in milk that enters the middle ear. Thirdly, the way a breastfed baby sucks and milks the breast tends to open up the Eustachian tubes, encouraging fluid to drain from the middle ears and making infection less likely – and this doesn't happen with bottle-feeding.

- In California, the DARLING study (1995) found that the rate of middle ear infections in exclusively breastfed babies was 19 per cent lower than in formula-fed ones, and the percentage of prolonged attacks (more than ten days) was 80 per cent lower. In the second year, any middle ear infections that did occur lasted nearly three days less in babies that had been breastfed.
- Dutch research (1994) reported that breastfeeding significantly reduced the risk of middle ear infection in the first four months. When a mother stopped breastfeeding, her baby's risk of ear infec-

tion gradually increased until twelve months after stopping, when the risk was the same as if that baby had never been breastfed.

- A Swedish study (1994) reported that breastfeeding decreased the risk of middle ear infection at two, six and ten months.

Urine infections

These are less likely in breastfed babies. One reason is that oligosaccharides (simple types of sugar) in breast milk make *E. coli* bacteria less able to cause trouble by sticking to the bladder lining.

Another reason is that a breastfed baby's urine contains more IgA, lactoferrin and lysozme than that of a formula-fed baby. These can't have come from breast milk as they aren't absorbed by a baby's gut, so they must have been made in the baby's urinary system. This means breastfeeding must encourage a better immune response in the urinary system.

- Welsh research (1994) noted that breastfed babies had higher levels of IgA antibodies in their urine at ten days.
- A Mexican study (1992) reported that preterm babies were five times more likely to have a urine infection if formula-fed.
- A Swedish study (1990) reported that children with a kidney infection tended to have been exclusively breastfed for a shorter time than healthy children.
- An Italian study (1990) reported that babies of up to six months with urine infections were nearly twice as likely to be formula-fed.

Sticky eye

Baterial infection of the front of the eye – conjunctivitis or 'sticky eye' – is common in newborn babies. Women in developing countries, including India, Jamaica, Brazil and countries in the Middle East and north Africa, often put a few drops of colostrum in their baby's eyes to counter this infection. This may reduce the need for antibiotic eye drops or ointment. Interestingly, an eighteenth-century London pharmacopoeia says, 'Breast milk . . . cureth Red Eye immediately'.

- Research from New Delhi (1982) reported that putting breast milk in the eyes reduces eye infections.

Meningitis

A study in 1986 found that breastfed babies of three months or younger are less likely to get meningitis.

Septicaemia

Breastfed babies are less likely to suffer from septicaemia (blood poisoning).

- A study in Pakistan (1991) reported that even partial breastfeeding was a great help in protecting against septicaemia.

Necrotizing enterocolitis

This rare but potentially fatal bowel infection is more common in babies who are preterm, tube-fed or formula-fed.

- Research in Cambridge, England (1990) found it was up to ten times more common in exclusively formula-fed babies than in exclusively breastfed babies. Babies fed both formula and breast milk had three times the risk of exclusively breastfed babies. The protection from donated and pasteurized breast milk was as effective as that from a baby's own mother's milk.

Researchers suspect that freshly expressed or pumped milk is more protective than frozen breast milk.

Better response to immunization

Breastfed babies make more antibodies when they are immunized, possibly because breastfeeding makes their immune system mature more quickly.

- A study in the *Lancet* (1990) which looked at antibody levels in babies immunized with *Haemophilus influenzae* type b vaccine (Hib vaccine) at two, four and six months found that at seven and twelve months breastfed babies had significantly higher levels of antibodies to Hib than formula-fed babies.

FEWER ALLERGIC DISEASES

Many studies, though not all, suggest that exclusive breastfeeding for the first few months helps prevent allergy. It may also help prevent the more common type of food sensitivity or intolerance that results from a non-allergic slow-onset immune response to food.

Food allergy and non-allergic food sensitivity

A food allergy involves the body producing protective IgE antibodies and leads to a rapid response to the food in question, with symptoms within hours. In contrast, a non-allergic immune reaction to food probably involves the production of IgG antibodies, and has a slow onset, with symptoms taking a minimum of two or three days and sometimes a week or more to appear after eating the culprit food.

Three factors encourage allergy:

1 **An inherited risk** – If there's allergy in the family – especially both sides of the family – a baby has an increased risk of eczema, asthma, hay fever and food allergy in general. Doctors call this sort of allergy 'atopy'.

2 **Diarrhoea** – Babies who develop food allergy have often had many more attacks of diarrhoea than non-food-allergic babies. Breastfeeding makes diarrhoea less likely.

3 **Allergy triggers** – A young baby's immune system is immature, and exposure to allergy triggers can sensitize a susceptible baby and make him prone to allergy then or later. Triggers include food proteins, house-dust-mite droppings, viral infection, smoky or

otherwise polluted air, and certain pollens and moulds. The trigger that first sensitizes a baby is called the primary allergy trigger.

Cows' milk protein – the most common primary allergy trigger

It isn't surprising that cows' milk protein is the most common primary trigger, as it's the first foreign food protein many babies get, and it's given in very large amounts.

- French research (1994) noted that cows' milk protein can act on the gut lining to stimulate an abnormal immune response, inflammation and diarrhoea.
- A Danish study (1990) suggested that 2 to 4 per cent of children are allergic to cows' milk.

In the US cows' milk allergy is said to affect at least 30,000 babies a year.

Knowing whether cows' milk protein is the primary allergy trigger can be difficult, because:

1. Formula occasionally sensitizes a baby without immediately provoking allergic symptoms.
2. Cows' milk antibody levels gradually fall after the initial sensitization, so aren't a reliable gauge of cows' milk allergy unless measured both before and immediately after the very first formula feed.
3. Breastfeeding women who drink a lot of cows' milk may have traces of its proteins in their breast milk, so cows' milk can be the primary allergy trigger even in an exclusively breastfed baby, though this is extremely unlikely.
4. Allergists believe that once a baby is sensitized, he then reacts more readily to other allergy triggers.

Reducing allergy triggers

All babies have to meet potential allergy triggers at some time, but it may be better to reduce or avoid them in early infancy.

- A Finnish study (1995) followed 150 children from birth to seventeen years. There were three groups: those breastfed for at least six months, those breastfed for one to six months, and those breastfed for less than one month or not at all. All those breastfed for six months or more, and some of those breastfed for up to six months, had three and a half months of exclusive breastfeeding. None had solids until three and a half months, or any fish or citrus fruits in the first year. Subsequently, the amount of allergic illness was related to the length of breastfeeding, and early formula-feeding was found to cause a higher risk of allergy than an allergic family history. Different symptoms peaked at different ages. There was most eczema at one year and most food allergy (rash, urticaria, lip swelling, aching lips and throat, or severe vomiting after certain foods) at three years. Asthma, wheezing and hay fever increased up to seventeen years. At one and three years there was least eczema, food allergy and respiratory allergy in children who'd been breastfed for more than six months. At least six months of breastfeeding – including three and a half months' exclusive breastfeeding – were needed to reduce the risk of eczema in the first three years. However, exclusive breastfeeding for just one month or more helped prevent food allergy and respiratory allergy. At seventeen years there was least respiratory allergy and dramatically less 'substantial atopy' (allergic symptoms of more than one type) in those who'd been breastfed for six months or more.

- In 1993 an Italian team studied 174 babies with an allergic family history. They were exclusively breastfed for six months (though allowed soya milk). Their mothers drank no more than 150–200 ml (5–7 fl oz) of cows' milk a day, and ate no more than two eggs a week. House-dust mites were eliminated as far as possible from the home; pets and smoking were avoided; and no babies went into day care until they were three years old. Cows' milk and other dairy products were gradually introduced after six months; eggs and fish after a year. The babies subsequently had a very much reduced likelihood of allergic illness compared with that predicted from their family history. This protection continued for at least five years.

A UK team conducted another study of high-risk babies. Allergy triggers were reduced or avoided in one group, while nothing was done in the control group.

The triggers reduced or avoided included:

For breastfeeding mothers

- Dairy products, eggs, fish and nuts.

For babies

- Cows' milk formula (all were breastfed for at least six months; only if necessary did they have hydrolysed soya formula supplements)
- All foods and drinks other than breast milk (or hydrolysed soy formula) for six months
- Cows' milk and unhydrolysed soya formula for nine months
- Wheat for ten months
- Eggs for eleven months
- Other dairy products, eggs, oranges, fish and nuts for twelve months
- House-dust mites.

By twelve months, 14 per cent of babies in the reduced allergy-trigger group had one or more allergic disorders, compared with 40 per cent of the controls.

How might breastfeeding protect against allergy?

1 The 'leaky gut' hypothesis – This suggests that foreign food proteins, for example from cows' milk formula, can pass through a young baby's gut into the blood and trigger food allergy (due to IgE antibodies) or the type of non-allergic sensitivity associated with a slow-onset immune reaction (probably due to IgG antibodies).

If the leaky gut hypothesis is correct, cows' milk protein may leak from a formula-fed baby's gut into the bloodstream and travel to other parts of the body where in a susceptible baby it could trigger an immediate allergic response or sensitize him to react to allergy triggers in future.

However, several substances in breast milk (including cortisone and epidermal growth factor) encourage a baby's gut lining to become mature and impervious to foreign proteins. They also encourage the immune system to become mature. And breast milk's immunoglobulin A (IgA) antibodies coat the gut lining, which is thought to help prevent foreign food proteins leaking from the gut into the blood. It takes several months for a baby to make useful amounts of IgA himself. This coating probably disappears fairly rapidly after a breastfeed, as there's a rapid turnover of gut-lining cells, so if breastfeeds were widely spaced and interspersed with bottles of formula, or solids, traces of cows' milk protein or other foreign food protein might enter the blood.

This is an argument in favour of exclusive breastfeeding for the first six months, especially for babies with a family history of allergy. Formula-fed babies lack protective IgA, because even if cows' milk's IgA were useful to them, it's spoilt by heat treatment during formula manufacture. Also, beta-lactoglobulin is the commonest potential sensitizer in cows' milk, but there's none of this in breast milk.

2 **Protection against diarrhoea** – Another way in which breast milk may protect against allergies and non-allergic slow-onset immune reactions is by influencing the population of micro-organisms in a baby's gut and thereby helping protect against diarrhoea. Repeated diarrhoea can be associated with damage to the gut lining, which in turn could encourage foreign food proteins to leak into the bloodstream.

3 **Protection against respiratory infections** – Breastfeeding also helps prevent respiratory infections, which is important as such infections can encourage respiratory allergy.

Eczema

Most recent studies suggest breastfeeding can help prevent eczema.

- An analysis (2001) of eighteen trials, in the *Journal of the American Academy of Dermatology*, found that exclusive breastfeeding in the first three months discourages eczema in children with a family history of eczema, asthma and hay fever (atopy).
- Finnish research (1995) suggested that exclusive breastfeeding can

delay the onset of eczema and make it less severe, especially if there's a family history of allergy.

- A study in the *Lancet* (1992) looked at breastfed babies with a family history of allergy. When mothers avoided eating milk, eggs, fish and nuts, and avoided giving their babies these foods, as well as soya, wheat and oranges, for up to twelve months, their babies were significantly less likely to have eczema at twelve months.

However:

- A large German study (2002) found the risk of eczema increased with each extra month of breastfeeding.

Asthma and wheezing

Most, but not all, studies suggest breastfeeding can discourage these conditions. The lack of agreement may be because many researchers call all wheezing 'asthma', rather than distinguishing between atopic ('allergic') asthma (wheezing associated with viral infection) and 'transient infantile wheezing'. It's possible that breastfeeding may help protect against wheezing associated with viral infection but not against allergic asthma.

- A study (2003) in the *Journal of Allergy and Clinical Immunology* reported that breastfeeding might either delay the onset or actively protect against asthma in children under two years.
- Australian research (2002) reported that exclusive breastfeeding for at least four months helped prevent wheezing and asthma.
- A review (2001) of twelve studies, in the *Journal of Pediatrics*, found that exclusive breastfeeding for at least three months reduced the risk of childhood asthma by one-quarter in all children, and halved it if there was asthma, eczema or hay fever in the family.

However:

- New Zealand research (2002) found breastfeeding did not protect children from asthma.

Hay fever (allergic rhinitis)

- A review (2002) of six studies, in the journal *Acta Paediatrica*, found that exclusive breastfeeding for at least the first three months offered substantial protection against hay fever in childhood, both in children with an allergic family history and in those without.

Food exclusion and challenge for a formula-fed baby

The only way to prove whether allergic symptoms result from cows' milk is to change the formula or, ideally, give breast milk, to see if the baby's symptoms disappear, and if so, then to reintroduce the original formula to see if they recur. This 'challenge' should be repeated twice.

If you are interested in doing this, *your doctor will advise what's best, and it's essential to have expert supervision by a doctor or state-registered dietitian to ensure your baby has adequate nourishment.*

Hydrolysed soya formula is one alternative, but one in five babies with cows' milk allergy can't tolerate soya milk either. As for goats' milk, it doesn't contain the right proportions of nutrients for babies (even if it's diluted); and about 30 per cent of babies who are sensitive to cows' milk are also sensitive to goats' milk.

Breast milk is the best food for a baby who is allergic to cows' milk. With time and patience, even if you've never breastfed, you can build up your milk supply to provide some or all of your baby's needs.

Allergy in breastfed babies

Babies breastfed exclusively for six months are much less likely to develop allergies. However, breastfeeding women should ideally avoid large amounts of cows' milk, egg, nuts, fish, citrus fruits and wheat, as traces of these in breast milk could trigger allergy in susceptible babies. Breastfeeding mothers of babies with a high allergy risk should avoid cows' milk, eggs, nuts and fish completely.

'Nature's immunization'

Some immunologists claim that traces of undigested foods in breast milk prepare a baby's digestive and immune systems for direct contact with these foods later. However, 'traces' come in many sizes. Some breastfeeding women, for example, drink vast quantities of milk – three, four or even five pints a day. Some believe this encourages their own milk production. Not only is this untrue but it may increase the amount of cows' milk protein that enters their breast milk.

Food exclusion and challenge for a breastfeeding mother

If you want to know whether your baby's symptoms could be the result of something you've eaten, do a trial of food exclusion and challenge. However, do this under the guidance of a doctor or registered dietitian to ensure your diet remains sound and neither your baby's health nor yours is put at risk.

When choosing what to avoid first, record in a diary whether your baby's symptoms relate to what you eat. Cows' milk is often high on the list because many women drink it so frequently and in such large amounts.

Avoid one food at a time, otherwise you'll be none the wiser, and avoid it for about a week. If your baby's symptoms improve, try adding the food back into your diet to see if his symptoms return. If so, repeat this 'challenge' twice to be sure.

LESS COELIAC DISEASE

Some children develop coeliac disease when they begin to eat foods such as bread, rusk and breakfast cereal that contain cereal grain. It results from sensitivity to a substance called gliadin in the cereal protein gluten found in wheat, barley, rye and, perhaps, oats. It represents a slow-onset immune response leading to the production of antibodies to gliadin. When the baby eats cereal-grain food, antibodies damages his gut lining. The symptoms include stomach ache, diarrhoea, wind, weight loss or failure to grow, a swollen abdomen and unpleasant-smelling motions. Other possibilities are seizures, mouth ulcers and pitted, discoloured teeth. Treatment consists of excluding gluten-containing foods.

It's preferable for babies to have no cereal-grain foods before six months, so as to avoid sensitizing them to gluten when their digestive and immune systems are immature. It's also best if you're still breastfeeding when you introduce these foods, and for a baby to eat them only in small amounts.

- Swedish research (2002) reported a 40 per cent reduction in the risk of coeliac disease in young children who were being breastfed when they first started eating cereal-grain foods; the lowest risk was in those in whom these foods were introduced only gradually. The researchers also found that the risk of coeliac disease was higher if a baby had large amounts of cereal-grain foods.
- A survey many years ago in western Ireland, where only 3 per cent of babies were breastfed, found that coeliac disease was about four times as common as in England, where many more babies were breastfed at that time.
- Scandinavian researchers reported in 1965 that cows' milk protein sensitivity could be a forerunner of coeliac disease.

LESS AUTOIMMUNE DISEASE

Autoimmune diseases, such as type 1 diabetes, juvenile rheumatoid arthritis, multiple sclerosis and Crohn's disease (see page 52), involve some kind of trigger (e.g., viral infection or stress) which makes the body produce rogue antibodies that then attack certain cells instead of being protective. Breastfeeding seems to reduce a baby's lifetime risk of autoimmune disease in general.

Diabetes

Studies strongly suggest formula-feeding can play a part in causing type 1 diabetes (the autoimmune sort, which comes on suddenly in young people).

- An Italian study (2003) reported that being breastfed for less than three months encourages type 1 diabetes.
- A study (1999) reported in *Diabetes Care* found that exclusive breastfeeding helped protect against type 1 diabetes developing in childhood.
- Australian research (1995) reported that formula-fed babies have half as much chance again as exclusively breastfed babies of developing type 1 diabetes.
- Canadian research (1992) reported that a cows' milk protein called bovine serum albumin (BSA) can trigger the production of BSA antibodies. In the first two years of their illness children with type 1 diabetes have seven times more BSA antibodies than do healthy children. In susceptible children BSA antibodies can trigger an autoimmune reaction in the insulin-producing cells of the pancreas, making them self-destruct. It's suggested that a viral infection sparks this destruction.
- US research (1988) reported that children who'd been breastfed for more than twelve months had only half the risk of type 1 diabetes compared with other children. They estimated that formula-feeding causes up to one in four cases of type 1 diabetes.

In addition, Canadian research (2002) found that being breastfed helps prevent type 2 diabetes in Native Canadian children.

Juvenile rheumatoid arthritis

Studies suggest that breastfeeding may help protect against juvenile rheumatoid arthritis – the sort that comes on in children.

Multiple sclerosis

Several studies suggest a link between formula-feeding and the later development of multiple sclerosis (MS); two others failed to show a link but didn't consider how long breastfeeding had continued.

- Italian research (1994) reported that adults with MS were less likely than healthy controls to have been breastfed; if they were breastfed, it was for a shorter time, an average of 8.4 months, whereas controls were breastfed for 12.5 months – nearly half as long again. Such a 'dose' finding is perhaps even more important than an 'all-or-nothing' finding. The researchers suggested several reasons why prolonged breastfeeding may have been protective, including the fact that breast milk and formula differ in their amounts and proportions of polyunsaturated fatty acids.
- Research reported in the *Lancet* (1992) stated that the grey matter in the brains of formula-fed babies had different proportions of fatty acids compared with those of breastfed ones.

It's possible, *though completely unproven,* that the fatty acid composition of a formula-fed baby's brain could allow easier viral damage, or make the fatty myelin in nerve coverings age faster. Breastfeeding also influences the developing immune system, and it's possible that this could encourage MS in later life by modifying a person's immune response to certain triggers.

LESS PYLORIC STENOSIS

This is a narrowing of the opening of the stomach into the gut. It can make a baby vomit and is reported to be less common in breastfed babies.

LESS LIKELIHOOD OF MECONIUM PLUGS AND MECONIUM ILEUS

These conditions can cause a blockage of a baby's gut that may need surgery. Both are less common and less severe in breastfed babies, because colostrum encourages the easy passage of a baby's sticky tar-like first bowel motions.

LESS APPENDICITIS

Breastfeeding may make appendicitis less likely in later life.

- Italian research (1995) found that being breastfed for at least seven months halved the risk of appendicitis in childhood.

LESS ULCERATIVE COLITIS AND CROHN'S DISEASE

These two inflammatory bowel diseases may be connected with infant feeding.

- A Canadian study (1989) found both formula-feeding and early diarrhoea made Crohn's disease more likely in childhood. The same researchers studied children with ulcerative colitis, but found no protective effect from breastfeeding. This contrasts with two studies of ulcerative colitis in adults, one of which found that people with ulcerative colitis were twice as likely as others not to have been breastfed.
- An Italian study (1998) found that not being breastfed increased the risk of ulcerative colitis and Crohn's disease.

LESS ACRODERMATITIS ENTEROPATHICA

Breast milk provides the only treatment for this rare disease, which is possibly caused by an inherited defect of zinc metabolism and is almost never seen in breastfed children. This may be because breast milk (and particularly colostrum) is rich in zinc, and zinc in breast milk is very efficiently absorbed.

FEWER COT DEATHS

Studies suggest breastfeeding is one of many factors that can help protect babies from sudden infant death syndrome – SIDS, or cot death.

Risk factors

Researchers think risk factors can have a cumulative effect. Known and suspected factors include:

1 **Mother being a smoker** – This is the most important, especially in the first weeks of life. If you are a smoker, you may multiply your baby's risk of SIDS fivefold. Having a father who smokes multiplies the risk too, but only by one and a half times. A study by US researchers suggests that breastfeeding reduces the risk of SIDS in babies of non-smokers, but not in those of smokers.

2 **The baby sleeping on his front** – European research (2004) attributed nearly one in two deaths from SIDS to this. So put your baby on his back to sleep – remember, 'Back to Sleep'.

3 **Overheating** – The danger comes from being wrapped up too warmly and/or being in too hot a place – there's no need for a baby to be in a room warmer than 18°C (64°F). However, being too warm during sleep seems to be a problem only for babies who sleep on their front, which isn't advisable anyway.

4 Mild infection – Some seemingly healthy babies seem to have an unusually powerful response to infection.

5 Being preterm.

6 Formula-feeding – Most studies record a higher risk of SIDS in formula-fed babies.

- Scandinavian research (2002) found that babies breastfed for less than one month were five times more likely to die from SIDS.
- Japanese research (2002) found that breastfeeding helped protect against SIDS.
- A UK study (1995) failed to find that formula-feeding was a significant risk factor. Breastfed babies had a lower risk of SIDS but were also more likely than formula-fed babies to have a non-smoking mother and a father in employment, to have been born at term and to sleep on their back, all of which are protective. However, the researchers considered only a small number of babies and said larger studies might be able to distinguish a small risk from formula-feeding.
- In the same year a New Zealand team criticized this UK work, claiming the statistics were misinterpreted and were actually similar to those of other large, well-controlled studies, which showed that breastfeeding halves the risk of SIDS. The UK researchers replied that their results still didn't suggest that breastfeeding had a strong independent protective effect. They also claimed that after extensive adjustment for maternal smoking, prematurity and sleeping position, only one other published study showed that breastfeeding offered significant protection.
- A New Zealand study (1993) found that babies who died of SIDS were less likely to have been breastfed, and those that were breastfed were breastfed for fewer weeks and were less likely to have been exclusively breastfed. Babies not still being breastfed on discharge from hospital were nearly twice as likely to succumb to SIDS. The conclusion was that breastfeeding had a significant association with a lowered risk of SIDS and this seemed to persist for several months.
- New Zealand research (1991) suggested three factors were particularly important: the baby sleeping on his front, a parent being a

smoker and the baby not being breastfed. Breastfed babies in this study were one-third less likely to succumb to SIDS than those who were formula-fed.
- A large US study (1988) reported that SIDS was twice as likely in babies formula-fed from birth.

7 **Post-natal depression** – At least two studies have found that having a depressed mother triples the risk of SIDS.

8 **Being a boy** – Three boys succumb to SIDS to every two girls. Fewer boys are breastfed than girls and breastfed boys are generally breastfed for fewer months than girls, which might help explain the gender factor if there really is a link between SIDS and formula-feeding.

9 **Lower socio-economic group** – This is probably significant only because of its association with other risk factors.

10 **An inherited factor** – An identical twin of a baby that succumbs to SIDS is at higher risk, suggesting a genetic factor may be involved.

11 **Alcohol** – A European study (2004) found the mother's consumption of alcohol was significant, but only if she shared her bed with her baby all night.

12 **Sleeping in a separate room** – If a baby who is in another room becomes distressed because he can't breathe, then unless he cries or makes some other loud noise his mother is less likely to know than if he's in her bedroom. (Though some mothers sense intuitively when their baby is distressed, wherever he is.) Having your baby nearby means you are readily alerted by his sounds or movements and can pick him up immediately if he is distressed.

- A European study (2004) attributed roughly 36 per cent of SIDS cases to the baby sleeping in a separate room.
- A New Zealand study (1996) suggested that room-sharing with a parent reduced the risk of SIDS, so the researchers recommended

that babies should sleep in the same room as their parents for at least six months.

13 Co-sleeping – Until recently SIDS was thought to be more common in babies who shared a bed with their mother only if she or her partner were smokers. Indeed, if you smoke, it's unwise to share your bed with your baby.

However:

- A European study (2004) reported in the *Lancet* attributed about 16 per cent of SIDS cases to bed-sharing. This took the form of a very small increase in SIDS in babies under eight weeks who co-slept, though if the mothers were non-smokers the risk was very small, and significant only in the first eight weeks. There was no indication of how the babies were fed, which could be important, because formula-feeding mothers probably aren't primed to be as sensitive as breastfeeders to a baby's needs when co-sleeping, so might not wake if their baby became breathless or otherwise distressed. Also, there was no record of where co-sleeping occurred, which is important, because babies who co-sleep on a sofa have a higher risk of SIDS than babies who co-sleep in bed.

14 Other factors under investigation – These include the possibility of a defect in the way some babies metabolize fatty acids. If proven, this could mean a supplement of certain fatty acids – given to the baby or his breastfeeding mother – might reduce the risk.

Breastfeeding certainly doesn't guarantee protection, but there are several reasons why it may be important:

Food sensitivity

It's been suggested that SIDS may, in some babies, result from a sudden overwhelming response to a foreign protein. Cows' milk protein is by far the commonest foreign food protein babies meet, and formula-feds consume a huge amount.

Viral infections

Another theory is that a baby succumbs to SIDS because he is unable to cope with a viral infection. Breast milk helps protect babies against some viral infections.

Inability to cope with long gaps between feeds

Babies who succumb to SIDS tend to have had a relatively long gap (more than six hours) between their last feed and the time of death. If this is important, it may be significant that most successfully breastfed babies have more frequent feeds than formula-fed babies, especially early on and especially at night.

Frequent sucking

- A New Zealand study (1993) reported that sucking a dummy (pacifier) may protect against SIDS, possibly because it helps keep the mouth and throat muscles active and 'toned', so keeping the airway well open. The researchers suggest that if this is confirmed, a dummy could halve the number of SIDS deaths.

It's possible that frequent breastfeeding might have the same protective effect as a dummy.

LESS DENTAL DECAY

Most studies agree that children who were breastfed have less dental decay than those who were formula-fed. Tooth decay in a child who was breastfed also tends to be less severe. There's a suggestion that this is because breastfeeding is more popular with women from higher socio-economic groups, who are less likely to give their babies sugary snacks. But this can't be the whole answer, because exclusively breastfed babies not yet on solids have less decay than formula-feds, and even partial breastfeeding gives some protection. So how might breastfeeding protect teeth?

Fluoride

An ample fluoride supply reduces dental decay by 50 per cent, and the amount in breast milk is relatively high in areas with plenty in the drinking water. Milk from cows that drink water in fluoridated-water areas doesn't show as great an increase, though its fluoride content is slightly higher than in cows in non-fluoridated areas. However, in non-fluoridated-water areas, although the amount of fluoride in breast milk and formula is nearly the same, breastfed babies still have reduced decay rates in early childhood, regardless of the amount of sugar they consume.

Experts recomend a fluoride supplement for both breastfed and formula-fed babies in areas with low fluoride in the drinking water (below 0.7 parts per million). However, the suggested starting age varies from one country to another, and it's important not to give too high a dose as this can cause mottling of the tooth enamel.

Defective enamel

Several groups of researchers claim decay is more common in front teeth showing signs of enamel hypoplasia. This shows up as horizontal lines of defective development which may be chalky-white, grey-yellow, brown or black, and are relatively weak and prone to decay, especially if associated with pits or grooves. It is more likely in babies who have been ill, or whose mothers ate a poor diet, or were ill in pregnancy – especially if they took antibiotics.

Family history

A genetic susceptibility to decay can pass from parent to child.

Diet

Teeth are more likely to decay in babies and young children who eat a poor diet including frequent snacks of foods containing sugar or refined cereal flour. This is because they have more plaque (a sticky layer of food residue and mouth bacteria, including lacto-bacilli and, perhaps, decay-encouraging *Streptococcus mutans*) on their teeth. Mouth bacteria produce acid as they feed on the sugar and refined starch in plaque; acid weakens enamel by removing minerals; and repeated acid attacks can lead to tooth decay.

A baby's teeth are most vulnerable to acid attack as they first appear and shortly after. This is when many babies are starting on other foods and drinks in addition to milk, so it's important to choose first foods thoughtfully. There's no need to give any foods containing added sugar on a regular or frequent basis. This rules out cakes, sweetened desserts, rusks and many breakfast cereals. As babies grow older and eat more solids, it's increasingly important that these contain enough tooth-protecting nutrients, such as vitamins A, C and D, calcium and phosphorus.

Pooling of milk round the teeth at night

Many babies sleep with their mothers and breastfeed when they wish. Some doze with the breast in the mouth on and off for long periods between feeds, having a few occasional gentle sucks. Several researchers have found that a tiny number of this group have early dental decay. However, this is rare and affects only an extremely small minority of those babies that sleep with their mothers and feed on and off at night. A few formula-fed babies who doze with a bottle in their mouths suffer in a similar way.

Babies who doze at the breast don't suck and milk the breast very much; they also produce less saliva to wash milk from the teeth. This means that a pool of breast milk may linger around the front teeth. Pooling of milk provides mouth bacteria with plenty of nourishment and encourages the thick film of plaque which makes decay more likely. Babies with defective enamel are at the highest risk.

However, many mothers and babies like to be together and to breastfeed at night, and this has many advantages to mother and baby. So let's see how breastfeeding mothers can protect their babies' teeth even further.

Cleaning your baby's teeth

Dentists suggest wiping away the plaque from a baby's teeth after a feed (though one expert prefers before) once a day to remove the layer of bacteria and food residues (plaque) that encourages decay. Use a cotton wool ball, a gauze square or a clean flannel (wash cloth) moistened in warm water, or, once your baby is twelve months old, a very soft brush. Even a paper tissue would do. Some experts recommend wiping away traces of milk from the easily accessible parts of the inside of the whole mouth as well.

Get into the habit of wiping clean your baby's mouth and teeth as soon as the first tooth peeps through. Even better, start wiping the gums before the first tooth appears.

BETTER JAW AND MOUTH DEVELOPMENT

Many specialists report fewer problems of jaw and mouth development in children who were breastfed. Indeed, in one survey only two of nearly 500 children with such problems had been breastfed!

Breastfeeding exercises the muscles of the mouth, jaw and face more strenuously than bottle-feeding, because it's harder work – using sixty times more energy! Also, different movements are involved in sucking from and milking the breast compared with sucking from a bottle. Over the months, as a baby's face and jaw grow, their shape is partly determined by the strength and balance of the repeated pull of the various muscles.

Some – but not all – researchers report that the longer babies are breastfed, the more likely are their jaw and palate to grow into an optimal shape. In contrast, formula-fed babies and those breastfed for four months or less seem more likely to develop a narrow dental arch (with less room for teeth to be properly spaced), and thus malocclusion, in which top and bottom teeth don't meet as they should.

LESS LYMPH-SYSTEM CANCER

Children with lymph-system cancer are more likely to have been formula-fed.

- An analysis of fourteen studies by US researchers (2004) found that babies who were breastfed had a lower risk of leukaemia later in childhood.
- Research from the United Arab Emirates (2001) revealed that children aged two to fourteen with a lymphoma or lymphocytic leukaemia had been breastfed for significantly fewer months than those in a healthy 'control' group.
- A large US study (1999) suggested breastfeeding reduced the risk of childhood leukaemia by 20 per cent, with the effect being strongest in those breastfed for more than six months.
- Chinese research (1995) reported that babies breastfed for more than six months had a lower risk of lymphoma (especially Hodgkin's disease before six years).
- An American study (1991) found that breastfeeding for longer than eight months protected against Hodgkin's disease.
- An American group (1988) reported that breastfeeding for longer than six months lowered the risk of lymphoma and some other cancers. Children who'd been exclusively breastfed for at least six months were only half as likely to develop cancer before fifteen than children who had been formula-fed.

MORE SUCCESSFUL KIDNEY TRANSPLANTS

Children with kidney failure who receive a kidney transplant from their mother, brother or sister (but not their father) have a dramatically better chance of the transplant taking if they were breastfed as babies.

BETTER BRAIN AND NERVE DEVELOPMENT

Earlier walking

Two studies have shown that breastfed babies walk earlier than formula-fed ones, even after allowing for differences in weight, and excluding babies whose mothers went out to work (because they might have had less encouragement to walk).

Better scores on intelligence and development tests

For many years some (but not all) studies have found breastfeeding is associated with higher intelligence. Before dismissing this because so many factors impinge on intelligence and how it's measured, it's worth remembering that the contents of human milk are different from those in formula, and it's likely that human milk provides optimal nutrient levels for the development of the human brain, which grows extraordinarily fast in the first year of life and fastest of all in preterm babies.

- An English study (2004) found that babies who were small for dates had a higher developmental quotient at nine months and at eighteen months if they were breastfed than if they were bottle-fed with either standard or 'enriched' formula.
- A Danish study (2002) found a strong link between how long a child was breastfed and subsequent intellectual performance as an adult.
- An English study (2001) found that breastfeeding for eight months

or more resulted in a significant increase in both verbal and performance IQ (intelligence quotient) scores at seven to eight years.

- An analysis of many studies (2000), in the *American Journal of Clinical Nutrition*, concluded that breastfeeding gave babies a three-point advantage in IQ over formula-fed babies.
- An analysis of twenty studies (1999), in the *American Journal of Clinical Nutrition*, revealed that breastfeeding was associated with significantly higher scores for cognitive development in adolescence. The benefit was strongest for low-birthweight babies.

Preterms

Breast milk is particularly important for nerve and brain development in preterms.

- Research in Cambridge, England (in 1988 and 1992) reported that preterm babies given breast milk had better development scores (measured by the Bayley mental development index) at eighteen months and a higher IQ at eight years, even allowing for the mothers' education, smoking (in pregnancy and after) and socio-economic status. Preterm babies given their own mother's milk had the highest scores. To put this increase in scores into context, the researchers said it was of about the same magnitude as the advantage of being first-born, a girl, or belonging to a higher socio-economic class. They pointed out that although any one baby's score has a limited capacity to predict his future mental ability, the average score of a group is likely to be more predictive. They also made it clear that although their results might indicate that something in breast milk promotes brain growth and maturation in preterm babies, there may (also or instead) be something about the mothers who choose to give their babies breast milk that benefits their babies.
- New data from the same researchers (1994) support the view that breast milk promotes neuro-development. They studied preterm babies given either donated mature 'drip' breast milk (milk that drips from the breast while a woman feeds from the other side) or preterm formula (alone or plus the mother's expressed breast milk), and found no difference at eighteen months in Bayley psychomotor

and mental development indices. This is interesting because drip milk is low in nutrients and calories compared with a preterm baby's requirements. And it's particularly important because the researchers previously found that preterm babies fed standard milk formula had lower Bayley psychomotor and mental development indices than preterm babies fed preterm formula. But preterm babies fed solely donated breast milk had significantly and substantially higher psychomotor development scores at eighteen months than babies fed standard formula. The conclusion was that there's something about breast milk itself which in this respect is more advantageous than standard formula to preterm babies. This may be its arachidonic (AA) and docosahexanoic (DHA) acids and its hormones and growth factors. Further work should ascertain whether preterm babies who receive breast milk might do even better were it supplemented with certain nutrients.

- Australian research (1992) reported a study of children born with a very low birthweight. The researchers did several tests (Bayley mental development indices, then Wechsler IQ tests) up to eight years old. The scores of the children who received expressed breast milk weren't significantly different from those of children who had no breast milk at all. However, children breastfed directly from their mother's breast had significantly higher scores. The researchers suggest it may not be breast milk itself that benefits the intellectual development of preterms, but something about the act of breastfeeding.

BETTER VISUAL DEVELOPMENT AND EYESIGHT

Breast milk is good for the eyes.

- An American study (2001) in the *Journal of Perinatology* found very low-birthweight babies were less likely to develop eye problems caused by retinopathy of prematurity if they received breast milk.
- Another American study (1998), reported in *Pediatric Research*, found breastfed babies had better eyesight than formula-fed ones.
- Research in Cambridge, England, discovered breastfed preterms had better visual development than formula-fed preterms.

- Australian research (1995) found formula-fed babies had similar visual development to breastfed babies only if they received milk formula enriched with docosahexanoic acid (DHA). Visual development in babies breastfed for less than sixteen weeks was between those breastfed longer than four months and those fed standard formula.
- A US study (1994) reported that the visual acuity of formula-fed full-term babies was similar to that of breastfed babies, suggesting DHA isn't essential for full-term babies.
- A US study (1993) reported that very preterm babies had significantly higher visual acuity if given milk formula enriched with DHA than if given standard formula. Also, three-year-old children who'd been full-term and breastfed were better able to match letters and to use both eyes together than were those who'd been formula-fed.

Further work suggests these outcomes are caused by the different fatty acid profiles of breast milk and formula. Many preterm and some full-term babies may be unable to manufacture certain omega-3 fatty acids (including DHA and arachidonic acid). Experts previously didn't think these fatty acids were essential but clearly for these babies they are. Following European recommendations, formula manufacturers are now adding certain fatty acids to some products.

LESS VITAMIN-A DEFICIENCY

In some developing countries, such as Bangladesh, long-term breastfeeding protects children from vitamin-A deficiency. This condition can cause xerophthalmia (dangerously dry eyes) and blinds a million children worldwide each year.

- One study (1986) found that children with xerophthalmia in Malawi, Africa, were more than three times as likely as others to have stopped breastfeeding before two years old.

DIFFERENT EMOTIONAL AND BEHAVIOURAL DEVELOPMENT

The influences on emotional and behavioural development in later childhood and adulthood are impossible to pinpoint with certainty. However:

- One study of seven-year-olds showed that those who'd been breastfed were less fearful, nervous, jealous and spiteful than their peers who'd been formula-fed. They were also more successful at school.
- Studies also show that breastfed babies spend less time in their cots and more with their mothers than do formula-feds.

In communities which not only allow but actively encourage unrestricted breastfeeding, mothers don't let their babies cry even for a short time, whereas in many developed countries babies are often left to cry because 'it isn't time for a feed' or 'they might be spoilt if they're picked up'. You could argue that the baby whose mother gives the breast for food or comfort whenever her baby cries or otherwise appears to need it might grow up feeling more secure that his needs will be met.

One researcher (Jean Liedloff) wrote of two neighbouring tropical islands whose inhabitants had very different child-rearing practices. In one, babies were carried or held by the mother or someone else almost all the time. They slept with their mothers and were virtually never left alone. When they were with their mothers they could breastfeed very frequently, pretty much as often as they wanted. As they grew up they scarcely ever cried and appeared much happier and less aggressive than the babies on the other island. These were reared in a way much more akin to the way in which many people in developed countries bring up their babies, neither carried nor held a great deal, and not breastfed on an unrestricted basis.

Research into a breastfeeding woman's behaviour before, during and after feeding shows it differs from that of a bottle-feeder.

A breastfeeder is more likely to kiss, rock and touch her baby, while a bottle-feeder is more likely to rub, pat and jiggle her baby and show much more concern over 'wind'. Breastfeeders also talk to their babies more than do bottle-feeders.

A baby breastfed on an unrestricted basis will rarely cry, because his hunger, thirst and need for comfort can immediately be satisfied by warm milk. In contrast, a formula-fed baby is more likely to have to wait until his mother considers it's time for his feed and then has to wait again while the formula is prepared and warmed. He may feel very real hunger and frustration by the time all this has happened.

ENABLES SPACING BETWEEN CHILDREN

The natural contraceptive effect of long-term unrestricted breastfeeding means that women using no other family planning methods have longer gaps between their children than if they were formula-feeding. In a developing country, having a longer gap between one baby and the next means a baby has a better chance not only of being healthy but also of surviving.

- Chinese research (1989) in the largely rural province of Shaanxi found the child-spacing effect of breastfeeding had a marked effect on survival in infancy and early childhood.

BETTER ATTACHMENT TO MOTHER?

Scientific proof of any increased attachment between a mother and her breastfed baby is hard to come by, but a closer relationship seems likely, if only because the baby depends on his mother for food. She's also likely sometimes to feed him to comfort him instead of just holding him or giving a dummy.

LESS HEART DISEASE?

We don't yet know whether early infant feeding affects the risk of heart disease in later life.

- An English study (2004) of children born preterm, showed that when aged thirteen to sixteen years, those who'd been fed on donated breast milk had a lower – and therefore healthier – ratio of low-density lipoprotein cholesterol to high-density lipoprotein cholesterol. This suggests a lower risk of heart disease in later life.
- Another English study (2001) found seven-year-olds had lower blood pressure if they had been breastfed; the longer a child had been breastfed, the bigger was the effect.

Cows' milk protein antibodies

Some susceptible formula-fed (and a few breastfed) babies are sensitized by cows' milk and develop antibodies to cows' milk protein, which may contribute to the later development of heart disease.

Cows' milk protein antibodies can mop up molecules of cows' milk protein and form 'immune complexes' (antigen-antibody complexes).

- Belgian research (1978) found that formula-fed babies have immune complexes in their blood, while breastfed babies have none. In adults, circulating immune complexes can damage arteries and make blood stickier and thrombosis (blood clots) in blood vessels more likely. Thrombosis in a coronary artery can lead to a heart attack; thrombosis in a brain artery to a stroke. By damaging artery linings, immune complexes make them more likely to attract fatty deposits and so trigger the gradual build-up of atheroma, which may sow the seeds for heart and other arterial disease in later life.
- A British study (1974) found that men under sixty who'd had a heart attack had higher than normal levels of cows' milk antibodies in their blood.

It has also been found that a heart attack is three times more likely to kill a man if he has any cows' milk antibodies at all. One study found cows' milk antibody levels eight times higher than average in one family with a great deal of heart disease, indicating that the tendency to make such antibodies may be inherited. Although breastfed babies can develop cows' milk antibodies if they drink cows' milk (or formula) later, there's evidence that their levels are lower than in people who were formula-fed as infants.

LESS NAPPY RASH?

One survey showed that formula-fed babies were twice as likely to suffer from nappy rash as were breastfed ones.

FEWER INGUINAL HERNIAS?

- A 1995 study found that babies with an inguinal hernia (a 'rupture' or weakness in the groin) were much more likely than other babies never to have been breastfed. The researchers suggest that hormones (such as gonadotropin-releasing hormone) in breast milk may help prevent inguinal hernias.

OTHER FINDINGS

- Dutch research (1994) reported that by nine years children who'd been exclusively breastfed as babies had half the number of minor neurological (nerve) problems of children who had received any formula. The researchers believed that the various polyunsaturated fats in breast milk (particularly arachidonic and docosahexanoic acids) accounted for this difference.

POSSIBLE DISADVANTAGES FOR BABY

Now let's look at the very few possible disadvantages of breast-feeding to a baby.

Lack of vitamin B_1 in babies of mothers with beriberi

In some countries women run the risk of developing a disease called beriberi, caused by a deficiency of vitamin B_1 (thiamine) if they eat large amounts of polished rice. The breastfed babies of women with beriberi can become acutely ill with infantile beriberi. Polishing brown rice in order to produce white rice removes the outer layers of each rice grain. Unfortunately, vitamin B_1 is lost at the same time. The solution is to eat unpolished brown rice.

Lack of vitamin B_{12} in the babies of some vegan mothers

Some strictly vegetarian or vegan women have too little vitamin B_{12} in their milk and their babies develop symptoms of deficiency. This is sometimes because the women have not grown up in a family that knows how to choose and prepare nutritious vegetarian or vegan foods. Expert advice about what to eat, together with extra vitamin B_{12} for vegan mothers, puts this right.

Malnourishment

If a woman is severely malnourished for some time and her diet is grossly deficient in protein and fat, her breastfed baby is liable to go short as well. The mother needs more food. The World Health Organization recently decided to concentrate famine relief monies on food for breastfeeding mothers rather than on formula for babies. This is because in famine circumstances formula-fed babies have a much greater risk of dying, as a result of the enormous risk of gastro-enteritis from unsterilized bottles and water. Mothers in such circumstances are also likely to give bottle-fed babies dilute feeds in order to save milk powder, in case they can't get or can't afford any the next day.

Insufficient milk

Babies who don't get enough milk can become dangerously dehydrated, and can starve.

It's vital to tell your midwife, doctor or, in the UK, health visitor, if your baby isn't feeding well, or doesn't have six to eight really wet cloth nappies or five to six really wet disposables a day from about the fourth day after birth, or whenever your milk comes in. Together you can work out how to increase your milk supply (see Chapter 10), and you should begin producing more milk within two or three days. However, if the health professional doesn't think your baby can wait, you'll need to give donated top-ups of breast milk or formula at the same time, to meet your baby's needs for fluid and nourishment.

Learning to cope with stress by eating?

Frequent feeds are important for young babies. However, as infants grow they may not always want the breast every time they fidget or cry. The only time it's ever sensible to cut down on breastfeeds is if you are giving very frequent feeds, your baby latches on properly and you let your milk down well, but you've got into the habit of misinterpreting restlessness or cries as signs that your baby wants the breast when he really needs attention of other kinds (for example, to be talked to, listened to, played with or simply accompanied when feeling grumpy). A crying or fidgeting baby will probably feed even if not hungry, so as to get attention. However, if milk isn't what he needs, this could be an early lesson in how to use food as a tranquillizer at times of stress.

Those of us who work with distressed and/or overweight adults know that many turn to food as a comforter in the face of stress or emotional pain that has little or nothing to do with being hungry for food and would be better met in other ways. A baby's experiences certainly affect behaviour in adult life and it's possible (though unproven) that early experiences at the breast could encourage eating disorders and other attempts to find solutions to emotional distress in later life.

So how best can we help babies grow up believing the world is a good place where they can get their needs met?

If a woman offers her baby the breast whenever he seems to need it, it's an excellent way of making him feel cared for. If he's hungry or thirsty or needs the non-specific comfort of sucking and being intimately close to his mother, then continuing to breastfeed is a good idea. But if your baby doesn't seem very interested, and you think he might need something else, interrupt the feed and see if you can find out what this might be. This way you'll teach a variety of methods of dealing with emotional situations such as being bored, lonely, angry, frustrated and so on. The sort of mothering that meets a baby's needs this precisely takes more thought and effort than simply pacifying him by indiscriminate breastfeeding, but may pay dividends over a lifetime.

Breast-milk colitis

A baby who has blood-stained bowel motions, perhaps with colic, may have a rare condition called breast-milk colitis. The cause isn't clear, though it may be associated with sensitivity to one of the proteins in breast milk – and possibly to traces of protein foods the mother has eaten and that instead of being digested have 'leaked' through the mother's gut into her blood and thence into her breast milk. Until researchers are more certain about what to do, the usual pathway at present is to stop breastfeeding. The symptoms then resolve within about seven to ten days, but recur if the baby again has breast milk.

More intussusception?

This is an infrequent emergency situation in which part of a baby's bowel telescopes into itself and requires surgery.

- An Italian study (1993) reported that intussusception was most common in exclusively breastfed babies, slightly less common in partially breastfed babies, and least common in formula-fed babies.

Overall, breastfeeding is clearly best for babies, partly because babies who are breastfed are healthier than those who are formula-fed. Next, we'll consider why breastfeeding is best for mothers too.

FOUR

Best for you

Breastfeeding has many advantages to mothers as well as babies. Before we go into these in detail, though, it may help to consider a woman's reproductive life from the biological perspective.

THE BIOLOGICAL PERSPECTIVE

Human females develop breasts when very young. Most mammals develop their mammary glands only in time to feed their offspring, but human breasts are well developed several years before child-bearing begins (even in hunter-gatherer and other traditional-living peoples), so they clearly serve other purposes, the chief ones being sexual attraction and arousal.

Humans have probably been on earth for about five million years, and until 10,000 years ago, when they started living in agricultural settlements, lived the life of hunter-gatherers and ate a predominantly vegetarian diet. It seems from the study of the few hunter-gatherer tribes remaining today that their reproductive life is very different from that of people living in developed countries and indeed from that of most people in the developing world.

Perhaps the best studied present-day hunter-gatherers are the !Kung of Botswana and Namibia. !Kung women start menstruating at about seventeen to eighteen, which is late by Western standards. They also have an earlier menopause, at about thirty-eight. So their reproductive span is only about twenty years, whereas ours – from an average age of thirteen to an average of about fifty-one

– is about thirty-eight. An average !Kung woman has six or seven children, some of whom may die young, leaving her with a completed family of three or four. Because she breastfeeds on an unrestricted basis for several years, she doesn't menstruate for much of her reproductive life. Such women become fertile, menstruate a few times, have their first child, breastfeed for several years and then, as they start breastfeeding less often, and therefore ovulate again, become pregnant again and repeat the cycle. To such women menstruation is not a regular monthly event but an uncommon one.

So hunter-gatherer women are either pregnant or breastfeeding for most of their reproductive lives and only ever have twenty to thirty menstrual cycles. This was the picture for all women until a mere 10,000 years ago, which is very recent indeed in evolutionary terms.

Biologically we are akin to these hunter-gatherers, yet over the past 200 years of industrialization we have dramatically changed our way of life. The average modern girl eats more and has a higher weight, so she starts menstruating much earlier. She also has very few pregnancies and breastfeeds for only a few months, if at all. This means that until the menopause intervenes she has a total of 400 to 450 monthly menstrual cycles, with their accompanying surges of oestrogen and other hormones, and it looks as if all this may cause her some health problems.

Obviously a few months or even years of breastfeeding won't transform a modern woman into a hunter-gatherer, but it can certainly have some advantages to her health.

LESS BLEEDING AFTER CHILDBIRTH

The hormone oxytocin is stimulated by breastfeeding and encourages the womb to shrink back to normal and therefore stop bleeding sooner than in a formula-feeding woman.

LESS BREAST CANCER

Several studies suggest that breastfeeding for a long time (estimated by totalling the number of months or years you feed each child) helps protect some women from premenopausal breast cancer. However, not all studies agree.

Breast cancer is a common women's cancer in developed countries. It's particularly common in the UK and the US. And it has become more common over the last 200 years. Yet in those parts of the world where women spend many years, in total, breastfeeding babies, breast cancer is rare.

Two out of three of the seventeen breast cancer studies that looked at breastfeeding before 1985 showed that *ever* having breastfed helped protect women against breast cancer. However, not all researchers define their terms in the same way, which makes their results difficult to compare. Some studies class women as long-term breastfeeders if they breastfed only one baby for a long time, whereas others add up the total number of months of breastfeeding in a woman's life and only then label her as either a long-term breastfeeder or not. 'Long-term' in itself means different things to different researchers.

Several studies since 1985 have looked at how many babies a woman has breastfed and for how long, and differentiated breast cancer before the menopause from that occurring afterwards. Their conclusions are largely in favour of breastfeeding having a protective effect. The US National Academy of Sciences reviewed all this evidence in 1991 and concluded that most epidemiological evaluations suggest that breastfeeding may be protective against breast cancer, but there is conflicting evidence.

Let's look at some studies that show a protective effect:

- A Korean study (2003) found a significantly reduced risk of breast cancer in women who had breastfed for a lifetime total of more than twenty-four months. Also, the greater the total duration of breastfeeding in a woman's lifetime, the lower was her risk.

- A re-analysis (2002) of forty-seven studies from thirty countries indicated strong links between breastfeeding and a reduced rate of breast cancer. Indeed, the relative risk of breast cancer decreased by over 4 per cent for every twelve months of breastfeeding.
- A UK study (2002) concluded that women could halve their risk of breast cancer by breastfeeding for longer.
- A Chinese study (2000) found a significant reduction in risk of breast cancer in women who breastfed for more than twenty-four months per child, when compared with those who breastfed for one to six months per child. There was also a significant reduction in the risk of cancer in those whose lifetime duration of breastfeeding was more than seventy-three months.
- A US study (1994) found that breastfeeding was associated with a significantly lower incidence of premenopausal breast cancer. This protective effect increased as the total number of months of breastfeeding in a woman's life went up. The researchers calculated that if all women in the US breastfed their babies for a combined total of two years or longer, the amount of breast cancer could be cut by nearly 25 per cent. Another startling finding was that women who breastfed for the first time when they were young had an even lower risk of breast cancer. If a woman was twenty or younger and fed her children for a combined total of six months, she had only half the cancer-risk of a woman who had never breastfed.
- The UK National Case Control Study Group (1993) concluded that breastfeeding helped protect women from premenopausal breast cancer. Breastfeeding for at least three months cut the risk of early cancer by half.

However, three studies did not find a protective effect:

- A large US study (1996) found no important association between breastfeeding and breast cancer. However, among women who gave birth only once, those who breastfed were less likely to get breast cancer.
- A Swedish/Norwegian study (1990) found no association between not breastfeeding and getting breast cancer, in women under forty-five.

- A Japanese study (1992) suggested there was either no protective effect from breastfeeding or only a marginal one.

What does all this mean? Clearly the effect on breasts from breastfeeding one or two babies for a few hours, days, weeks or months is very different from feeding one or two babies for many months or even years, and different again from feeding more children for two, three, four or more years each. Today most women breastfeed very little, if at all, which robs their breasts of their main function. When a woman is neither pregnant nor breastfeeding, her body prepares itself each month to welcome a fertilized egg. Her breasts, womb and ovaries undergo profound changes, many involving new cell growth and the stimulation of genetic material (RNA) in cells. One theory is that the repeated monthly multiplication of breast cells may be one reason behind the high levels of breast cancer in developed countries.

There are two other theories on how breastfeeding may help protect against some breast cancers. If correct, these may act together or separately.

1. Milk left stagnant in the breast (because a woman is letting it dry up) may increase the usual breast-cell multiplication rate and the numbers of atypical cells, causing a state not far off that required for cancer to begin. This is because stagnant milk is slightly less acidic than recently produced milk from frequently emptied breasts. This slight decrease in acidity may be important, as test-tube studies show that cells are more likely to multiply rapidly and become abnormal in a relatively less acidic environment. Interestingly, the Tanka boat-women of Hong Kong who feed only from their right breast are very unlikely to get cancer in this breast; however, their risk of cancer in the left breast is relatively high, being similar to that of women in the US.
2. Milk production and the removal of milk from the breast by breastfeeding may flush out foreign chemicals that are potentially carcinogenic (cancer-causing). Once some of these have entered the breast (for example, from food), they can remain in its milk glands or ducts unless flushed out.

So what should you do? Choose to breastfeed on an unrestricted basis, don't give your baby solids for the first six months and breastfeed each child for at least a year. This usually prevents ovulation for many months, which delays the return of the monthly disruption of breast cells. There's some evidence this may reduce the risk of breast cancer.

LESS OVARY CANCER

Ovary cancer is most common in industrialized countries and kills more women than any other cancer. The risk factors are similar to those for breast cancer. For example, years of repeated monthly ovulation make it more likely. The sort of breastfeeding most likely to suppress ovulation for a long time is outlined later in this chapter. The more children a woman has, and the longer she breastfeeds each one, the lower her risk of ovary cancer is likely to be.

LESS CYCLICAL BREAST PAIN?

Anecdotal evidence suggests women are less likely to suffer from this each month after they have breastfed a baby.

DOING WHAT NATURE INTENDED

Breast milk is the food nature intended for your baby. You can do no better!

CLOSER RELATIONSHIP WITH YOUR BABY?

According to one large British survey, one in four women planning to breastfeed their first baby believed it would give them a closer bond with their baby.

SATISFYING?

There's something wonderful about being able to nourish your baby yourself, body to body. Being able to give the baby the pleasure of being at your breast is rewarding too, as is the ability to comfort a crying baby almost immediately. Women who breastfeed successfully for as long as they want report being very satisfied, even if they are unaware of the health advantages to their babies.

A survey of recently delivered women found those greatly pleased with their babies were much more successful at breastfeeding than those who were indifferent towards them.

- In a survey (1987) of long-term American and Canadian breastfeeders, 98 per cent considered the benefits of breastfeeding to their babies to be emotional security, happiness and earlier development of independence. They also commented that breastfeeding enhanced the love between a mother and her child.

ENJOYABLE?

Overall, most breastfeeding women enjoy doing it. There's something very special about having a baby at your breast staring up at you and perhaps stopping sucking every now and then to break into a gummy smile. And the sight of a baby's tiny, dimpled, star-shaped hand resting on the breast as he feeds is among the magic moments of mothering.

Many women enjoy talking to their baby, especially towards the end of a feed when he isn't concentrating so much on drinking. And breastfeeding mothers around the world love speaking in baby talk. Researchers note that their voices all have a similar lilting, adagio rhythm. This is a delightful interlude when the levels of endorphins (natural 'feel-good' chemicals in the blood) are high, but those of stress hormones (such as adrenalin and cortisone) low.

FULFILLING?

Another often expressed feeling is that breastfeeding is one of the things only a woman can do. In today's world of sexual equality this feminine fulfilment is valued not only by the naturally maternal but also by the career woman who sees her enjoyment of breastfeeding as symbolic of her womanliness.

The oneness many breastfeeding women feel with their babies is often quoted as the major advantage to breastfeeding mothers. Certainly they often seem particularly at ease with their babies.

EMPOWERING?

A woman who breastfeeds for as long as she or her baby wants gains in confidence and self-esteem.

- A US study (1993) found that breastfeeding women of low economic means had more confidence in their skills as mothers and their ability to meet their children's needs. This lasted well beyond the time they breastfed.
- Another US study (1988) found that young (average age sixteen) pregnant women from poor socio-economic backgrounds thought breastfeeding would make them feel important.

CAN REDUCE STRESS AND BOOST MATERNAL FEELINGS

Breastfeeding women benefit from increased prolactin, which encourages calmness. They also have a less intense response to the stress hormone adrenalin.

- A Japanese study (2002) reported that oxytocin – a hormone produced while breastfeeding – stimulates an area of the brain called the hippocampus; researchers say such stimulation dramatically boosts mental ability and short-term memory, and may make a woman feel more maternal.

HELPS YOU GET YOUR FIGURE BACK

Three months after her baby is born a breastfeeding woman is more likely to be losing weight without dieting than one who is formula-feeding. Breastfeeding uses up some of the fat stored in pregnancy and helps a woman get back to her pre-pregnancy shape and weight, provided she doesn't overeat. If her breasts change shape, they probably do so because of pregnancy, not breastfeeding. Women report that their breasts are variously either smaller, larger or droopier after breastfeeding, but there's no general trend. However, breasts tend to return to their previous shape and size about six months after weaning.

CONVENIENT

A big practical bonus is that breastfeeding is more convenient, even at home, with no bottles and teats to wash and sterilize and no feeds to prepare. Breast milk is always ready at hand. And going out is easier, as you have no equipment to collect, prepare and take with you. Holidays and all forms of travel become much more practical. Not for you the cooling of a bottle of hot milk by holding it out of the car window at great speed! And no spilt milk powder in the car, train or plane.

A breastfeeding woman needs only her baby and a clean nappy to go anywhere, and it takes only a little ingenuity and forethought to breastfeed anywhere without embarrassment to you or anyone else.

Another advantage is that it's nearly always possible to comfort an infant with the breast easily and quickly, anywhere and any time, without overfeeding, whereas a formula-fed baby often isn't comforted by sucking a bottle of water or a dummy, yet may get too much milk if allowed to suck freely at a bottle. This means a breastfed baby may be more contented than a formula-fed baby.

CHEAPER

Breastfeeding is cheaper than formula-feeding. In the UK, for example, breastfeeding saves a family about £450 a year. However, the relative cost isn't usually very important in developed countries, where a few pennies here or there don't influence the average woman either way, even when taking into account the costs of formula, bottles, teats, and sterilizing tablets or fuel to boil the equipment.

A breastfeeding woman many need to consider the cost of any extra food she eats, which can be an extra 300 to 500 calories a day over and above her non-pregnant and non-breastfeeding intake. The baby takes more than this but the difference is made up by calories from fat stored in pregnancy. However, breastfeeding women use energy from food more efficiently than do formula-feeders, and may not need much extra at all. Obviously the cost of any extra food depends on a woman's preferences – if she takes her extra calories in the form of best steak and asparagus, it will be more expensive than if she eats cheese-and-tomato sandwiches.

But if she simply eats a little more of everything that she would normally eat, the cost of her extra food will probably be less than the cost of formula. This is vitally important in developing countries, where some mothers can't afford enough formula but can afford a little extra food for themselves.

CAN PROVIDE BIRTH CONTROL

The contraceptive effect of a certain type of breastfeeding can be as efficient as better-known contraceptive methods such as the Pill. It's the only contraception available to many of the world's women, in developing countries it has two vitally important effects.

1. Breastfeeding spaces children more widely apart. In parts of the world a child born less than two years after an older brother or sister has more than twice the risk of dying young compared with one born after a longer gap.
2. Breastfeeding does more to contain the global population explosion than does any other sort of contraception.

Using data gathered from over 4,000 women in more than fifteen countries, an international group of experts stated in December 1995 that the contraceptive effect of breastfeeding in certain circumstances – when used as part of the lactational amenorrhoea method (LAM – see below) – is very safe and more than 98 per cent effective.

No popular contraception is 100 per cent reliable, but the contraceptive effect of LAM is the same as that of the Pill and the condom and it is very useful as a temporary family-planning method after childbirth.

So what is LAM and under what circumstances is breastfeeding a safe contraceptive?

The lactational amenorrhoea method (LAM)

If a woman breastfeeds fully (that is, exclusively) or nearly fully (with at least six and preferably many more feeds well-spaced throughout the twenty-four hours), and hasn't yet had her first period after childbirth, she has a better than 98 per cent chance of avoiding pregnancy. In other words, LAM depends on:

- Your baby being under six months old.
- You breastfeeding exclusively (giving your baby no other drinks or food) or nearly exclusively.
- Feeding frequently, with no long gaps between feeds (N.B. feeding very infrequently, with fewer than six feeds a day, allows the prolactin level to fall to levels seen when women are ovulating, see below).
- Your periods not yet having returned.

Scientists aren't completely clear why conception is less likely during the sort of breastfeeding necessary for LAM, but know the hormone prolactin is involved, as is some combination of vigorous sucking and milking by the baby and frequent breastfeeds with no long gaps night or day. There isn't a direct relationship between prolactin and the absence of periods. However, LAM helps prevent the prolactin level dipping low enough to allow ovulation. A high prolactin level seems to prevent ovulation by discouraging the ovaries' response to follicle-stimulating hormone, a hormone which in non-pregnant, non-breastfeeding women allows an egg to ripen each month.

As time passes, a breastfeeding woman's prolactin level falls until eventually it's no longer high enough to prevent ovulation. In *exclusively breastfeeding women* this doesn't happen until the tenth week after childbirth at the very earliest, and only one exclusively breastfeeding woman in twenty ovulates before the eighteenth week. The contraceptive effect of breastfeeding differs from woman to woman, even if they breastfeed in similar ways. But the type of breastfeeding makes a very big difference to the return of fertility. The average time before the first period in women who breastfeed exclusively and on an unrestricted basis for six to eight months, then introduce solids but continue to breastfeed frequently for drinks and comfort, is over fourteen months! A woman breastfeeding like this can expect an average gap between babies of two to three years, which means ovulation returns, on average, after fifteen to twenty-seven months, the exact timing depending on personal factors.

By contrast, *formula-feeding women* ovulate on average eight to ten weeks after giving birth, which means one in two risks becoming pregnant before her baby is eight to ten weeks old if she resumes sexual activity without contraception.

Partially breastfeeding women ovulate on average later than bottle-feeding women but before exclusively breastfeeding ones.

If a breastfeeding woman menstruates in the first six months after delivery, her menstrual cycles are likely to be anovulatory (without ovulation), which is why most women can rely on LAM until their first period after childbirth (but remember LAM is only for women with babies up to six months). *However, this certainly doesn't mean you can't become pregnant while using LAM – just that you have only a 2 per cent chance of doing so.*

As the months pass after delivery, ovulation before the first period becomes increasingly likely. One woman in twenty ovulates before her first period, which is one reason LAM isn't 100 per cent effective. However, there are several ways of discovering when you're about to ovulate (see 'Other contraception', below).

Many studies suggest that breastfeeding's contraceptive effect is more powerful and lasts longer in developing countries. There are several possible reasons, including poor nourishment and taboos against sex with lactating women. But undoubtedly the main reason is that many breastfeed in an unrestricted way, with frequent feeds day and night, whereas in developed countries women many breastfeed only five or six times in twenty-four hours, with very few or no feeds at night.

Women in developing countries also tend to allow more non-nutritive suckling, putting their babies to the breast for comfort and pleasure as well as 'proper' feeds. This means that even if their babies have solids or bottle-feeds, they still spend a lot of time at the breast, which helps prevent ovulation.

The first eight weeks – If using LAM, you need no other contraception. It's *exceedingly* unlikely even for formula-feeding women to ovulate now.

After eight weeks – Ask yourself three questions:

1 Are you content with 98 per cent reliable contraception from LAM (which is better than most women settle for most of the time)?
2 Are you breastfeeding exclusively or nearly exclusively?
3 Are you still without periods (defined as a recognizable period or two consecutive days of bleeding or spotting)?

If you answer 'no' to questions 2 or 3, breastfeeding alone will give you nowhere near 98 per cent reliability and you need other contraception.

But if you answer 'yes' to all three, LAM can be your only contraception until your baby is six months old or until such time as your answers change.

However, if you feel strongly that you don't want to get pregnant again quickly, then in case you are among the one in twenty exclusively breastfeeding women who ovulates before their first period after childbirth, you may like to take one or two other precautions. These include:

- 'Extra-safe' LAM.
- Additional contraception compatible with breastfeeding and recent childbirth.

Extra-safe LAM – You can delay ovulation and help detect the unlikely event of ovulation before your first period by stimulating your milk supply more. Do this by:

- Breastfeeding frequently, with no long gaps day or night.
- Checking your baby is well positioned at the breast.
- Allowing non-nutritive suckling as well as 'proper' feeds.
- Avoiding a dummy.
- Delaying solids and bottles of formula, juice or water until your baby is six months old. Once a baby starts solids, LAM's reliability falls from 98.5 to 96 per cent.

If you or your baby don't want to or can't breastfeed frequently (for example, if your baby is unwell or disinterested, or you're not with each other) you can mimic the effect of breastfeeding to some extent by hand-expressing (or pumping) a little milk every two to three hours by day and every four hours or so at night.

- A study (1992) found that once periods had returned, frequent breastfeeding (an average of nine feeds in twenty-four hours) prevented ovulation in seven out of ten women, whereas less frequent feeds (an average of six in twenty-four hours) prevented ovulation in only three out of ten women. The more frequent feeders had a higher average prolactin level.

Other contraception compatible with breastfeeding and recent childbirth

When you resume having sex, you could use a *condom* or a *diaphragm* with spermicidal jelly. If you've used a diaphragm before, you may need to be refitted after having a baby because you'll be a different size inside. This can be done at your six-week post-natal visit to your doctor. Another idea is to have an *IUD* (intrauterine contraceptive device) fitted. Researchers say that while the combined Pill is inadvisable (because it decreases breast milk production), the *progestogen-only Pill* does not interfere with breastfeeding or affect the breastfed baby.

According to the World Health Organization, the advantages of monthly hormonal *contraceptive injections* for breastfeeding women during the first six weeks after delivery outweigh the disadvantages. However, doctors in India discovered that women who had contraceptive injections lost minerals from their bones, leading to lower bone density. They suggest these injections are unsafe for breastfeeding women.

The *sympto-thermal method* is a natural form of birth control. An analysis of five studies shows that when used carefully it's 96.8 per cent effective. (When used imperfectly it's only 86.4 per cent effective.) It involves:

- Being aware of the bodily changes (including changes in the amount and nature of vaginal mucus, and body temperature) that herald impending ovulation and the fertile time of your cycle. The average woman ovulates on the twelfth day of her cycle, counting the first day of her period as day one. However, ovulation may occur at any time between the tenth and fourteenth days or even, in a few women, outside these times. Most women are especially fertile for the six days before – and on the day of – ovulation.
- Avoiding sex (or using a condom or diaphragm) if you recognize you're entering a fertile time.

The sympto-thermal method can help you recognize the unlikely event of ovulation before your first period after childbirth. It can also help you to identify whether or not newly returned periods are associated with ovulation. It becomes easier to use as the months pass and you settle back into ovulatory menstrual cycles.

However, it's wise to get expert help if you want reliable contraception from a combination of breastfeeding and the sympto-thermal method, as many women find the signs indicating their fertile time are less obvious while breastfeeding. When using the sympto-thermal method, a simple, small *saliva microscope* (see page 418) can help you identify the fern-like pattern in your saliva that precedes your fertile time. *Ovulation prediction kits* (see page 419) that test hormone levels in a few drops of urine are another useful aid.

BETTER FOR BONES

Two studies suggest breastfeeding reduces the long-term risk of osteoporosis.

- Australian research (1993) reported that among 311 women over sixty-five, those who'd had a baby but never breastfed had twice as many hip fractures as those who had breastfed. Also, the longer a woman breastfed each baby, the lower her risk of hip fracture in later life. Breastfeeding each baby for more than nine months lowered a woman's risk of hip fracture to one-quarter of that of women who had never breastfed.

- A South African study (1992) showed that breastfeeders had a higher bone mineral density in later life than women who formula-fed. And women who developed osteoporosis were four times less likely to have been breastfeeders.

However, it's possible that if breastfeeding does protect against osteoporosis, as these studies suggest, it does so only if done for a cumulatively large number of months or even years. Long-term breastfeeding delays the onset of ovulation after each baby. This means a woman's supply of eggs lasts longer and she can then go on ovulating longer into middle age. The longer she has menstrual cycles, giving her high levels of oestrogen and progesterone, the later is her menopause and the further away the time when low hormone levels encourage osteoporosis.

LESS RHEUMATOID ARTHRITIS?

Studies into this are inconsistent. However, a suggested mechanism for any possible reduction in the risk of rheumatoid arthritis (RA) is that women who have ever breastfed for twelve months or more have significantly increased levels – persisting past the menopause – of the anti-inflammatory hormone cortisol.

- Norwegian research (1994) looked at the records of 63,090 women, 355 of whom had died from RA. They found an association between the total time a woman had breastfed and her chance of dying from RA. Those who had breastfed for a total of twenty months or more had a particularly low risk.

However:

- North American research (1995) reported that in a small group of susceptible women, breastfeeding *increased* the risk of developing RA; they are currently investigating whether there is a genetic basis for this. One theory is that prolactin may in certain circumstances provoke the immune system to turn against the joint linings.

POSSIBLE DISADVANTAGES FOR YOU

Many women decide not to breastfeed and it would be foolish to pretend there are no drawbacks to breastfeeding. However, many perceived disadvantages can be overcome and other concerns may disappear when well aired.

Embarrassment

Our society equates breasts with sex, and some people think women who reveal their breasts while breastfeeding are immodest or provocative. Yet the idea that women should breastfeed only at home or in a private place is clearly untenable. Babies need nourishment when they need it! And breastfeeding is a human right.

Most women breastfeed in public discreetly, partly for personal reasons and partly to avoid anyone staring or even being unpleasant. You can easily learn the knack of feeding without exposing your breast, though a few babies tend to attract attention by making loud sucking noises, kicking in delight, or choking or spluttering when the milk lets down.

Breastfeeding in public is accepted without question in many developed and developing countries and is becoming more and more acceptable in countries such as the UK. Public acceptability always advances when a celebrity talks about herself breastfeeding or a TV or film director features a breastfeeding actress.

However, the fear of embarrassment deters many women from breastfeeding. They may feel anxious at the thought of feeding not only in front of strangers but even in front of relatives. Indeed, for some, it's the main thing that puts them off choosing to breastfeed. Obviously it's no good telling a woman she needn't be embarrassed, especially if she's breastfeeding for the first time, or is shy and retiring by nature, or sexually inhibited. But perhaps she could use her confidence that she's doing the very best for her baby to strengthen her resolve.

Also, we should all have the courage of our convictions and explain to anyone who makes things difficult for a breastfeeding woman that what she's doing is normal, natural and best.

Being tied?

Some women choose not to breastfeed because they don't want to be tied to the method or to their baby. Certainly if a woman is to breastfeed successfully and exclusively for at least four to six months, she'll find it far easier if she's with her baby. However, some women learn the knack of expressing enough milk for someone else to give (by cup, spoon or bottle) when they are out; others give their babies the occasional bottle of formula – though even occasional bottles of formula are unwise before your milk supply is well established.

Outings other than to people's homes may have to be limited in the first few weeks because very young babies can't last long between feeds. This can be overcome if you feed in a parked car, on a park bench or in a cafe with helpful staff.

Some breastfeeding support groups have lists of shops and other public places which support breastfeeding. (For example, Sainsbury's, the UK food retailer, provides facilities for breastfeeding customers.) If no such list is available to you locally, why not consider compiling one and sending it to your local paper or baby clinic? It could be excellent publicity for supportive shops.

Rather than worry about never being able to leave your baby, it helps to be positive about taking the baby with you when you go out. There are very few places you can't take a baby, especially a very young, easily transportable one. Even a woman brought up to believe anyone can take her place as a mother may decide to think of her baby as an extension of herself, for a few months at least. A baby loves to be with his mother, and once this becomes a reality to you, you may not want to go out alone.

No one else can feed the baby

This isn't true. A breastfeeding woman can leave milk for someone else to give her baby if she collects enough by expressing it after each of several feeds. However, a large survey in Britain in 1990 showed that nearly one in two pregnant women who planned on formula-feeding gave as one of their reasons the fact that other people would be able to feed their baby.

Expecting to return to work

One in twenty women said they planned to formula-feed because they were expecting to return to work soon, according to the large survey mentioned above. However, very few women in fact return to work when their babies are very young. And even if they do, they can continue breastfeeding.

Friends aren't doing it

A woman's friends have a big influence on her choice of infant feeding. If she has a lot of formula-feeding friends, she is more likely to formula-feed herself, and vice versa. It takes a courageous person to break out of line.

Pain?

Some women who have never breastfed imagine it will be painful; indeed, many breastfeeding women do occasionally have sore nipples, especially in the early days, and a few have other painful breast conditions. However, sore nipples, for example, are temporary and often avoidable to some extent, and there's a lot you can do to make them better.

Can't see how much he's getting

Our society is obsessed with measuring things, and we have been brainwashed into thinking it's important to know how much milk a baby takes. In reality it very rarely is important, especially if the baby is healthy and thriving. No two infants are alike and each needs different amounts of milk at different times of day. Properly managed breastfeeding is a perfectly balanced demand-and-supply system, with the emphasis on the supply – the more and better you stimulate your breasts by breastfeeding (or expressing or pumping), with no long gaps and with the baby feeding well, the more milk you'll make.

If ever you fall into the trap of test-weighing your baby to find out how much he's getting, remember breastfed babies thrive on smaller volumes of milk than formula-fed babies, partly because breast milk is perfectly digested.

Unfashionable?

To a certain extent humans have a herd instinct and like to copy each other's behaviour. Midwives often remark that if one mother is breastfeeding successfully, others tend to copy her, but if she fails, they're likely to stop too.

When formula-feeding first became fashionable, only the relatively wealthy could afford it, but gradually the habit spread, with the middle classes leading the way.

Today, women in low-earning families and those with the least education are the ones most likely to formula-feed. In many hospitals the majority of women start breastfeeding. Once back at home, though, many stop within a few weeks.

Unsexy?

Some women imagine breastfeeding will make them less sexy, both in their own eyes and those of their partner. But many find the opposite.

Your breasts will sag?

Studies show that pregnancy can change the shape of the breasts. However, this is just as likely to happen to formula-feeders as to breastfeeders.

Breastfeeding won't make your breasts sag if you wear a properly fitting, supportive bra by day and night. This prevents heavier than usual breasts stretching the skin's elastic fibres and the breasts' supportive connective tissue. If you look after your breasts, then although they may appear rather shrunken when you stop breastfeeding and the milk-producing tissues shrink, they'll fill out with repositioned fat over the next few months.

The other important things to guard against are engorgement and getting fat from overeating, as both can stretch breast skin and make your breasts more likely to sag later.

Disgusting?

A few women are disgusted by breastfeeding, even seeing others doing it, and either refuse to breastfeed or give up after a day or two because it seems 'animal-like'. One way to help prevent girls growing up with such deep-rooted feelings is to introduce lessons at school mentioning breastfeeding as a natural and beautiful part of childcare. In some schools teachers ask a woman and her breastfeeding baby along to these classes so children can watch and ask questions directly.

Risk of failure

A number of women are so afraid they'll fail at breastfeeding that they actually do. They then feel deeply disappointed. Some health workers don't like to use the word 'failure', but the fact is that many women do see it as a failure. So great can this feeling be that some doctors and nurses refuse to tell women about the benefits of breastfeeding for fear they'll be unable to succeed at it and then feel guilty. This is tragic, because babies are denied their natural food and women their natural right – and all for nothing, because failure rarely needs to happen. Nearly every woman *can* breastfeed for as long as she wants if she understands how to make enough milk and has enough help. And taking steps to increase the milk supply generally works within a few days. But having said this, there are a very few women who are indeed unable to provide enough breast milk whatever they do and whatever help they get. Rather than castigate themselves and allow their babies to go without adequate nourishment, it's essential that they put their pride to one side and give their baby formula as well as their breast milk.

Broken sleep

Breastfeeding helps babies get off to sleep, but breastfed babies tend to sleep rather less on average than bottle-feds and also tend not to sleep quite as long, especially if they sleep with their mothers and feed at night.

> Breastfeeding has many very real advantages for women as well as for babies. The next chapter explores how to prepare for it during pregnancy.

FIVE

Preparation and pregnancy

You can do a great deal during pregnancy to prepare for breastfeeding. First and foremost, look after your health and well-being so you feel at your best and your baby gets a good start. You may want to learn about breastfeeding, discuss it with your partner and find out who will be able to help if you have any difficulties. It's sensible to prepare yourself and your home so things run as smoothly as possible when the baby arrives. And you need to choose the best place to have your baby.

Let's start by considering how to look after yourself.

WHAT TO EAT

Eat a healthy, balanced diet with five helpings of vegetables and fruit a day, noting that several nutrients, including folate (called folic acid in supplements), calcium, iron and fibre are particularly important in pregnancy.

Have plenty of foods rich in the B vitamin *folate*, especially early in pregnancy, as this discourages certain congenital deformities (including spina bifida and cleft palate). Folate-rich foods include most vegetables (especially dark green leafy ones), fruit, eggs, wholegrain foods, beans, peas, lentils, fish, nuts and yeast extract. Some breakfast cereals and white breads are fortified with folic acid – check on the packets.

Many experts advise a folic-acid supplement as an extra precaution for women who want to become pregnant or are so already. The recommended amount is 0.4 mg (400 micrograms) a day, starting before conception and continuing for the first three months of pregnancy. This is twice the amount in the average woman's diet. Some experts, however, point out that a supplement is necessary only for women who eat an unhealthy diet or have a poor appetite and as a result don't eat much at all. If you have already had a baby with spina bifida or a cleft palate, you need a bigger supplement of 5 mg (5,000 micrograms) of folic acid a day.

You also need plenty of foods that contain *calcium*, as this mineral strengthens a baby's developing bones. When you are pregnant you automatically absorb more calcium from the foods you eat. But if your diet is low in calcium, your bones may supply it preferentially to your developing baby, which will weaken them. Calcium-containing foods include peas, beans, lentils, wholegrain foods, cabbage, watercress, fish, milk, yoghurt, cheese, nuts and seeds. The soft bones of tinned salmon and sardines are another good source of calcium.

Many people believe milk is essential for a pregnant woman but this is not so, as long as she gets enough calcium from other foods. Anyway, some women can't drink milk without getting stomach ache, bloating, wind and diarrhoea, because they have lactose intolerance, caused by a deficiency of lactase – the enzyme that breaks down milk sugar (lactose) in the gut. Lactose intolerance affects one in twenty people of northern European descent and up to nine out of ten people of Afro-Caribbean, Chinese, Mediterranean and Middle Eastern descent. If you are lactose-intolerant yet would like to drink more milk, you can buy lactase from pharmacies and add it to milk to pre-digest the lactose.

About one in ten pregnant women has iron-deficiency anaemia, and this is almost always due to a poor diet. To guard against it, you need foods containing *iron*, including meat, egg yolk, dark green leafy vegetables, peas, beans, lentils, wholegrain foods, apricots, raisins and prunes. Eating foods rich in vitamin C (for example, citrus and other fruit, fruit juice and vegetables) at the same time helps you to absorb iron. However, avoid drinking tea with a meal as its tannins reduce iron absorption.

The World Health Organization says there is no need for women in developed countries to take iron supplements provided they eat well. Routine blood tests (usually at the first antenatal clinic visit and again at thirty-two weeks) detect anaemia early enough for treatment with iron supplements to begin well before the baby is born.

A good balance of *omega-3s* and *omega-6s* helps keep you healthy and discourage depression after childbirth. Omega-3 fatty acids are found in green leafy vegetables, broccoli, beans, tofu, walnuts (a particularly rich source) and their oil, pumpkin seeds, linseeds (flax-seeds – the richest source), rapeseed (canola), soya and olive oils, meat from grass-fed animals, fish (especialy oily fish) and shellfish. Omega-6s are in avocados; beans; corn; seeds; rapeseed (canola), sunflower, safflower, sesame, peanut (groundnut) and soybean oils; margarine; cereal and other grain-based foods; eggs; meat from corn or cereal-grain fed animals. However, many of us eat too much omega-6 in comparison with omega-3, so consider whether you need to right the balance. If so, the most effective ways are to eat:

- Less cereal-grain food (e.g., bread, biscuits, breakfast cereal), grain-fed meat, and margarine and other processed food containing sun-flower oil.
- More green leafy veg and fish. If using olive oil, don't fry with it as this spoils its omega-3s.

Eating vegetables, fruit and wholegrain foods gives you plenty of *fibre*, which helps you avoid the common pregnancy problem of constipation.

Vegetarians

If you're a vegetarian, make sure you eat enough foods rich in iron, calcium, zinc (found in nuts, wholegrain foods, peas, beans, root vegetables and garlic) and vitamin B_{12} (eggs, milk, cheese, seaweed). If you are a vegan and eat no food of animal origin, you need a supplement of vitamin B_{12}.

Avoid foods most likely to be infected with *Listeria*

Many experts recommend avoiding soft cheeses such as Camembert and Brie, blue cheese, unpasteurized cheeses and insufficiently reheated pre-cooked chilled foods in pregnancy, because of the risk that they contain an overgrowth of *Listeria* bacteria. These bacteria are normally harmless but in some pregnant women they cause a flu-like infection which damages their unborn baby.

Avoid liver and liver pâté

Many experts recommend avoiding these because they contain high levels of vitamin A, which could, at worst, damage an unborn baby.

YOUR WEIGHT

Most women eat no more food than usual during the early months of pregnancy and only about 100 calories a day more in the last few weeks. However, if you are very active, or go into pregnancy underweight, you may want, or need, to eat more. If you have pregnancy sickness you may feel like eating less than usual, though your appetite should increase again later.

The average woman gains 7–18 kg (15–40 lb) in pregnancy. This weight gain represents the baby, the placenta, the amniotic fluid, the increased size of the womb and breasts, the increased volume of blood and other body fluids and about 2–3 kg (4–7 lb) of extra fat – which is deposited in the body's fat stores. After childbirth, a woman who bottle-feeds may have trouble losing this extra fat. But in a woman who breastfeeds it should gradually disappear (as long as she isn't overeating), as it's used to make breast milk. Indeed, a woman's pregnancy fat stores contribute up to 300 calories a day to breast milk for three or four months. Since a baby needs only 600–800 calories a day, the mother's fat stores provide up to half her baby's requirements and she needs to eat only an extra 300–600 calories a day on top of her usual intake in order to produce breast milk without depleting her body of nutrients.

However, you don't have to store fat in pregnancy to be able to breastfeed. If you don't lay down much extra fat, all you need to do when breastfeeding is eat more; millions of women in developing countries lay down no fat in pregnancy, yet breastfeed successfully for very long periods if they have enough to eat. Also, note that gaining too much weight encourages swollen ankles, varicose veins, backache, fatigue and heartburn.

ALCOHOL

Experts can't say exactly how much, if any, alcohol is safe in pregnancy, but the official guidelines in some countries, including the US, Australia and New Zealand, are to have none. Many other countries, including the UK, recommend limiting the amount. If you drink, it's probably sensible to limit it to one unit of alcohol a day, which means having no more than one small glass of wine, a half-pint of beer, a quarter-pint of strong lager, a small glass of sherry or a measure of spirits a day. It's also wise to have two or three alcohol-free days a week. And it's particularly important not to binge on alcohol.

GOING OUTSIDE

Go outside in bright daylight each day, because bright outdoor daylight on your skin enables your body to make a significant amount of vitamin D. This helps keep your bones strong during the time you are breastfeeding, and helps supply your unborn baby with vitamin D too.

CHOOSING WHERE TO HAVE YOUR BABY

Once you know you are pregnant, book into a hospital for the delivery unless you plan on giving birth at home. Choose carefully, because some hospitals are much more helpful than others with breastfeeding.

This checklist may help you decide:

- Ask your doctor if the hospital you are considering has a 'Baby Friendly' award (see opposite), meaning its practices match criteria set by the World Health Organization and UNICEF, or is seeking one, or at least encourages baby friendly policies.
- If the doctor doesn't know, ask friends and local women whether the staff in the hospital they went to were helpful with breastfeeding.
- Ask each hospital you are considering to supply you with a copy of its breastfeeding policy, and ask whether most women who want to breastfeed manage to do so.
- Ask whether you'll be allowed – and, preferably, encouraged – to labour in an upright position if you want to, rather than on your back. Labouring upright can speed up labour, make contractions less arduous and increase a baby's oxygen supply; it also tends to make labour easier and quicker, and childbirth safer. And because both mother and baby are more likely to feel well afterwards, breastfeeding is more likely to get off to a good start.

With good information, support and help if necessary, being in hospital need not load the dice against successful breastfeeding, even though breastfeeding is more likely to be successful at home. A hospital environment, after all, does little to encourage the establishment of the let-down (page 125). One newly delivered American woman logged the number of intruders into her hospital room each day: it came to between fifty and seventy. So many intrusions could hardly be said to be relaxing! Some hospitals employ midwives whose main job is to encourage and advise breastfeeding mothers.

Baby Friendly Hospitals

More and more hospitals around the world are changing their policies to become eligible for Baby Friendly Hospital status, awarded by UNICEF.

Baby Friendly Hospitals use 'Ten Steps to Successful Breastfeeding'. This means they:

1 – Have a written breastfeeding policy that is routinely communicated to all health staff.
2 – Train all health care staff in the skills necessary to implement this policy.
3 – Inform all pregnant women about the benefits and management of breastfeeding.
4 – Help mothers initiate breastfeeding within half an hour of birth.
5 – Show mothers how to breastfeed and how to maintain lactation even if they are separated from their infants.
6 – Give newborn infants no food or drink other than breast milk, unless *medically* indicated.
7 – Practise rooming-in (when mothers and infants remain together) twenty-four hours a day.
8 – Encourage breastfeeding on demand.
9 – Give no artificial teats or pacifiers (dummies or soothers) to breastfeeding infants.
10 – Foster the establishment of breastfeeding support groups and refer mothers to them on discharge from the hospital or clinic.

There are three Baby Friendly awards. The Global Award means a hospital has adopted all ten steps and at least three out of four women are still breastfeeding when they leave. The Standard Award means a hospital has adopted all ten steps, is working towards continued improvements and at least one in two women is still breastfeeding when she leaves. And the Certificate of Commitment means a hospital has adopted steps 1, 7 and 10 and is working towards the rest.

By March 2002 Canada had one Baby Friendly Hospital (though many other hospitals were working towards an award), Japan had 14, Australia 17, the US 25, China 6,312, Africa and the Middle East 2,752 and India 1,250.

Focusing on the UK, the Royal Bournemouth Hospital became the UK's first Baby Friendly Hospital in 1995 and now over fifty-four health-care facilities have full Baby Friendly accreditation, and eighty maternity units and community services have a Certificate of Commitment. This still leaves many with neither.

UK Hospitals wishing to apply for Baby Friendly status can contact the UNICEF UK Baby Friendly Initiative at Africa House, 64–78 Kingsway, London WC2B 6NB; or call 020 7312 7652, or visit www.babyfriendly.org.uk. Other hospitals should write to UNICEF Baby Friendly Hospital Initiative, Palais des Nations, 1211, Geneva 10, Switzerland.

MAKING A BIRTH PLAN

A birth plan should ideally be discussed and agreed with the hospital staff during pregnancy and include your ideas of how you want to give birth, feed and care for your baby. For example, you might say you would like to hold your newborn baby immediately after birth and to offer the first feed when the baby is ready. You might want to point out that you want your baby to have *only* breast milk and not be given bottles without your personal permission. And you could say you would prefer not to have pain-relieving drugs such as pethidine too close to the actual birth, as these might make your baby too sleepy to feed well at first.

PLANNING FOR WHEN YOU GO HOME

If you and your baby are well, plan on returning home from hospital as soon as you can after the birth. Women who leave hospital within forty-eight hours are more likely to breastfeed successfully than those who stay in longer. This is scarcely surprising, as most of us relax better in our own environment and therefore produce more milk and let it down more reliably. Also, the loving, constant emotional support and encouragement you need can best be supplied by family and friends.

If you've been unlucky enough to give birth in a hospital where babies are kept in a nursery at night, you'll have to wait until you get home to be able to have your baby with you all the time. Once home, you can breastfeed on an unrestricted basis day and night, which will help you get off to a good start.

Well ahead of time, arrange for a relative, friend or paid person to be at home to help out when you return after the birth, if possible. This will ensure you get the rest you need, have time to enjoy your baby and learn to breastfeed successfully.

INVOLVING YOUR PARTNER

Talk with your partner about breastfeeding and what it will mean for him. Tell him what you know about its advantages and suggest he goes to the fathers' night at your antenatal class, where he can discuss any queries. He might be interested in reading parts of this book too; chapter 16 is written specially for fathers.

He'll probably be pleased to support your decision to breastfeed, especially once he understands how important breastfeeding is and how valuable he can be as protector and encourager. Researchers say the partner's attitude is the single most important influence on a woman's decision on how to feed her baby. Partners of women who plan to bottle-feed usually don't know about the health benefits of breastfeeding; they also tend to imagine that breastfeeding makes a woman's breasts sag (which isn't true provided you give your breasts adequate support) and will spoil their sex life (though fatigue is a far more common culprit after childbirth).

Discuss practical matters, such as how he'll get home from work if you usually pick him up but happen to be breastfeeding at the time; how he can sometimes cook supper or why, if you cook, you'll need to be flexible about mealtimes; and how it'll mean you both get more sleep if the baby sleeps in your bedroom so you can easily breastfeed at night – though your partner may sleep even better if he decamps to another bedroom.

Some women choose to bottle-feed so that their partner can sometimes enjoy giving the baby a bottle of formula. But no mother need feel guilty about depriving a man of this experience. He can enjoy cuddling his baby as much as he likes any time other than during a breastfeed.

CHOOSING HOW TO FEED YOUR BABY

Many factors influence a woman's decision on how to feed her baby. A survey of expectant mothers in the UK in 1990 discovered some interesting ideas underlying their choice of feeding:

%	*Reasons for planning to breastfeed first babies*
85	Breastfeeding is best for the baby
34	Breastfeeding is more convenient
23	Closer bond between mother and baby
21	Breastfeeding is cheaper
14	Breastfeeding is natural
13	Breastfeeding is best for mother
13	Mother loses weight more easily
4	Infiuenced by medical personnel
4	Influenced by friends or relatives

%	
3	History of allergies/illness in the family
3	No particular reason

(Percentages don't add up to 100 as some women gave more than one reason.)

%	*Reasons for planning to bottle-feed first babies*
29	Other people can feed baby with bottle
27	Didn't like idea of breastfeeding
7	Can see how much baby has had
7	Expecting to return to work soon
6	Other reasons
5	No particular reason
4	Would be embarrassed to breastfeed
2	Medical reasons for not breastfeeding
2	Bottle-feeding is less tiring

(Percentages don't add up to 100 as some women gave more than one reason.)

(Both tables from *Infant Feeding* 2000, HMSO)

What's so fascinating is that many of the women who chose bottle-feeding gave reasons *against* breastfeeding, not *for* bottle-feeding. In contrast, most of those who chose breastfeeding were positively *for* breastfeeding, not *against* bottle-feeding. So the bottle-feeders gave negative reasons, the breastfeeders positive ones. Perhaps, then, a more thorough discussion in antenatal classes of the imagined disadvantages of breastfeeding, preferably with inputs from at least one successfully breastfeeding woman, might help women who would have chosen bottle-feeding overcome their perceived negatives about breastfeeding. Also, as the number one choice breastfeeders give for breastfeeding is that it's best for babies, this fact must be well aired – and not hushed up to allay guilt in those who don't want to breastfeed and the very few who can't.

Your feelings about breastfeeding

If you strongly dislike the idea of breastfeeding, consider doing some emotional spadework to discover why, perhaps using the information on page 209. This may enable you to make a freer choice about feeding by allowing you to become more emotionally aware.

Sources of information about breastfeeding

Find out as much as you can about breastfeeding before you start to do it. Even if you have breastfed successfully before, read about it or discuss it because each baby is different and the way he feeds will be different too. If you understand how breastfeeding works, you'll be aware of what might happen, be more confident and know when to get help for any problems.

ANTENATAL CLASSES

Hopefully the session on baby feeding will focus on breastfeeding. By making friends now with other women who want to breastfeed, you can become 'bosom buddies' when you have all had your babies – encouraging each other, giving extra information or advice and generally caring for each other.

Researchers find that antenatal education about breastfeeding makes successful breastfeeding more likely. Giving information about breastfeeding and the care of a newborn baby – including an idea of the large number of breastfeeds and nappy changes, the lack of a predictable schedule and the possibility of setbacks – gives pregnant women a more realistic idea of their future role as breastfeeding mothers. Women who aren't taught about breastfeeding may waste time blaming their baby for breastfeeding problems instead of focusing on factors under their control.

Other researchers have found that women are more likely to

plan on breastfeeding if the antenatal-class leader favours breastfeeding. So it's wise for people running such classes to make it clear that breast is best. It's also a good idea for the leader to invite a breastfeeding woman to talk and demonstrate. This is because quite a few young women have never seen anyone breastfeeding, yet doing so can often be a very potent influence on making the decision to go ahead with breastfeeding – more important for many women than knowing about its health benefits.

INFORMATION PAMPHLETS

Be vigilant about the source of booklets and leaflets about pregnancy and baby feeding, such as those available in some clinics and surgeries. The way information about breastfeeding is put across in booklets sponsored by milk-formula companies may be much less helpful and encouraging about breastfeeding than information sponsored by non-commercial bodies.

Interestingly, one pamphlet sponsored by a large milk formula company some years ago had a photograph of a woman breastfeeding with her sweater pulled down to expose her whole breast. No successfully breastfeeding woman would do this – she would pull her sweater *up*, giving her baby access while exposing little or no breast to the outside world. Given that the idea that they might have to expose their breasts puts many women off the whole idea of breastfeeding, this photograph makes one question the company's motives.

HEALTH PROFESSIONALS

If you live in the UK you may meet your health visitor at the antenatal classes. She will be your official breastfeeding adviser once you part company with the community midwife (which happens within the first four weeks after the birth – normally after ten days) and her support and advice could be invaluable. You can contact her at your baby clinic in person, or by phone. Ask local women expecting second babies whether the local health visitor's breastfeeding advice is good. If she has the reputation for advising bottles of formula too readily, get in touch with an NCT breastfeeding counsellor or LLL leader as well (see below).

Learning together

Some health professionals are wonderful, in that they go on learning about successful breastfeeding alongside women doing it. The very best helpers know they can always learn more.

Some breastfeeding women are willing and confident enough to learn about successful breastfeeding independently, and to teach and encourage their midwife, doctor and, in the UK, their health visitor, as they learn themselves. This requires an eagerness to learn, together with intellectual humility, on the part of the health professional, but some brave breastfeeding women and helpers team up with excellent and mutually rewarding results. Many such professionals have gone on to help many other women. People with this generosity of spirit light the way for others and deserve warm congratulations and gratitude.

There's a section especially for health professionals on page 403.

BREASTFEEDING SUPPORT GROUPS

Many countries have national breastfeeding support organizations with local groups. In the UK, for example, the National Childbirth Trust (NCT) organizes courses of antenatal classes. An NCT breastfeeding counsellor usually gives a talk during each course and you can contact her if you need help once you've had your baby, whether or not you are a member of the NCT. These counsellors are volunteers who are well trained in helping with breastfeeding problems on a mother-to-mother basis, and have breastfed babies themselves. Some NCT branches arrange post-natal meetings and support groups too.

La Leche League International (LLLI) is a worldwide organization of women who are breastfeeding or have breastfed and want to encourage and help each other with breastfeeding. Anyone interested is welcome to attend local LLL branch meetings. Your nearest LLL leader will give you her telephone number so you can contact her if you need help. League leaders are volunteers with an excellent training in assisting and encouraging breastfeeding women; they have all breastfed babies successfully for long periods and can discuss things on a mother-to-mother basis. LLL group meetings are open to anyone, whether pregnant, breastfeeding or neither.

BRAS

When your breasts start growing, from about the fifth month of pregnancy or even before, you'll need a bigger bra, though you may be able to make do for a while by using simple extenders to increase the chest size of your existing bras (available from NCT Maternity Sales, see page 420).

You'll need several bras when breastfeeding, because they'll require frequent washing, especially early on when you're bound to leak. Some people think cotton 'breathes' better than synthetic fabrics. It's important to wear a bra that supports and fits well, yet doesn't squash your breasts or nipples.

Many women wear an ordinary bra and either undo it or pull it up or down to breastfeed; only 40 per cent of breastfeeding women wear a special bra. Pulling the cup down to free the breast works well if the bra is not too built up, but make sure it supports you well enough, is large enough, and doesn't squash any part of the breast when pulled down, as this could lead to a blocked duct. If you have small breasts, you may not need a bra at all.

If you buy a nursing bra, note that they can have drop-down

cups or zipped cups. Drop-down cups are easier to use, but go for ones with one hook per cup, rather than rows of tiny hooks and eyes which make frequent feeds difficult and are awkward to do up and undo discreetly in company. The NCT Maternity Sales catalogue has a good selection, including a style going up to an HH cup size. In the UK women can be measured and order bras from local NCT branch bra agents. Choose bras no earlier than around thirty-six weeks of pregnancy, or if possible wait until after your baby is born, so they fit well.

Wearing a bra at night

Pregnancy is a time to be especially careful about looking after your breasts. It's sensible to wear a bra in bed during the last three months of pregnancy to support your increasingly heavy breasts and help prevent your skin stretching. Maternity bras sold as sleep bras are usually too insubstantial to provide much support.

CLOTHES

Good clothes to have ready for breastfeeding include loose T-shirts, sweatshirts, jumpers, blouses and almost anything you can pull up from the waist. These make for easy breastfeeding and allow you to feed without showing everything. Indeed, feeding a baby with your top pulled up just enough looks as though you're simply having a cuddle, which makes it easy to feed in public. Dresses that undo in front are fine for breastfeeding at home when you don't need to be discreet. If you're wearing a blouse when you're out, pull it up to feed rather than undoing the buttons. Some women alter existing clothes to make them more suitable. Check you have several changes of clothes to wear while breast-feeding because being in the same things day after day can be depressing. There are lots of nighties that undo in front, and pyjamas are fine.

Clothes should be washable because apart from your milk leaking, your baby may bring up small amounts of milk and you won't want huge dry-cleaning bills.

FURNITURE AND EQUIPMENT

You'll probably want your baby near you so you can hear him, so you'll need a crib, a cot on wheels, a carrycot or a pram to use during the day. Similarly, if you want your baby by your bed at night for easy feeding, it's a good idea to have a readily movable cot. You can buy a cot with a removable side, so the baby's mattress is level with yours, making it easy to slip the baby into your bed for a feed and back again (see page 418). Babies sleep anywhere if tired, warm and full, and in the early days, before they are old enough to roll over or wriggle and fall, they can sleep on a sofa or easy chair. However, this isn't always a good idea. Your baby may sick up some milk on the upholstery; someone may accidentally sit on him; a sibling or pet is more likely to interfere with him; and the day will come when he will roll for the first time. Note too that it's probably unwise to drop off to sleep by your baby on a sofa, since cot death in a baby sleeping with his mother is more likely on a sofa. Some sort of cot is safer for a sleeping baby who isn't in your arms.

Think about where you'll sit to breastfeed, since a comfortable place will help you relax and so reduce the risk of aching shoulders and arms after a feed. A good nursing chair is low, so your lap is flat enough to support the baby well, and has arms or a place to put cushions to support your elbows at the right height. Experiment before you have the baby. A rocking chair can be pleasant and many women are comfortable sitting on a sofa or bed with their feet up. Lying down to feed is most relaxing of all.

SHOPPING AND HOUSEWORK

Store as much food as possible before you have your baby. Stock up with tinned and dried food and if you have a freezer fill it with prepared meals so you and your partner can rustle something up quickly if you are too tired to cook. Convenience food is a great help early on, though it's better to eat fresh food when possible.

If you can afford it, buy stocks of washing powder, disposable nappies or cloth-nappy sterilizing solution, and basic household goods. Shopping with a very young baby can be a headache as he may want feeding so often that there isn't time to be out for long. You might like to find out whether any local shops or supermarkets accept phone or Internet orders and deliver to the door. Your partner could go late-night shopping, or a relative or neighbour might do some shopping for you until your baby is old enough to go for longer between feeds.

The laundry generated by one small baby is a big surprise to many first-time mothers. It's worth preparing for this in advance. If you don't have a washing machine, see if you can possibly afford one now as it'll make all the difference, especially if you use cloth nappies. Otherwise, think about sending bed linen, towels and other big things to a laundry for the first few weeks. This is especially important if you have your baby at home, or come home within forty-eight hours, as you may soil bed linen in the first few days. An alternative is to use disposable absorbent mats (e.g. Pampers Care Mats) in your bed early on. If you don't have a machine, buy a few boxes of disposable nappies, even if you intend to use cloth nappies eventually, since washing nappies will tire you in the early days. You may consider disposables too expensive, or environmentally damaging, to continue using after the first week or so, but they'll give you an easy start.

HELP AT HOME

Consider arranging for someone to come in to help you in the house when you get home with your new baby, as you'll need to take things easy for a few weeks. It's even more helpful with a second or third baby because there's more work with a family this size. If you haven't any willing relatives nearby, you might want to pay for domestic help for an hour or two each day if you can. Many partners take a week or two off work to help, especially if there are other children. Whatever happens, you'll need time if you are to breastfeed successfully, especially at first when the baby needs very frequent feeds, so don't expect to be a superwoman.

BREAST AND NIPPLE CARE

The advice some expectant mothers are given about caring for their breasts and nipples puts them off breastfeeding. The average modern woman doesn't want to push and poke her breasts and nipples for months before her baby is born. Anyway, there's no convincing evidence from surveys that any antenatal preparation – such as rolling nipples, rubbing them with a rough towel, putting on lanolin, cream or alcohol and expressing colostrum – makes successful breastfeeding any more likely than doing nothing at all. The only reasons for rolling nipples, for example, might be to make them less sensitive (though that will happen anyway once your baby starts feeding), or to get you used to handling your breasts.

However, some women find it helps to go without a bra during pregnancy, or cut a small hole in the centre of each bra cup, since the nipples then rub against their clothing and become less sensitive.

Three other things can be valuable – knowing more about

nipple shape and nipple cleanliness and learning the basics of how to express milk.

Nipple shape

Some nipples are *flat* or *inverted* (turned inwards), because short milk ducts tether the nipples down. Some antenatal clinic staff routinely check the shape of pregnant women's nipples, but to see if nipples are flat or inverted it's no good just looking – they must do the *pinch test*. To do this yourself, pinch your areola (the darker skin around the nipple) between your finger and thumb to see if the nipple comes out. If it does, it's unlikely your baby will have any difficulty. Also, if your nipples usually come out when you feel cold or sexually aroused, you shouldn't have a problem.

Between 7 and 10 per cent of pregnant women who want to breastfeed have truly inverted nipples (which won't come out at all) or *poorly protractile* nipples (which don't come out much). The good news is that nipple shape and protractility often improve in pregnancy, probably because of the action of oestrogens on the tissues behind the nipple. Inverted or poorly protractile nipples are said to hinder one woman in twenty feeding a first baby, one in fifty feeding a second, and none who've fed two or more. However, a great many women with nipples like this manage perfectly well, especially if a skilled carer helps them position their babies and reminds them not to limit the number or length of breastfeeds or give bottles of formula.

Some people think *breast shells* help inverted or poorly protractile nipples, though no studies have shown this. These are hollow, plastic or glass, saucer-shaped devices with a circular hole on the inner surface for the nipple. Wearing shells inside a bra is supposed to encourage the nipples to protrude through the holes and gradually improve their shape in pregnancy, but nipples that improve with shells would probably have improved anyway.

One study (1995) looked at 463 pregnant women in England and Canada who had inverted or non-protractile (not protruding half a centimetre with the pinch test) nipples and intended to breastfeed. They were divided into four groups, one rolling their nipples twice a day, one wearing breast shells, one using rolling and shells, one using neither. In each group 45 per cent were still breastfeeding six weeks after childbirth. So whatever they did antenatally made no difference.

Breast shells are probably more useful after a baby is born, when using them for a short while before a feed helps poorly protractile nipples protrude for long enough for the baby to latch on well (get a good mouthful of the nipple and areola). After a few seconds the nipple returns to its original shape, so the baby has to catch hold fairly quickly. The disadvantage is that the pressure of the shell can obstruct milk ducts and encourage engorgement. Also, the skin under the shell can become moist and swollen and more liable to soreness and cracks. In the US you can buy a breast shell (made by Medela) with numerous openings on the rounded dome to allow more air to circulate around the skin. If ordering or buying breast shells, note that some people wrongly call them breast shields or milk cups.

Avent Niplettes (see page 416) are suction devices which look like little clear plastic thimbles and are said to help bring out inverted or flat nipples by encouraging short milk ducts to lengthen. To use them, you hold one on your nipple, then use the syringe (already attached to a valve on the Niplette) to suck out the air between the nipple and Niplette. When the nipple comes out, you let go of the Niplette and remove the syringe. You can leave the Niplette on all day under loose clothing, and overnight if you wish – either as well as during the day or instead. When your nipples have lengthened to fill the Niplettes, you gradually stop wearing them. Two to three months of use should lead to a permanent result. Niplettes are designed to be used during pregnancy, not while breastfeeding. One small trial found that each of six pregnant women with inverted nipples had normal-looking nipples after two weeks of using Niplettes, and all found them easy to use.

If you still have inverted nipples at the end of pregnancy, and breast shells make no difference, your baby may still be able to suck efficiently if you 'make a biscuit' of your areola and nipple with your thumb and forefinger and offer it to him. Engorgement is the number one enemy of successful latching-on in women with inverted nipples, so avoid this at all costs.

Nipple cleanliness

Tiny protruberances around the areola, called Montgomery's tubercles, produce an oily fluid which keeps the areola and nipple supple and kills bacteria. If you wash this away with soap, your skin is much more likely to become sore when you breastfeed. So avoid soap for the last few weeks of pregnancy and just wash your nipples with warm water. There's no need to use any ointment or cream to prepare for breastfeeding, because nature's own lubrication is best. Similarly, there's no need to remove the yellowish grains of dried secretions you may see on your nipples – a simple water splash is enough.

Expressing milk

There's no need to express milk in pregnancy to remove colostrum or 'clear the ducts'.

> With everything prepared for breastfeeding you can concentrate on looking forward to your baby's birth. The next chapter looks at how breastfeeding works.

SIX

How breastfeeding works

This chapter includes basic information about how breastfeeding works. Let's start by looking at the breasts themselves.

THE BREASTS

Changes in the shape and size of the breasts, nipples and areolae begin a year or so before a girl's periods start and continue until her late teens. After this the breasts stay much the same until she gets pregnant, always supposing her weight remains steady. Breasts also have a sexual role in courtship that isn't seen in other mammals, and in the developed world in particular this helps colour our attitudes to breastfeeding. Humans are the only mammals whose breasts enlarge before pregnancy.

The increase in size of the breasts during adolescence results from fat being laid down and milk ducts lengthening and branching. There's very little glandular tissue now, but little collections of cells begin to form that will later develop into milk glands.

The breast has fifteen to twenty segments, each containing a gland leading to a main duct which opens at the nipple. The openings look like little crevices and if you stop a moment while feeding your baby, you'll notice drops of milk coming from them. Sometimes you'll see fine sprays or drops of milk coming from several ducts at a time. Some ducts may merge within the nipple, in which case there are fewer openings at the nipple than there are ducts.

In a pregnant or breastfeeding woman the glandular part of

each segment of breast is rather like a bunch of grapes on a stalk. Each 'grape' is a milk gland (alveolus) and has a tiny duct leading to the 'stalk' or main milk duct. The milk gland is lined with milk-producing cells, each bordering the tiny duct. The milk they produce flows from this tiny duct to one of the fifteen to twenty larger ducts and thence to the nipple. Around each gland is a branching network of star-shaped muscle cells, which can contract and squeeze milk from the cells into the ducts.

The main duct from each breast segment widens under the areola, forming fifteen to twenty milk reservoirs (lactiferous sinuses). These distend as they fill, a full reservoir's diameter measuring half to one centimetre (quarter to half an inch). Their role is to store milk ready for the beginning of a feed. Their storage capacity increases after several weeks of breastfeeding, which is why leaking often stops after six to eight weeks.

BREAST CHANGES IN PREGNANCY

During pregnancy many women notice tingling and fullness of their breasts as early as their first missed period – indeed, these sensations are often the first sign of pregnancy. Little prominences (Montgomery's tubercles) around each areola become more noticeable from around six weeks. These contain glands that produce an oily substance that lubricates and protects nipple skin. Some women produce milk from one or more tubercles, since anatomically they resemble tiny breasts.

By five months of pregnancy, most women need a larger bra; in a first pregnancy the nipples and areolae begin to darken; and even if you lose your baby you'll produce milk from now on.

All these changes are caused by hormones, some present only in pregnancy.

Breast size in pregnancy

By the end of a full-term pregnancy each breast weighs an average of 650 g (1½ lb) more than at the beginning, mainly because of the development of milk glands and the proliferation of milk ducts.

In women of healthy weight, the size of their breasts before pregnancy has little bearing on their ability to breastfeed. Indeed, some small breasts contain more milk-producing glands than do some large ones. However, the relatively large, fatty breasts of an overweight or obese woman can affect her milk supply. According to one study (2004), this is because such a woman makes less prolactin, the hormone that stimulates milk production, when she feeds her baby. The solution is not to diet during pregnancy or while breastfeeding, but to get good quality help with your breastfeeding technique.

However, women with very small breasts may be at a slight disadvantage early on in breastfeeding because their breasts can become overfull more quickly than larger breasts and may leak unless offered to the baby more frequently. However, this becomes less of a problem as their storage capacity increases during the first few weeks.

This said, the increase in size of your breasts during pregnancy is quite a good indicator of your ability to feed easily. As a general rule, if you need a bra one or two sizes larger by the end of pregnancy, you should have little trouble getting off to a good start. One reason why women having their first baby relatively young tend to produce more milk at first is because they have a larger than average increase in breast size.

BABIES' BREASTS

The commonly observed enlargement of newborn babies' breasts, both boys' and girls', results from maternal hormones travelling across the placenta into the baby's bloodstream before birth. Sometimes milk comes out of them in boys and girls. This is sometimes called witches' milk. Both the swelling and the milk eventually disappear, sometimes over several months or longer.

NIPPLES

A woman's nipples become larger and more protractile (able to be lengthened) during pregnancy, which makes it easier for the baby to latch on – to take the nipple and areola into his mouth. In a few women the nipples don't change much and a good latch may be more of a challenge.

MILK PRODUCTION

The fall in the progesterone level immediately after childbirth helps trigger milk to come in (be produced more copiously) over the next few days. Other hormones involved in milk production include prolactin, growth hormone, corticosteroids, thyroxine and insulin. Each gland is surrounded by a fine network of blood vessels whose blood conveys these hormones and provides the milk-producing cells with the materials they need to make milk.

As milk glands produce milk after a feed, the milk-producing cells gradually enlarge and become round and full. Pressure from the increasing volume of the milk in the glands makes it trickle continuously into the milk ducts and on into the reservoirs under the nipple. As the reservoirs fill with milk they gradually expand because their walls are elastic. The fullness and slight lumpiness you may feel before a feed is caused by these swollen milk glands with their laden cells and by the swollen ducts and reservoirs.

Prolactin

The level of this hormone increases from the eighth week of pregnancy, peaks at the birth, then gradually decreases during the time a woman breastfeeds. During pregnancy it stimulates breast growth, but other hormones (oestrogen, progesterone and human placental lactogen) prevent it producing milk in any volume.

After a baby is born these brakes disappear and high prolactin levels trigger milk production. Prolactin 'turns on the taps'. It also stimulates casein and lactose production. Colostrum is present from the beginning. Mature milk usually starts to be produced ('comes in') between the second and fourth days after delivery but can begin earlier in women feeding their babies frequently and in an unrestricted way from birth, and in those having second or subsequent babies. Milk usually comes in slowly, but some women have a deluge.

Prolactin is produced by the pituitary gland in the brain. Nipple and areola stimulation during a feed sends messages along nerves to this gland to tell it to make more prolactin. It's the baby's milking action (rhythmic squeezing and milking, or 'stripping') that stimulates the nipple, rather than its suction. This is why an electric breast pump may not be as good at boosting prolactin. A baby who sucks and milks strongly may raise his mother's prolactin more than a baby with a weaker sucking and milking action.

One researcher has noted that newborns 'write their signature with their sucking rhythm', since each one has a constant unique pattern in the number of sucks and the intervals between sucks per minute. This helps explain why some babies take longer over a feed than others.

Nipple stimulation immediately boosts prolactin; it reaches a peak within thirty to forty-five minutes of starting a feed and gradually falls to its resting level over the next two hours. The more a baby is at the breast the more milk a woman makes, and each time he feeds he effectively places an order for more milk to be ready for the next feed. Waiting longer between feeds doesn't produce more milk because it doesn't increase prolactin. Prolactin levels fluctuate by day and are highest at night and in the early morning.

Research suggests that early and frequent stimulation of the nipple and areola encourages the development of tiny prolactin receptors in milk-gland cells. These receptors capture and remove prolactin from the blood, enabling it to increase milk production. This may explain why the prolactin level in the blood isn't directly related to the amount of milk produced and why, if a woman breastfeeds only or mainly from one breast, as a few do (page 181), the milk in the little-used or unused breast gradually decreases, or even dries up, despite high prolactin levels in her blood due to stimulation of the other breast.

— Put another way, nipple stimulation is necessary for breasts to respond to prolactin and to make milk, and the more frequently a woman feeds from a breast, the more sensitive and responsive to prolactin does that breast become.

The response of prolactin to suckling is at its most sensitive in the first week of breastfeeding, which is partly why it's so important not to restrict feeds then.

So far we've considered only the milk-producing effects of prolactin, but it may have other actions too. For example, many breastfeeding women experience feelings of happiness and tranquillity, which is why some people call prolactin the 'mothering' or 'happiness' hormone. These emotions are boosted by an increase in endorphins – hormone-like substances also stimulated by breastfeeding; research shows these help reduce the effects of stress in lactating rats, and this may be true in humans too.

Foremilk and hindmilk

If you look at your nipple during a feed or when expressing milk, you may see different looking drops from different duct openings at the nipple. Some may look bluish-white and relatively thin, others creamy-white and thicker, others somewhere between. There are four reasons for this:

1 The composition of the milk in a drop from any one reservoir depends on whether it's leaving the breast early or late in a feed. Some drops may contain milk that was already in the ducts and reservoirs at the beginning of the feed, others milk let down during the current feed, others a mixture of let-down milk and the milk that was already there.
2 A baby empties different reservoirs at different rates, depending on his position at the breast.
3 The segment of breast from which a drop comes may not have been completely emptied during the last feed.
4 Milk ducts sometimes merge within the nipple, so there may be fewer openings than reservoirs. If some segments of the breast were emptied more thoroughly than others at the last feed, and their ducts merge, the combined milk may look neither thin nor thick.

— At the beginning of a feed most drops contain bluish-white thinner milk (foremilk); towards the end most contain creamy-white thicker milk (hindmilk).

Two things are vitally important to successful breastfeeding. One is the let-down reflex; the other is the principle of demand and supply.

THE LET-DOWN REFLEX

When a woman feeds her baby, the pituitary gland in her brain produces oxytocin, which quickly releases milk from the milk glands' milk-producing cells into the ducts. This is the let-down reflex; without it the milk stays put in milk-gland cells and the baby gets only the milk that's already trickled into the reservoirs and ducts.

Oxytocin

This hormone is responsible for the let-down reflex (also known as the milk-ejection reflex). An experienced breastfeeder automatically releases oxytocin from her brain's pituitary gland into her blood when she knows her baby is ready for a feed, sometimes even before the baby gets to the breast, because her let-down reflex is conditioned by past experience. The baby's presence is a powerful stimulus, but many women find their let-down is triggered simply by the sight, sound or even the thought of their baby (or even someone else's baby!), particularly if they haven't breastfed for some time. Stimulation of the nipple skin and the tissues under the areola during suckling is another important trigger for oxytocin. Messages travel along nerve pathways from the nipple to the pituitary, where they trigger the release of oxytocin.

Once released, oxytocin travels to the breasts, where it makes muscle cells around the milk glands contract and squeeze milk into the ducts, which expand so they can contain it. This cycle of suckling (or other triggers listed above) – messages to the pituitary gland – oxytocin release – contraction of muscle cells around milk glands – and squeezing of milk into the ducts is why the let-down is described as a 'reflex'.

The let-down reflex usually takes some weeks to become reliable, and when people talk about establishing breastfeeding, they are referring to the establishment of a reliable let-down reflex.

The time needed to let down milk varies from woman to woman and also depends on many other factors, including a woman's surroundings and how she feels. From when a baby is put to the breast, the let-down can take a minimum of thirty to fifty seconds to work but often takes longer. Some women need two to three minutes of nipple stimulation before maximum milk flow occurs. This means a hungry or thirsty baby may finish the milk in the ducts and reservoirs before any more milk is let down. This can be frustrating.

The let-down is fairly sensitive and, especially in the early weeks, can easily be disturbed. If her baby cries and becomes restless, perhaps turning away or 'fighting' at the breast, an inexperienced mother may become so anxious that she won't let down her milk. Being anxious, over-stressed or embarrassed can inhibit the let-down in two ways. First, it can prevent oxytocin from causing contraction of the muscle cells around the milk glands; second, it can prevent the pituitary from releasing oxytocin.

The let-down is usually a pleasant feeling, described as something between a sneeze and an orgasm. Let-down milk spurts through the ducts so quickly it may spray or drip from the nipples. Any one let-down consists of a series of spurts of milk, with a gap between each, and there may be up to eight let-downs during each feed. This explains why oxytocin rapidly rises and falls in waves during a feed. The first let-down of a feed is associated with a higher oxytocin level than subsequent let-downs. The oxytocin level falls extremely rapidly after the start of a let-down and is all gone within about four minutes.

In the early days it's often easy to know when your let-down is working because your breasts feel tingly, tense and warm; you leak, drip or spray milk; and you get rhythmical womb contractions (which are one cause of 'afterpains'). Many women report welcome relief as their baby removes let-down milk and the emptying breast becomes less tense. Other women have none of these sensations yet have a very good let-down, and any individual can experience different let-down sensations from one baby to the next. Others say the sensations change or disappear throughout the months or years of breastfeeding. One woman described the sensation of the let-down in the first few weeks of breastfeeding as being like cold water trickling down her breastbone; later she had tingling throughout her breasts; later still, itching beneath each areola.

Leaking

Warmth from a hot bath or your baby's mouth can cause leaking. This is because the muscle fibres in the nipple and areola are usually contracted, keeping duct openings closed. Warmth lengthens them, releasing their tight hold on the ducts and allowing milk to escape.

If your breasts are full of milk, leaning forward or sideways can cause leaking, as can sexual arousal.

HOW YOUR BABY GETS MILK

A baby obtains milk by a combination of sucking, milking and allowing let-down milk or leaking milk to drip or spray into his mouth.

Holding the breast in his mouth

A baby holds the breast between his tongue and upper gums, the tongue covering the lower gums. To do this he sticks the front of his tongue out beneath the nipple and as far as his lower lip, curls it up slightly, then pushes the back of his tongue up against the nipple and areola. He then sucks to help hold the breast in place.

Sucking

When the nipple touches the baby's palate in the roof of his mouth, he automatically starts sucking by working his cheek muscles to draw the nipple and areola well into his mouth and keep them there. This sucking reflex is instinctive and strongest twenty to thirty minutes after birth. If a baby isn't put to the breast then, this reflex temporarily becomes much weaker, but after forty hours or so it becomes stronger again. A delay of eight hours or more before the first feed after childbirth reduces the chance of breastfeeding successfully; specifically, a delay of more than twelve hours increases the likelihood of stopping breastfeeding in the first two weeks because of insufficient milk. But if you want to breastfeed, even delays such as these won't stop you.

When milk is flowing fast, the baby sucks slowly, strongly and purposefully at a rate of about one suck per second. When milk isn't flowing, he sucks faster and less strongly, in short sharp bursts of 'flutter sucking' at a rate of about two sucks per second. Both sorts of sucking help stimulate the production and let-down of milk, but stronger sucking is more effective.

A sucked nipple is about twice as long as usual and the nipple and areola together form a teat shape in the baby's mouth. As a baby's cheeks suck they create a vacuum which draws milk into the mouth and encourages milk reservoirs to refill. However, 'milking' is very much more important.

Milking

The main way a baby gets milk is by milking – or 'stripping' – the nipple and areola with his tongue. To do this, he takes them into his mouth, presses his tongue up against them, and moves it backwards. The tongue contracts rhythmically in transverse waves of movement (peristalsis) which squeeze milk from the reservoirs. Meanwhile, the baby's jaws open and close vigorously to help his tongue compress the nipple and areola. The further the baby draws the nipple and areola into his mouth, the better he empties the reservoirs.

If you could see inside your baby's mouth during a feed, you'd see your nipple and areola go as far back as where his hard and soft palate join. You'd also see a furrow down the length of the upper surface of the tongue. The teat made from the nipple, areola and reservoirs fills this furrow. The baby's milking action stimulates your let-down reflex, which ejects milk from the nipple in fine jets towards the back of his mouth. All he needs do is to swallow.

Many babies start a feed with continuous rapid sucking and milking for around thirty seconds. They then settle into a rhythm of bursts of slow deep sucking and milking interspersed by pauses, according to the number of let-downs during a feed. As a baby pauses between let-downs, his lower jaw drops, releasing the tongue's pressure on the nipple and areola and allowing the reservoirs to refill with let-down milk.

The swallowing reflex

This enables a baby to send milk from his mouth into his stomach.

All three feeding reflexes in babies – the rooting reflex (page 139), sucking reflex and swallowing reflex – may be temporarily absent in pre-term babies, or impaired in infants with brain damage, jaundice or an infection. Mechanical problems such as a cleft palate may also interfere.

DEMAND AND SUPPLY

This is the second principle of successful breastfeeding. All the time a baby feeds, he stimulates the nipple and areola, which boosts his mother's prolactin and oxytocin levels. In general, the more your baby is at your breast, the more prolactin you'll make and the more milk you'll have. And the more often you feed him, the more reliable your let-down becomes.

'Supply and demand' isn't an appropriate term, because demand produces supply, not the other way round. However, while 'demand and supply' is the right way round, there are two reasons why the word 'demand' isn't particularly appropriate either.

First, many babies let their mothers know they're ready for a feed by becoming slightly restless or nuzzling at the breast, making their needs known gently, rather than in a demanding way (though if they aren't fed quite soon they start to cry). A mother quickly gets to know her baby's cues that he is ready for a feed, which is why the term 'cue feeding' has been suggested instead of 'demand feeding'.

Second, a few babies don't make their needs known, especially if they've often been left to cry in their mother's mistaken belief that feeds should be at set times. These babies become quieter and quieter even though they're in desperate need of milk. Without attention to their needs they can starve, and they also learn that the world is an unfriendly place that makes them unhappy.

Every time your baby gives the cue he's ready, you can offer a breast. This doesn't mean you should feed only when he asks – you may want to because your breasts feel full, you want the pleasure of a close cuddle, or it's a convenient time. Neither does it mean you have to feed at the slightest sign of a cue, since many babies can wait a while, especially if you distract them.

Successful or natural breastfeeding puts no rules or limits on suckling time, provided a baby is latched on properly – if not, he may keep asking for feeds simply because his poor feeding position means he can't get enough milk. 'Suckling', by the way, is something a mother does to her baby. A mother suckles, a baby sucks, and a baby is sometimes called a suckling.

Babies allowed to feed as often as they need take very variable numbers of feeds during the twenty-four hours. In the early days some ask for a feed every hour or so, with the greatest number of feeds often occurring on the fifth day after birth. In one study many years ago in Sheffield, 29 per cent of babies allowed to feed when they wanted had eight feeds on the fifth day and 10 per cent had more than nine.

A medical textbook published in 1906, when successful breastfeeding was the norm, recommended the following number of feeds:

First day	4
Second day	6
Rest of first month	10
Second and third months	8
Fourth and fifth months	7
Sixth to eleventh months	6

Some years later, many hospitals recommended a breastfeeding schedule of every four hours for a large baby, every three hours for a small one. Unfortunately, with the increasing medicalization of childbirth and mother and baby care, and the tight control exerted over women and babies in hospitals, this bad advice remained widespread for decades and is still given today in some out-of-date, non-baby-friendly hospitals.

Both women's experiences and scientific research agree that any schedule that restricts the number of feeds produces poor results.

— Any woman who wants to breastfeed successfully should discard any schedule restricting the frequency of feeds.

One sure way of reducing the number of feeds your baby asks for (and thus decreasing your chances of breastfeeding successfully) is to keep him apart from you. In countries where mothers carry or hold their babies by day and lie next to them at night, the babies spend very much more time at the breast. Babies allowed virtually unrestricted access to their mother's breasts are almost always breastfed fully and successfully for a long time, the milk supply continuing for an average of three years until the baby no longer wants to be at the breast.

One study in Africa in which researchers watched mothers sleeping with their babies found that no baby went longer than twenty minutes without feeding. Contrast these lucky babies with the many in developed countries who are rationed to one feed a night at most until their mother's milk dries up – which isn't long.

A word of warning. Never compare your baby with that of any other woman. Each baby is unique and we should let them be so. Some settle into a self-created routine of six feeds a day within a few weeks, but this is not a goal to aim for, just one of many patterns your baby may adopt in time.

Another word of warning. One expert says that in her experience if a baby has five or fewer feeds a day, the likelihood is that his mother's milk will dry up within a month through lack of stimulation of the breasts.

LENGTH OF FEEDS

The length of a feed is a matter for the individual baby and mother, and shouldn't be dictated by health workers. The average time a baby spends at one breast is about ten minutes, but averages are worked out from many babies – some get all they need in five minutes while others need twenty or more before they are satisfied.

Feeding times vary for several reasons. First, the let-down may be slow to work so a baby doesn't get let-down milk for some minutes. Second, some babies are hungrier than others (perhaps always, or perhaps because they are going through a growth spurt), so suck and milk the breast more strongly and get all they need faster. Third, some babies – especially in the early days – may not be very alert and so need to take time over a feed.

'FEEDS'?

Talking about the periods of time a baby spends at the breast as 'feeds' makes us think of them as times to get milk down in as businesslike a way as possible. Many babies, however, especially in the early days, like to drink in a leisurely way, snoozing between bouts of sucking and milking. While resting this way, they may let go of the breast, only to wake again in a short while, or may hold the nipple in their mouth and give an occasional gentle, 'fluttering' suck for minutes at a time. It's not uncommon for a young baby sometimes to spend hours at the breast in this fashion, if allowed. Such behaviour, which can be perfectly normal, makes counting feeds meaningless, because many such encounters involve very little actual 'feeding' at all.

It's important not to curtail feeds in the first few days particularly, because you could take the baby from the breast before the let-down starts. Many hospitals insist on very short suckling times in the first few days, to prevent sore nipples, but this is fallacious, as we'll see later. Short suckling times often prevent or delay the establishment of successful lactation and benefit mother or baby only in very occasional circumstances (page 257).

Now we've taken a look at the breasts and how breastfeeding works, the next chapter will focus on the early days of breastfeeding.

SEVEN

The early days

This chapter is about breastfeeding your newborn baby in hospital or at home.

CHILDBIRTH

A good midwife or obstetrician is a safe one who stands back while a woman labours, intervening only if necessary.

There's mounting evidence that labour is safer for babies and easier for women if they labour in an upright position. They are also less likely to need painkilling drugs or an episiotomy (a cut to widen the opening of the vagina). This is important for breastfeeding because the better a woman feels after labour, the easier it is for breastfeeding to get off to a good start.

Pain relief in labour

If a woman has the painkilling drug pethidine in the second stage of labour, it can make her baby sleepy, which may mean he is slow with feeds for a day or two. This makes some women become dispirited and give up breastfeeding, though there are ways of coping with this (page 315). A similar drug, meptazinol (Meptid) has a weaker analgesic effect but is less likely to make a baby sleepy.

If you need pain relief (especially towards the end of labour), it's better from the point of view of making a good start with breastfeeding if you choose another method, such as breathing 'gas and air', having mild electro-stimulation of your lower back with a TENS (trans-cutaneous electrical nerve stimulation) device, asking your birth companion to do light, rapid 'butterfly' massage towards the bottom of your spine, or having an epidural anaesthetic (an injection to numb the nerve roots that carry pain messages into the spinal cord).

THE FIRST FEW MINUTES

The moment of birth comes after nine months' wait and hours of labour. Not surprisingly, most women are relieved, excited and tired. Pride in producing a baby that a few hours ago was nothing more than a wriggling bump mingles with fatigue, curiosity and elation. A few women are so exhausted that all they want is rest.

If all is well, you'll be able to hold your baby for a time before the routine weighing, washing and labelling. While you're having a cuddle, the staff will stand by while your placenta is delivered, and do any necessary stitching. It takes a single-minded woman to put her baby to the breast amid all this, but it's a good idea if you can because it helps your womb contract and speeds delivery of the placenta. Some women find immediate suckling the most natural thing to do. Others aren't really sure and feel awkward if the baby seems disinterested, as some are at first.

Let your baby nuzzle your breast and feed if he wants, but don't be discouraged if he isn't very interested. He doesn't know what to do yet, but he'll like the smell of your breast skin, and when he tastes the sweetness of your colostrum he'll probably be much keener.

Ideally, put your baby to the breast within the first half-hour, as his sucking reflex is at its height soon after birth. If he doesn't want to feed, hold him close and touch his lower lip with your nipple from time to time.

WHY EARLY SUCKLING IS A GOOD IDEA

The oxytocin you produce when you put your baby to the breast the first time makes your womb contract, helping expel the placenta and reduce bleeding. Early suckling means you may not need a routine injection of Syntometrine (oxytocin plus ergometrine) to make your womb contract, dislodge the placenta and push it out. This could be helpful as some doctors suspect ergometrine sometimes reduces the milk supply.

- A study in Singapore (1994) found that breastfeeding immediately after birth makes the womb contract nearly as much as an oxytocin injection.

If you put your baby to the breast before the cord is cut, your womb contractions give the baby an extra surge of blood and therefore of iron. There is no need for your midwife or doctor to cut the cord until the placenta has separated.

Another good reason for early suckling is that a baby's sucking reflex is strongest in the first thirty minutes after birth. After this many babies become tired and disinterested for forty hours or so before they're keen to suck again.

Your placenta may take up to half an hour to come out and during this time you can be getting to know your baby. Many women aren't a bit sleepy and want to be with their baby, and most studies agree that being with her baby makes a woman more likely to breastfeed successfully and for longer. She is also more likely to sleep well later if she has time to cuddle and suckle her baby and isn't anxious about where he is and what's happening.

Have a good look at your baby and enjoy your first meeting. You may not feel a rush of motherly love – this often takes time to come – but you'll probably be curious to examine and touch your baby. Newborn babies have a very distinctive smell, which many mothers find delightful.

Self-attachment

For the first feed – if you have the opportunity, your baby is in good condition and the room is warm – try letting him get to the breast by himself. Lie down with him lying naked on his tummy, on top of your naked tummy. After a while, as you relax, he may start wriggling up towards your breast, then hunt for the nipple and latch on of his own accord.

PUTTING YOUR BABY TO THE BREAST

Sit up in bed or sit on a chair – either choosing a low chair or raising your feet (on some books, for example) so your lap is flat. Get as comfortable as possible, preferably with your elbow supported on the chair arm or on one or more cushions so your arm doesn't have to take all the baby's weight (which could make your back and shoulders ache). Sit upright, perhaps slightly leaning forward. If your breast is tense, soften it before a feed by expressing a little milk (see page 159), as this makes latching on easier. It may help to put the baby on a pillow on your lap.

A good way of holding your baby is to put him in the crook of your arm with your hand under his bottom, and use this arm to position him so his face, chest, tummy and knees all face your body (remember, 'tummy to mummy') and his ear and shoulder are in a straight line; that way he won't have to turn his head to the breast to feed. You can either have his head resting on your arm or support him with your other hand around his shoulder. Some mothers prefer to hold their baby with their other arm, with his bottom in the crook of their arm and their hand cradling the baby's head; some babies, though, dislike having their head cradled this way and push back against it, away from the breast. If necessary, tuck his lower arm around your side to keep it out of the way. His neck should be extended (meaning his chin is up and his head not bent down).

Move him towards your breast (but don't push his head, or his rooting reflex – a searching movement that's natural in newborns – will make him turn his head away from the breast). Move him if necessary so his upper lip and nose are at the same height as your nipple, his chin is against your breast and his bottom is no further away from you than his chest is.

He may automatically open his mouth wide; otherwise, stroke his lower lip with your nipple until he opens his mouth wide (don't tickle his upper lip, though, as this would mean he wouldn't open his mouth as wide; don't tickle both lips either, as he'd probably find this confusing). Check nothing else is touching his mouth, such as a sheet or clothing, as this could trigger his rooting reflex and make him turn towards it. Some babies get excited and lick the nipple, perhaps even starting to feed; others hold it in their mouths and don't latch on properly and start sucking and milking until later. They aren't in any hurry and simply gaze at their mother.

There's no need for most women to hold their breast. However, if your breast is very big you may need to hold it back so it doesn't obstruct his nose – though be careful not to squeeze it too much as this could obstruct the milk ducts. Some women find it helps to support the breast gently from underneath with the flat of their upturned hand, but avoid lifting or squeezing as this can obstruct the milk ducts.

LATCHING ON

When your baby's mouth is really wide open, and his tongue is down over his lower lip, quickly and gently bring him to your breast so his chin and lower lip meet it first and take in as much of the breast as possible. Hold his whole body close to you.

He should take some of the areola as well as the nipple into his mouth, so his tongue's milking action can empty the reservoirs. If he takes in only the nipple, or only a small part of the areola, it means he's poorly latched on and he'll only be able to 'nipple-suck' – meaning he'll get only the milk he can suck from the reservoirs, or swallow if it's spurting or flowing fast. When he realizes he isn't getting enough, he'll suck more strongly, which will make your nipple sore. Another problem with nipple-sucking is that it doesn't stimulate the breast well, which means there isn't such a boost to prolactin and you might not make enough milk.

If the baby is positioned so he can milk your breast efficiently, his lips will be splayed out around the mouthful of breast, his bottom lip will be pressed back against his chin and there will be more of your areola visible above his upper lip than below his lower one. His lower jaw should be be tucked well in towards your chest. (If it isn't, his lower jaw will be tipped away from the breast and an observer will see more of your areola below his lower lip, instead of more above his upper one.)

Note that he shouldn't drag your breast downwards.

If the baby finds it difficult to latch on, try holding your breast between finger and thumb (or index and middle fingers – the cigarette hold) to make the nipple and areola a little easier to latch on to. Don't squeeze hard, though, or you'll obstruct the milk ducts, and release this hold as soon as he starts feeding well.

As he latches on, aim your nipple up towards his nose to ensure it's high in his mouth and won't get hurt as he sucks.

You should see his lower jaw and cheek muscles working hard (though hollowed cheeks may suggest he isn't latched on well). Within half a minute or so he'll start doing slower, deeper sucks.

Try to relax, as this helps your milk let down more readily. Your baby may like something to hold while he's feeding – your finger will do.

When your baby has finished he'll come off the breast of his own accord and you can offer the other one either straight away or after a break – though he may not want it.

Being unsure of what to do is normal, especially with a first baby. Animal studies show they too need time and experience to feed their young, and some zoo animals need to be taught by their keepers.

In Chapter 12 there is information for women who have had a Caesarean section or are dealing with other special situations.

Ideally, if you, your birth partner and baby are content, the staff will leave you alone for half an hour or so. You can have a wash and put on clean clothes afterwards.

DIFFERENT POSITIONS

During the day you'll probably usually breastfeed sitting up, but it's well worth feeding lying down on one side by day sometimes, or using the 'football' hold. At night it's often easier to lie down.

Feeding lying down

Roll on one side and lay your baby on his side by you, so his head faces your breast. Move him towards you with your hand on his back, and stroke his lower lip with your nipple until he opens his mouth wide, roots for your nipple, takes it in his mouth, and latches on.

The 'football' hold

This is a useful feeding position to use sometimes, and it's particularly useful for mothers of twins. Hold the baby so his legs point backwards under your arm on the side you're feeding from. Support his body with a cushion if necessary.

WATCHING YOUR BABY FEED

You may notice your baby doesn't feed continuously, like a bottle-fed baby does, but every so often takes short pauses between bouts of sucking. This is because let-down milk spurts into the ducts and from the nipple in an uneven flow. After several spurts there's a short pause before they begin again. Your baby is simply adapting to your milk flow.

WRAPPING YOUR BABY

If your baby goes to sleep after a feed and you want to put him down, wrap him snugly in a shawl (though not so he gets too hot). This way he's less likely to wake with a start. Towards the end of pregnancy the walls of your womb held him fairly tightly; being wrapped up now may remind him of the security of the womb. Babies carried next to their mothers in the firm hold of a sling seem to like it.

RELAXING AND ENJOYING YOUR BABY

Relaxing helps you enjoy your baby as you feed. If you're happier with curtains drawn around your bed, ask someone to draw them. Be encouraged by positive comments about you breastfeeding, but if anyone says anything negative, listen and just say calmly that you've all the time in the world to learn.

Your newborn may stare at you from the breast from time to time, or even all the time. Having a baby gazing up at you is a wonderful feeling, so take time to let it sink in. You may sometimes like to hold your naked baby close to your naked body to feed him, with the room warm and a nappy to soak up any leaks from you or the baby if necessary.

You may also like to cuddle, wash and even feed him while you are having a bath. Hold him securely and he'll probably like it much better than being in a baby bath, because of having you so close. Make sure the room is warm and the water temperature is suitable and ask your partner to come and take him when you're finished.

Some women enjoy massaging their babies all over with warm oil, and babies nearly always enjoy this too, but note that it's safest to do it on a towel on the floor where his oily body can't come to any harm if it slips between your fingers.

Remember there are no limits to how much time you and your baby spend together. Babies thrive on lots of body contact, love and attention.

WHAT'S YOUR BABY GETTING?

At first your baby gets colostrum. He doesn't need much to drink for the first few days as nature intended him to have only small amounts. These small volumes of colostrum are worth their weight in gold. So valuable is colostrum in protecting newborns against infection (among other things) that some experts believe every bottle-fed baby should have a 'colostrum cocktail', and farmers have been giving colostrum to ready-weaned but valuable calves for years, to stop them getting 'the scours', or diarrhoea. Don't doubt your ability to nourish your baby in these first few days. Your colostrum may not look much, but cows' milk formula, in however large a volume, cannot compare for goodness.

Colostrum's relatively high protein level enables many newborns to go longer between feeds than when the mature milk comes in. This may be nature's way of ensuring that newly delivered women get more of a chance to sleep.

The more a baby feeds during the first few days, the sooner the breasts produce mature milk, which is made in larger amounts than colostrum. This is known as the milk 'coming in', but there's no sudden alteration in content. The phrase 'coming in' leads some people to think the breasts are empty until this happens, which, of course, they aren't. Women who've had more than one baby find their milk comes in sooner than it did with their firstborn. The milk may come in on the second or third day if a woman feeds her baby frequently, but not for four or five days if she feeds infrequently. The sooner your milk comes in, the sooner your baby will have plenty to drink.

HOW OFTEN SHOULD YOU FEED?

Feed your baby on an unrestricted basis – whenever he cries, when he seems to want a feed, when your breasts are full and if you want or need to for reasons of your own. *Don't* count how many feeds you give, or feed on any sort of schedule. The more schedule-feeding there's been over the last century, the less successful breastfeeding has become.

Studies strongly suggest that women who breastfeed in an unrestricted way not only produce more milk and continue breast-feeding for more months than schedule-feeding women, but are also less likely to develop sore nipples. And their babies put on more weight and are less likely to become jaundiced.

Breast milk is so well digested that it stays in a baby's stomach for a maximum of an hour and a half (compared with nearly two and a half hours for formula), which is partly why breastfed babies need frequent feeds.

Demand-feeding – when a baby 'demands' a feed by crying – can work well but is sometimes a disaster. This is because some babies simply don't demand enough feeds, so they don't give the breasts the stimulation they need to make milk and the supply dwindles. Best of all is a successful, natural way of breastfeeding that meets both mother's and baby's needs and desires.

- A large UK survey (1990) found that one in ten mothers in hospital were told to feed at set times. However, this was an improvement on the 19 per cent who had to feed at set times in 1985.

Women who feed on an unrestricted basis aren't concerned when their babies want more feeds some days than others – they simply give them what they want, trusting their baby to know what's best for him.

Growth spurts

Babies may suddenly want more feeds because they are having a growth spurt (see also page 228) – growing faster for a while and therefore needing more milk. Common ages for growth spurts are three weeks, six weeks and three months, though they may occur at any time, depending on the individual baby. Don't think that because your baby suddenly seems dissatisfied you don't have enough milk. During a growth spurt you may very temporarily not meet his needs, but two or three days of extra feeds will boost your supply.

Successful breastfeeding

Knowing you don't have to wait until your baby cries before you breastfeed him means you are well on your way to breastfeeding successfully for as long as you want.

You can feed baby, for example, when:

- He seems ready (perhaps being fidgety or nuzzling your breast).
- Your breasts are full and you want to relieve the pressure.
- You want to go out soon.
- He is jaundiced, affected by drugs given in labour, ill, preterm, small-for-dates or apathetic for some other reason – and unlikely to ask for a feed.
- You want to.

The only time to watch the clock is if your baby doesn't ask for feeds very often (see page 276). Even if he's sound asleep, it's probably better not to leave a young baby unfed for more than three hours at the longest. Too many longer gaps could endanger your milk supply and mean he doesn't get enough. Some babies go four to five hours between some feeds, but this generally isn't sensible in the early days until you are more confident with breastfeeding and your milk supply is well established.

Babies gain weight better with frequent feeds because these stimulate greater milk production. Frequent suckling from a well latched-on baby also encourages the development of prolactin receptors in the milk glands; these attract prolactin and allow it to get to work making milk.

The number of feeds each day

This varies according to each mother–baby pair, depending on:

- The maturity of the milk – babies need more frequent feeds of mature milk than of colostrum.
- Your breasts' milk-producing capacity.
- Whether the baby is latched on properly ('well attached'), so he can suck and milk optimally; if not, he'll only get relatively low-fat low-calorie milk, which leaves the stomach quickly and won't satisfy him for long; also, he won't stimulate his mother's prolactin and milk supply optimally, which means she may not be making enough milk and he may go hungry.
- How strongly a baby sucks and milks. (The more vigorously he does so, the more prolactin – therefore the more milk – you make. However, a baby who doesn't suck and milk very strongly may simply get what he needs by taking longer over each feed, the exception being a small or poorly baby who needs frequent short feeds as he lacks the energy to take a long time.)
- Whether a baby is allowed to feed as long as he wants at the first breast, and continue at the second breast if he wants (if not, he may not get enough relatively high-fat, high-calorie milk and will be hungry sooner).
- Whether a baby is allowed to be at the breast for comfort as well as for milk (since any stimulation helps increases prolactin, which increases milk production).
- The baby's preferences and needs.
- The woman's culture, lifestyle, preferences and needs.

It isn't wise to compare yourself with other breastfeeding women because while it may be interesting to know how many feeds someone else gives, you may find yourself competing over whose baby lasts longest between feeds. The lack of competition at home is partly why many women breastfeed more successfully if they leave hospital soon after delivery.

Some women feed their babies as many as thirty to forty times in twenty-four hours (in some cultures mainly in the evening and night), others as few as six. However, six times a day gives the breasts very little stimulation; five usually makes the milk supply fail; and eight is probably the absolute minimum for very young babies and almost all need more – probably at least twelve.

Babies also need different numbers of feeds from day to day, depending on how they're feeling, how fast they're growing and how well they are.

To help put frequent feeding into perspective, remember that until your baby was born he was 'fed' continuously by your placenta. In fact, a breastfed baby of under nine months has been dubbed an 'exterogestate fetus', implying he is so immature that he has to rely on being attached to his mother's breast much of the time.

Women differ as to how much breast stimulation they need to make enough milk for their baby, but the vast majority find their milk supply increases if they feed more often. Breastfeeding tends to be much more successful in cultures where women feed frequently.

Frequent breastfeeding is good news for midwives too. Indeed, research in one Oxford hospital found the midwives' workload fell dramatically when they no longer insisted on schedule-feeding.

Babies allowed completely unrestricted feeds – for example, those carried next to a naked breast all day in developing countries – don't have to cry before they are fed, and feed *very much more often* than most Western breastfed babies.

Anthropologists can predict how often any mammal's young need to be suckled by the amount of protein and fat in the milk. If there's a lot (as in cow and rabbit milk), the young need infrequent suckling – perhaps only once a day. However, if the milk is low in protein and fat, the young need frequent suckling. Human milk has very little protein and along with other animals with low-protein milk we are grouped as '*continuous contact mammals*'. Human babies suck on and off much of the time, given the chance, which seems to be what nature intended. We automatically reduce the frequency of feeds our babies ask for by not carrying them next to our naked breasts all day and not sleeping naked next to them at night. But if we make feeds too infrequent, we run the risk of reducing our milk supply through too little breast stimulation. We also run the risk of separating our babies from ourselves so much that we can't give them enough physical and emotional comfort.

Waking your baby

Some women worry about waking their baby for feeds during the day. But this is the right thing to do if it's a long time since a feed or your breasts feel full. If you don't wake him or express some milk, your breasts will become tense or engorged (swollen) and your milk production will slow down. Never go so long between feeds that your breasts feel tense and lumpy. Remember, you are part of a nursing pair – sometimes you feed for your baby's benefit, sometimes for your own.

Mothers who breastfeed on an unrestricted basis are only half as likely to get sore nipples and engorged breasts as those who schedule-feed their babies.

One breast or two?

When your baby finishes what he wants from the first breast, he'll almost certainly stop spontaneously. This is generally better than switching him to the other breast after some arbitrary time, as it means he's more likely to get a good helping of fat-rich hindmilk from the first breast. Have a short break if you want, perhaps to change his nappy or bring up wind, then offer the second breast. If you're trying to boost your milk supply, aim to feed from both breasts, or the unemptied one might not produce as much milk as it could. This is partly because of the pressure of the remaining milk on its milk-producing cells, and partly because milk contains a hormone that reduces further milk production if some is left behind.

Which breast to start with?

If you fed from both breasts during the last feed, start the next feed with the breast you fed from last, as this will probably be less well emptied. If you fed from only one breast during the last feed, start with the other one next time. The let-down is more efficient early on in a feed, and a baby sucks more strongly at the first breast, which means the first breast is usually emptied more effectively than the second.

Note that your baby may sometimes want to go back to the first breast after finishing the second.

Some women find they or their babies prefer feeding from one side. This is often the left side. It's been suggested that the sound of the mother's heartbeat (which is on the left) soothes her baby. Most women have one breast that is bigger than the other. If the difference is mainly caused by fat, the baby may find it easier to feed from the smaller one, but if the difference is in the amount of glandular tissue, the baby may prefer the larger one. Some women only ever feed from one side. However, in this case it's wise to express milk (though not necessarily after every feed) from the unused breast, in view of the differing rates of cancer in the used and unused breasts of Hong Kong's Tanka boat women (see page 78).

HOW LONG SHOULD FEEDS LAST?

Let your baby feed till he's had enough. Different babies feed for different times, depending on:

- How hungry they are.
- How strongly they suck and milk.

- How fast the milk flows.
- Whether they feed from one breast, or two, or go from one to the other several times.
- How much they need the comfort of being at the breast.

Any one baby takes different length feeds at different times.

Babies, like adults, sometimes want different amounts of food from day to day, and at different times of the day. Sometimes a baby wants a snack, other times a feast. Research in South Africa showed that a baby feeding on demand took feeds of very different volumes at different times – one feed sometimes being ten times as big as another.

Some women's milk flows faster than others, and their babies tend to get what they need more quickly.

Some babies suck and milk the breast so enthusiastically that they stimulate several let-downs in rapid succession and thus get the milk they need very quickly. In one study one baby got all he needed in four minutes from just one breast, while another took nearly twenty-two minutes (and fed from both breasts). But most were in between. And in my experience, many babies take longer – sometimes much longer – than twenty minutes or so for a feed.

Gentler or weaker babies may run out of steam sooner and have to wait a while before they have the energy to suck hard enough to stimulate another let-down. You may be able to help to stimulate a let-down yourself by massaging your breasts as if expressing milk (see page 159).

You may be told, wrongly, to feed your baby for a specified number of minutes each side and to increase this time each day to ten minutes a side on the fifth day.

— Restriction of feed length is completely unnatural. It hinders milk from coming in, may not give your let-down time to work and become established, prevents your baby getting as much colostrum as he could, and encourages sore nipples.

All this has been known for years, but a few hospitals or individual health workers still enforce out-of-date rules. Ideally you should question such rules openly, so as to give any unknowledgeable hospital or staff the chance to learn better, but if you find it difficult to question authority, especially just after having a baby, simply go ahead and suckle as long as you and your baby want.

- UK researchers reported in 1981 that 80 per cent of women who decided for themselves how long feeds should be were still breastfeeding at the end of the first week, compared with 57 per cent of women who were told how long to feed.

How to tell when he's had enough

Many babies show they've had enough by falling asleep and coming off the breast; others come off while still awake. A baby nearing the end of a feed may relax his fists, smile, or arch his back. Accept your baby's judgement. Lots of babies, especially in the evening or if preterm, like to have frequent small feeds with short gaps of, for example, ten to fifteen minutes, or doze on and off during a feed. This can make it difficult to know when they've had enough milk, and when they are simply enjoying being at the breast. But after a while you'll get to know how much he's had by feeling your breasts.

What about stopping a feed?

Some babies have to be gently removed from the breast or they'd be there all day. If your nipples are sore, you may need to limit the length of feeds for a day or two – but don't do this for longer unless you express some milk after each feed to give your breasts more stimulation, or your milk supply will diminish.

Never pull your baby off the breast while he's feeding as suddenly breaking the strong vacuum in his mouth could damage your nipple. It's better to put the tip of your little finger gently in the corner of his mouth and push the nipple sideways to allow air in. Your baby will then come away easily without hurting you.

Why won't he stop feeding?

Some babies who don't want to stop feeding aren't latched on properly, so they persist in order to get enough milk. Others may have got into the habit of using the breast as a dummy to help them drop off to sleep or provide comfort.

ROOMING-IN

In hospital it's best if your baby rooms-in – stays by your bed day and night – and the good news in the UK is that increasing numbers of hospitals now facilitate this practice.

- Large surveys in the UK showed that rooming-in increased from 17 per cent of mother–baby pairs in 1980, to 63 per cent in 1990, and to 79 per cent in 2000.

Most women sleep better and are more content with their babies by them, and studies show that women who have their babies with them are twice as likely to breastfeed successfully as those whose babies go to another room at night.

It's wise to sleep with your baby in your bed only if you did not have painkilling drugs in labour (as these might make you sleep so deeply that you won't wake up if you roll on to him), if you're not a smoker, and if you can put a hospital bed's 'cot sides' up, or, at home, position a heavy chair by the side of the bed to prevent him falling out.

In general it's fair to say that no hospital has enough staff to give a baby the love and care his mother can, so it's scarcely surprising that babies who room-in are more contented than those who don't.

Even if you're in a large, open-plan ward, you can have your baby by you at night, provided you pick him up as soon as he needs a cuddle or a feed, to avoid waking other mothers. Rooming-in makes life easier for staff and more pleasant for mothers and babies, and leads to less noise because babies don't have to cry for long, if at all, to get attention. And women sleep better because they don't worry that their babies are crying unattended in the nursery or being given bottles.

Many women remember going through agony when they could hear their baby crying yet weren't allowed to be with him. A woman doesn't know the sound of her own baby's voice this soon after birth and may worry it's her baby every time any baby cries. She'll have far more peace of mind if she's with him. And her milk will come in far sooner if she picks him up for a feed not only whenever he 'asks' for one, but also whenever she wants to.

If you'd like your baby with you at night and there's no good reason not to, but the hospital staff aren't keen and you're too tired to be assertive, ask your partner to have a word.

BREAST MILK ONLY

If your baby has to be apart from you for any reason, make sure hospital staff know you want him brought to you as soon as he needs a feed, and you don't want him given anything to drink, even water or sugar water – except in the unlikely event that it's medically essential (for example, if he has low blood sugar that doesn't respond to frequent breastfeeding).

Giving breastfed babies anything other than breast milk is unnecessary for the vast majority. It's also unacceptable, as it can interfere with the establishment of successful breastfeeding. Don't be fobbed off with excuses. He's your baby and feeding frequently and on an unrestricted basis is the best way to establish successful breastfeeding. If he has anything else to drink he won't want to breastfeed as often as he otherwise would, and unless you express your milk frequently to make up for him wanting relatively few feeds, your milk supply will diminish.

Unfortunately, some hospital maternity units are so out of date that breastfeeding mothers are routinely given bottles of formula to 'top up' their babies after a feed.

- Large British surveys found that 45 per cent of breastfed babies received bottles of formula in hospital in 1990, which was slightly better than the figure of 50 per cent in 1985. However, by 1995 this figure had fallen to 36 per cent and in 2000, to 28 per cent. This ongoing improvement is good news and, although there's still room for improvement, hospitals can rightly give themselves a pat on the back, for the stark fact is that mothers who give their breastfed babies bottles of formula are much more likely to give up breastfeeding before they are ready.

If someone asks why *your* baby is not allowed to drink formula, sugar water or boiled water at night, when other babies have it and seem all right, reply that there are many reasons why breast milk alone is best for almost every baby.

Why breast milk alone is nearly always best

- The more your baby feeds, the sooner mature milk comes in.
- Frequent breastfeeds help you make plenty of milk.
- Colostrum gives your baby the correct proportions of nutrients, supplies protective antibodies and other substances not present in formula and encourages his bowel to expel the sticky early motions (meconium).
- Formula satiates a baby's appetite for several hours, making him less likely to want to breastfeed. This, in turn, reduces breast stimulation, which may decrease the milk supply. Bottle-fed babies go longer between feeds than breastfeds because it takes longer to digest formula.
- Formula contains foreign proteins which (especially if your baby has an allergic family history) might increase his risk of allergic and autoimmune diseases in later life.
- Sugar water is nearly always unnecessary for full-term, healthy babies, because breast milk provides all the sugar and water they need. A high-calorie drink satiates his appetite and makes him less

likely to want to breastfeed. A sudden slug of sugar is unnatural and best reserved for only when medically essential (see page 312).

- Properly and exclusively breastfed babies don't need extra water. Breast milk provides enough even in the early days and in hot countries. Research at the University of Rochester in New York showed that breastfed babies given water or cows' milk formula complements lost more weight in the first few days and were less likely to start gaining before they left hospital than were exclusively breastfed babies.
- It's better for a young baby not to feed from a bottle. A bottle teat is too easy to drink from and a baby used to bottles has to work harder to get milk from the breast, which may put him off. If your baby can't breastfeed, or in the unlikely situation that he really needs something extra (for example, if he has a low blood sugar level or excessive weight loss that don't respond to frequent breastfeeds), it's better for him to have whatever's necessary from a cup or spoon (or, if very premature, a tube). Preterm babies are more likely to have trouble breastfeeding if they've had bottles, as are other low-birthweight babies, babies whose mothers had a difficult labour, and babies who are unwell. Some women want a babysitter to give bottles of expressed breast milk (or formula), so are keen for their babies to get used to the bottle. But giving occasional bottles (especially to young babies) can interfere with successful breastfeeding, so it's better to wait a few months. Most older babies readily get used to feeding from a cup, if not a bottle.

Is it a good idea to give bottle-feeds of formula at home?

The subject of giving your breastfed baby bottles of formula may come up again when you get home – either because you think it's a good idea or because someone else suggests it.

However, *giving bottle-feeds of formula is nearly always bad news for a breastfeeding woman and her baby.* They reduce the supply of breast milk, because a baby full of formula doesn't want frequent breastfeeds, yet breast stimulation is essential for milk production.

Women who want to breastfeed successfully should not allow

their babies to have formula. As one mother said, 'How can demand and supply work if you suppress half the demand?'

— If bottles of formula are recommended because your baby doesn't seem to be thriving, you can almost certainly avoid them simply by increasing your milk supply – for example, by feeding your baby more often.

- A large survey in the UK (2000) found that 35 per cent of breastfed babies aged three to six weeks also had bottles of formula, along with 44 per cent of breastfed babies aged three to five months. This is a pity, because experts advise that exclusive breastfeeding for six months is better both for babies and for their mothers. Many of their mothers would undoubtedly have preferred to go on breastfeeding exclusively – and if only they had been told how and received enough skilled support and encouragement, they almost certainly could have done.

Doctors and midwives may refer to drinks of formula as 'complements' or 'supplements'. Some people make no distinction; for others, a complement is a drink (in a bottle or cup) of formula given after a breastfeed, and a supplement is one given instead of a breastfeed.

SLEEPING AND NIGHT FEEDS

During your hospital stay it's best for your baby to be by you at night, and it's worth mentally gearing up for night feeds because you'll be doing plenty of them. Night feeds may become less frequent from two months or so onwards, but many babies continue wanting them for a long time.

Young babies have more periods of light, REM (rapid eye movement) sleep than do older children and adults, and are most likely to wake for a feed during these times, which helps explain night waking. As your baby gets older, he will have longer periods of deeper sleep and wake up up less often.

Try to get as much sleep as you can between feeds, especially in the early days, as you'll probably be tired after giving birth and broken nights take their toll.

Midwives may suggest you rest on your tummy for an hour or so every day. If your breasts are at all full, you can make yourself comfortable by lying with your head on one pillow plus another one below your breasts to make a sort of bridge.

You may be too excited to sleep much soon after you've had your baby. It's a common feeling to want to live through the birth experience over and over again in your mind, as though you were 'learning' it.

Some mothers dream very little in the first few days or even weeks after the birth, probably because their sleep patterns are broken by their baby waking. Sleeping with your baby by your side means you soon get used to snoozing and resting during breastfeeds, even though you are not properly asleep.

If your baby goes into a hospital nursery at night, tell the staff on duty each night that you are breastfeeding. Although they should know, it's easy for an inexperienced person, a new agency nurse, or a nurse who thinks she's doing you a favour, to give your baby a bottle of formula, sugar water or water, along with all the bottle-fed babies. Some women tie a card to their baby's cot saying, 'I am breastfed, please take me to my mother when I cry.' This will probably make it easier for you to get what you want but isn't infallible.

When you feed your baby at night, aim to do so as calmly and quietly as possible, and make the light level in the room as dim as possible too. This helps your baby learn from an early age that night-times aren't times to play and talk.

BREAST AND NIPPLE CARE

This is very simple. There's no need to wash your breasts before a feed. There's no need to wash your breasts after a feed either, though you can rinse them with water if you want. When you have a bath, don't use soap. If you put salt in the bath water to help heal an episiotomy, splash your breasts with plenty of plain water to remove the salt before you dry them. Don't soak your nipples in water as this will make them more likely to become sore and cracked. Nipples readily become soggy and liable to crack if left moist inside a bra. Avoid this by changing breast pads frequently and leaving your bra off sometimes to give your nipples some air. This may be easiest at night.

There's generally no need to put anything on your nipples. Although lanolin, cocoa butter or vitamin E oil won't hurt, they are usually unnecessary, as the Montgomery's tubercles around your areolae produce a protective oily liquid. Your baby will prefer to taste you, not anything else. And the smell of your milk, though imperceptible to outsiders, will attract your baby when you next put him to the breast. If he's a reluctant feeder, this could make all the difference to his desire to suck.

Many experienced breastfeeders say that expressing a little milk after a breastfeed and rubbing it gently into their nipples helps prevent nipple soreness.

So all you usually need do is wash your breasts with water when you want, avoid getting soap on your nipples, and keep your nipples dry between feeds.

Nipple soreness and pain

If you look after your nipples in the way I've described and feed naturally, taking care to position your baby well, you may be able to prevent soreness. However, quite a few women have sore nipples at some time in the first week or perhaps later. Unfortunately, poor advice – or no advice – on how to make this better and prevent it happening again leads many women to give up feeding. So if you get soreness, turn to page 255 to see what really helps.

Engorgement

Your breasts will swell as you start making mature milk some time in the first week after the birth. Some swelling is normal, but to avoid letting your breasts getting too full and becoming painfully engorged, simply carry on breastfeeding on an unrestricted basis. Research shows that women feeding on a schedule are twice as likely to become engorged as those feeding more frequently.

Women who have a large increase in the size of their breasts in the first week, often think their milk supply must be failing when their breasts become smaller as the days go by. However, this isn't so, provided they are feeding frequently; it's just that breasts tend to get smaller once their milk supply becomes established and matches the baby's demand.

See page 252 for what to do if your breasts become engorged.

EXPRESSING

There are several reasons why expression can be a useful technique to learn. If your breasts become tense, it may be difficult for your baby to latch on, but expressing a little milk softens them enough to make it easier. You may need to get rid of some milk by expressing it in the first few days while your baby's needs catch up with your supply. Mothers of preterm babies who can't yet take milk from the breast can provide their babies with milk and keep their milk supply going by expressing. If you get a cracked nipple, regular expression keeps your breast empty yet allows the nipple to heal. And some women need to express milk to leave for someone else to give by cup or spoon.

Before expressing, wash your hands (and if in hospital, rinse with disinfectant solution). Get a small plastic bowl or jug ready; this should be sterilized first if you intend storing your milk in a fridge or freezer. Then make yourself comfortable.

Gently massaging or stroking to your whole breast from the

outside towards the nipple for a minute or two encourages your milk to flow.

Feel where the milk reservoirs are – in a full breast they may feel like peas or little grapes under the areola.

Put the flat of your thumb over the upper reservoirs, the flat of your index finger over the lower reservoirs. Some right-handed women find it easier to use their left hand for both breasts and to collect the milk in a container held by the right hand.

Move your hand firmly backwards towards your chest, but don't let your finger and thumb slide over the skin. Now move your hand away from your chest, pressing the finger and thumb together but not pulling the breast forward, so you gently squeeze milk from the reservoirs to the nipple. Keep repeating these movements, getting into a rhythm, and after a while you'll see drops of milk slowly coming from the nipple, or, once milk is let down, faster dripping or even repeated sprays.

Carry on expressing once the milk lets down, even in the intervals between sprays. Move your hand from time to time to empty the other parts of the breast (using your other hand if necessary) and change to the other breast several times if the flow slows.

Let-down milk drips or sprays from both breasts, so if you're collecting milk for your baby you may want to collect the milk from the other breast too. Some women who are feeding their own baby and donating milk to a milk bank, collect only milk that drips from the other side, though this tends to have a relatively lower fat content. One easy way of collecting drip milk is to put a sterilized breast shell inside your bra, positioning it with the tiny hole uppermost so you don't get drenched! Pour the collected drips into a sterile bottle or other container you can cover.

Expressing is easy once you acquire the knack. The first few times you'll probably get only a few drops. Even later it's normal to express only a little – most successful breastfeeders never express more than two to four tablespoonfuls (28–56 ml or 1–2 fl oz). Be reassured that babies absorb energy more easily from breast milk than from formula, so they need less of it.

If you want to collect enough milk to leave a feed for someone else to give your baby you'll need to express after each feed for a couple of days. Alternatively, express or pump from one breast while your baby feeds from the other. Leave the bottle in the fridge between times and the small volumes will soon mount up.

Pumping

Some mothers prefer to pump their milk (see page 299); various pumps are described in the Appendix (page 412).

STORING MILK

Wash your hands, then express (or pump) your milk into a sterilized plastic container – plastic is better than glass as some of the immunological components of milk stick to glass. Label the container with the date you collected the milk.

Your milk will separate into layers as it stands but these will soon disappear when you warm it up later.

Expressed or pumped breast milk contains many anti-infective factors and if you collect it in a clean (not necessarily sterilized) container and cover it, you can safely leave it at room temperature (19–22°C, or 66–72°F) for up to six to eight hours, some experts say up to ten.

- A Nigerian study (1988) found no significant bacterial growth in expressed colostrum left at high room temperatures 27–32°C (81–90°F) for twelve hours.

Fridge

You can keep expressed or pumped milk in the fridge for up to three days (though this is very much on the safe side; a 1987 study found it was safe in the fridge for up to five days, a 1994 study up to eight days). If you want to keep it for longer, freeze it immediately you've expressed it.

Freezer

Freezing has little effect on milk's antibodies but can harm its living cells, so don't freeze it unless you have to; however, previously frozen breast milk is better for a baby than formula.

Freeze only small amounts of milk, for example, in the compartments of an ice cube tray, because once it's been thawed it shouldn't be refrozen (though you can put leftover milk in the fridge as long as you use it within twenty-four hours). You can always thaw more if necessary. If you want to add another batch of expressed or pumped milk to a container of already frozen milk, cool the new batch first in the fridge.

You can store your milk in a freezer for three to six months (the higher its 'star rating', the longer you can keep the milk).

If using an ordinary freezer compartment in a fridge, store milk for only up to one month.

If using a frost-free freezer compartment in a fridge, store milk for only two or three weeks.

Thawing milk

Thaw frozen milk quickly by holding the container under running water – first cold, then gradually warmer until the milk is all liquid; alternatively, stand the container in a jug of hot water.

Warming milk

Gently warm a container of expressed or pumped breast milk that has been refrigerated, or frozen and thawed, by putting it in a pan of water on the hob. Shake the container to get the milk to an even temperature. Milk at body temperature (slightly cool to your skin) is the most pleasant for a baby. Preterm babies should never have cold milk.

Microwaving?

It is preferable not to thaw and warm breast milk by microwaving.

- US researchers (1992) found that microwaving expressed breast milk at high temperatures (72–98°C, 162–208°F) reduced its protective anti-infective properties; microwaving at cooler temperatures (20–53°C, 68–127°F) had no significant effect on the total amount of antibodies, but reduced the amount of lysozyme and antibodies against certain potentially harmful *E. coli* gut bacteria.
- Also, Austrian researchers report that microwaving breastmilk alters the structure of some of its amino acids, which could mean a baby wouldn't digest or use them properly.

Don't simply microwave the container you use to store expressed or pumped milk, as the temperatures reached in a microwave aren't high enough to kill concentrations of bacteria reliably. However, it's fine to use a microwave sterilizer.

COLLECTING DRIP MILK

Some breastfeeding women collect the milk that drips from the opposite breast while their baby is feeding, or while they are expressing. They do this either to keep themselves dry, in which case they discard it, or to give it to their baby later by cup or spoon (preferably not by bottle). Collect drip milk easily by putting a breast shell inside your bra, with its hole or spout (if there is one) uppermost.

VISITORS

This can be a vexed subject. While you'll want to show your baby to relatives and friends and talk about the birth, you may feel shy about feeding in front of people, yet won't want your baby to go hungry, and an hour may be too much with some visitors but not enough with others. However, you'll probably feel left out if you don't have visitors when everyone else does.

There are several ways to cope. One is to ask your partner to vet the people who want to visit you in hospital. If you wouldn't feel happy feeding in front of them, ask him to put them off tactfully. When people visit you at home you can go to another room to feed if you're embarrassed or think they will be.

NAPPY CHANGING

You may be advised to change your baby's nappy before a feed, because some babies don't feed well with a wet or dirty nappy and others are woken by being changed after a feed. This is all right if he isn't crying, but if he is, wait till afterwards, otherwise you may get stressed and not let down your milk. A crying baby may also swallow air, then regurgitate more milk. After a good feed, though, many babies are so content and full that not even a nappy change wakes them. Changing after a feed also saves nappies because babies often wet or fill their nappy during a feed. However, if your baby won't feed with a dirty nappy, you'll have to change it straight away. The good news if you have a baby who falls asleep halfway through a feed is that a nappy change may wake him enough to take the second breast.

YOUR BABY'S BOWELS

A breastfed baby's motions gradually change during the first week from the dark green meconium of the first day or so to bright yellow, liquid motions which may just leave a stain on the nappy. Young breastfed babies tend to pass bowel motions more often than do bottle-fed ones, and in the early days of breastfeeding almost every nappy may have a yellow stain. Breastfed babies tend to pass motions less frequently as they grow older, and after three or four weeks some go only every week or so, and some even less. For example, there's one story of a healthy breastfed baby who passed no motions for twenty-seven days between seven and eleven weeks old. When eventually passed, the motion was soft and vast!

A breastfed baby's motions are usually bright yellow, though perhaps occasionally green. And their smell is not unpleasant, unlike a bottle-fed baby's motions, which smell foul.

Babies often open their bowels during a feed, so it's sensible to change the nappy after a feed, unless your baby is one of those who won't feed in a wet or dirty nappy.

WIND

Many breastfed babies don't need winding – they simply bring up any wind spontaneously or pass it out the other end. If you think your baby is windy, cuddle him after a feed in a fairly upright position, for instance against your shoulder, to let the wind come up. If he doesn't usually burp, lay him down to sleep after a feed if you want. Some people seem almost obsessed with wind, but in many countries, including certain European ones, women don't recognize it as a problem so do nothing about it, with no obvious ill effects.

Some babies are obviously uncomfortable after a feed but drop off to sleep when they've brought up some wind. These babies sometimes frown or even go momentarily cross-eyed. The skin above a windy baby's upper lip may be slightly blue and he may cry or fidget. If you think your baby is windy and putting him upright doesn't do the trick, sit him on your lap with one of your hands rubbing his back gently and the other holding his chest. If you then bend him slightly in the middle, some air often comes up, perhaps with a little regurgitated milk. If at night after feeding your baby lying down, he doesn't settle easily and you think he's windy, you may need to sit him up in bed to get rid of the swallowed air.

CRYING

There's a lot going on in the average maternity ward, with trolley shops, paper rounds, meals, visitors, bed-making and room cleaning, plus doctors' and nurses' rounds, baths, talking to your neighbour in the next bed, letters to write, phone calls to make, and, if you're lucky, presents and flowers to deal with and letters and cards to open. Amid all this it's easy to let your baby come second and not feed him when he's ready.

At first you may not know why your baby is crying, but as the weeks go by some women – not all – learn to distinguish between hungry, tired, lonely, angry and wet- or dirty-bottom cries. Some babies cry very little, if at all, as their mothers are able to recognize, anticipate and meet their needs so well.

However, some babies cry much more than others. Indeed, midwives and women who have had many children say babies behave very differently and have different characters from the start. Some are quieter, more placid and content, and easier to look after; others make much more noise and are more demanding, less easily satisfied and more challenging to care for.

Babies cry for many reasons. Hunger and thirst are by far the most common. Others include feeling tired, lonely, angry, afraid, tense or too hot or cold; having wind, colic, a sore bottom or something poking into or rubbing them; sensing their mother's anxiety or haste; hearing a sudden loud noise; reacting to something the mother has eaten; breathing smoky air; and being ill.

The first things to do

You'll usually be able to stop your baby crying by putting him to the breast and/or attending to his other needs. Babies who breastfeed successfully and on an unrestricted basis, who are carried around for much of the day and sleep with their mother at night, scarcely need to cry. And babies whose mothers respond to their needs promptly and feed them as often as they want tend to cry much less than other babies.

- A study in the US (1988) revealed that babies whose mothers breastfed them frequently and responded to their needs quickly cried less, both at two months old and at four months.

No woman likes to hear her baby cry, because crying usually suggests unhappiness. Also, her baby's cries will probably upset her, which may prevent her letting down her milk.

It's sensible to comfort a squawling newborn infant straight away as this will encourage him to think the world is a good place. This won't spoil him. If you were left to yell for hours for your food, you'd become dispirited or angry: babies are no different. Many mothers notice that babies who are fed and comforted at the breast whenever necessary grow up to be happy, independent, loving children, not demanding, unhappy and spoilt.

— Being able to comfort a crying baby at the breast is one of the great rewards of breastfeeding. A woman who limits suckling time denies this pleasure to herself and her baby. Breastfeeding is not only a means of getting milk: it's also a way of being close to a warm, soft, comforting mother.

If your baby cries at the beginning of a feed

He may be frustrated, afraid or angry if your milk takes time to let down. Try encouraging your let-down before putting him to the breast, and consider waking him and/or offering the breast before he cries, so he doesn't get so hungry he has to cry. If he gets so upset he can't feed, try rocking him from side to side to calm him enough to settle at the breast.

If your baby cries after a feed

In a young baby this probably means he's still hungry, either because he hasn't had enough and needs to go back to the breast, or because you didn't let him stay at the first or second breast long enough.

Try to calm him enough to stop him crying temporarily, since crying makes a baby's tongue pull right back inside the mouth (look and you'll see this happen), which makes it harder to latch on properly. Then put him back to the breast and let him go on feeding until he drops off spontaneously.

If your baby often cries in the evening and you think you may not have enough milk for him by then, try expressing some milk after the first big morning feed next day. Store this and give it in a cup or in a supplementer (see page 302) next time he cries after a feed in the evening.

When your baby won't stop crying

Some babies go on and on crying. If you leave your baby crying for long he'll get tired out, because it uses a lot of energy. After crying for a long time he probably won't feed well because he'll be too exhausted.

The commonest cause of continued crying is schedule-feeding. Exhaustion from long periods of crying is one reason why schedule-fed babies don't get enough milk and why their mothers often can't breastfeed successfully. A baby who wakes an hour 'early' and is left to cry until the clock says it's time for a feed may not be hungry when feed time arrives – just tired out and angry or frightened because his tummy hurts and he's been alone. A few days of this and his mother's breasts will lack stimulation and her milk supply may diminish.

Could it be colic?

Real colic is intermittent pain caused by muscle spasm of the walls of a hollow organ such as the bowel. It nearly always improves after the first three months.

However, many babies cry for long periods in the first three months, especially in the evenings, for no apparent cause, and this is traditionally put down to colic. It is sometimes called evening colic or three-month colic, even though it's highly likely it isn't real colic at all. Many people assume crying results from air passing through the bowels, but there's no evidence for this; indeed, X-rays show that colicky babies have no more air in their bowels than do other babies. Having said this, some babies cry less from 'colic' if they have a bowel-calming medicine.

The vast majority of studies show that whether a baby is breastfed or bottle-fed makes no difference to whether or not he has colic. However, one study showed that colic was more likely in babies who started solids before three months. And some women believe vitamin drops give their babies colic.

Causes of colic

Some babies get real colic, and there are several causes:

- Not latching on well, so he doesn't milk the breast properly and encourage the let-down of higher-fat milk; he then goes to the second breast to fill up with even more relatively low-fat milk, so as to get enough calories. (Conversely, a well-attached baby gets some relatively higher-fat milk from the first breast, therefore gets the necessary calories from a lower volume of milk.) Low-fat milk tends to leave the stomach quickly, and because there's such a lot of it, there's a large amount of lactose (milk sugar); this then ferments in the gut and produces gas, or wind, which causes colic and, perhaps, a sore bottom.

- Being moved to the second breast before he's finished at the first breast has the same result. This is particularly likely with a mother who makes a lot of milk and is trying to curtail feeds.
- Breathing smoke-filled air, or drinking the nicotine-containing breast milk of a mother who smokes.
- Having one of variety of medical conditions that can cause colic, including food poisoning, gastro-enteritis and an obstructed bowel. For this reason, if you don't know why your baby is crying a lot, or his cry is worryingly unusual, or there are other abnormal signs, you should consult a doctor.

Other reasons for continued crying

These include:

- Swallowing too much air while trying to drink fast-flowing milk.
- Not being given attention and cuddles when he wants them.
- Being sensitive to traces of foods in your milk (for example cows' milk, eggs, peas, onions, garlic, citrus fruit, cauliflower, broccoli, brussels sprouts, beans, cabbage, tomatoes, bananas, apples, oranges, strawberries, rhubarb, spices, chocolate, coffee, alcohol), so try avoiding eating a lot of any one of these.
- Not having had enough satisfying milk, because you haven't yet had your main meal of the day.
- Being upset because he senses you are overwrought (perhaps with an evening rush of things to do).
- Reacting to your stress. A Finnish study (1993) reported that mothers who suffered from stress or physical problems in pregnancy, were dissatisfied with their sexual relationship, or had negative birth experiences, were more likely to put their baby's crying down to colic. The researchers suggested it might be a good idea to learn stress-management and parenting skills.

TEN WAYS OF CARING FOR YOUR CRYING BABY AND YOURSELF

1 – Feed him as much as he wants.

2 – Let him finish one breast before he goes to the other.

3 – Check for simple things like a cold, wet or dirty nappy.

4 – Sit and cuddle him if he's happier like that – or get your partner to do the cuddling, as some colicky babies are calmer with someone else. Alternatively, carry your baby around in a sling while getting on with other things; your movements plus your warmth, sounds and closeness may be comforting, and you can talk or sing to him as well.

5 – Gently massage his tummy in a warm room, using a little warmed oil and circling his tummy with slow, rhythmic, clockwise movements.

6 – Consider whether you've eaten or drunk anything that could upset him (for example, cabbage, onions, unaccustomed spicy food or alcohol) and avoid it or have less of it in future.

7 – Eat healthy, enjoyable, regular, balanced meals, plus something nutritious in each gap between breastfeeds.

8 – Try holding your baby in different positions after a feed, for example, with him leaning slightly forwards and bending to the right, with your arm pressing against his abdomen. He'll assume this position if you hold him with his back to you, your arm round his right side, and your right hand supporting his crotch.

9 – Consult your midwife, health visitor, doctor or breastfeeding leader or counsellor.

10 – Last, but by no means least, look after yourself by relaxing and resting more and asking for help to ensure your needs are met.

REGURGITATION

Many babies, especially small ones, regurgitate milk during and after a feed, particularly if the milk flows so fast that they swallow air as they gulp it down, or if they drink too much. Sometimes a baby brings up so much milk that he wants more.

There's no need to worry about any of this as long as your baby is thriving. However, if your milk flows very fast early in a feed, you could try expressing some beforehand to prevent him having to swallow a lot quickly to keep up.

If the brought-up milk has been in your baby's tummy some time, you'll notice it's been changed into fine curds and whey.

AFTERPAINS

When you let down your milk, you may have low tummy pains caused by oxytocin making your womb contract. These contractions encourage the womb to return to its former size. Other signs you're letting milk down are tingling in your breasts, dripping or spraying milk, lessening of any nipple pain as milk reaches the baby, and the regular 'glug-glug' of your baby swallowing.

SORE PERINEUM

There's nothing like the nagging pain of a sore perineum to put the dampers on the let-down. Try having a hot bath and ask the hospital staff for a rubber ring to sit on to take the weight off your most tender parts. If you still need a ring when you get home, buy or hire one from a surgical supplies shop, or buy or hire a Valley Cushion, available in the UK through the National Childbirth Trust (see page 420). If necessary, take some suitable painkillers.

LEAKING

You'll leak if you let down your milk before you put your baby to the breast, but leaking can occur from full breasts without the let-down, especially if you're warm and you lean forward. Leaking means your breasts are ready for your baby. To relieve the pressure you can either suckle your baby or express a little millk. If in the first few weeks your breasts are full too long, they're highly likely to become engorged.

If you leak, don't immediately think you're producing too much milk and decide to breastfeed less often, because leaking is normal, especially in the early days. Don't reduce your fluid intake either, as this won't prevent leaking. Mop up leaking milk by tucking into your bra a pad of soft clean material such as a hanky or an old cloth nappy cut into squares; alternatively, use commercial breast pads or a folded 'one-way' nappy liner. To avoid soaking your other nipple in soggy material while feeding from the first breast (as this can make soreness and cracking much more likely), uncover the second breast and let any leaking milk drip on to a cloth nappy or pile of paper tissues. A trick many women discover is to put the heel of one hand over the nipple and push it firmly towards the breast. This often stops leaking like magic.

WEARING A BRA AT NIGHT

Wearing a bra at night prevents leaking over the bedclothes in the early days and makes heavy breasts more comfortable. However, going without a bra in bed discourages nipple soreness, as it lets air get to them; placing a cloth nappy loosely over your breasts soaks up any leaks, and a waterproof sheet over your mattress prevents leaks soaking through. It's also much easier to breastfeed at night without a bra!

BREAST PADS

Cloth or paper pads tucked in your bra will soak up any leaks. You can buy purpose-made paper nursing pads from pharmacies, supermarkets and babycare shops; the cheaper ones are flat, the more expensive ones cone-shaped; washable breast pads are also available (for example, from Boots and the NCT Maternity Sales catalogue, see the Appendix, page 420). Don't use paper tissues or cotton wool because these dry on to the nipples and can be difficult to remove without washing them off. Some women use squares of soft absorbent material such as pieces cut from an old cloth nappy or towel, or a nappy roll. Plastic-backed pads sound like a good idea but prevent air getting to the nipples and make the skin wet, soggy and more likely to become sore or cracked.

HOW YOU FEEL

Many newly delivered women feel weepy and emotional around the fourth day; this often coincides with their milk coming in and may result from changing hormone levels. This happens just as often, if not more, in bottle-feeding women. Unfortunately, if a woman is having any trouble feeding her baby, this temporary depression may be the last straw that makes her decide to give up. Apart from hormonal changes, it isn't surprising that a newly delivered woman feels particularly emotional. Giving birth is both a crisis and a rite of passage in her life, and the accompanying excitement and loss of sleep can disturb the calmest person. It isn't uncommon for one mother in a ward to start crying and all the others to follow suit. All the more reason, then, to learn how to cope with breastfeeding problems before you have your baby so you won't have this to worry about.

Any hospital procedure that institutionalizes and regiments women – such as insisting on scheduled breastfeeds – does little to help a new mother's fragile emotional state, and depression is sometimes made worse if her baby goes to a nursery.

Kindness, encouragement and empathy from post-natal ward staff matter a great deal when you've just had a baby. Similarly, the slightest criticism can hurt a lot.

NORMAL WEIGHT LOSS IN BABY

A newborn's body has enough fluid to tide him over the first few days when he is getting small volumes of colostrum, and as he uses up this extra fluid it's normal for him to lose weight. Most healthy newborn babies lose 6 per cent of their birthweight, and some lose as much as 10 per cent.

BABY'S WEIGHT GAIN

The speed at which a breastfed baby regains his birthweight depends partly on how often he is fed. Babies fed frequently tend not to lose much weight in the first week, then gain more rapidly than babies breastfed on a three-hourly schedule (who, in turn, gain faster than those on a four-hourly one). Some babies take up to three weeks to regain their birthweight, a few perfectly healthy ones take even longer.

On average, breastfed newborns lose 5 to 7 per cent of their birthweight in the first few days of life, and there's a need for concern only if they lose more than 10 per cent.

- An Italian study found that 8 per cent of exclusively breastfed newborns lost more than 10 per cent of their birthweight in the first three to five days. In three out of four of them this was because either the mother or the baby hadn't yet learned a good breastfeeding technique.

In the old days a woman wasn't allowed to take her baby home from hospital until it had regained its birthweight, and this still sometimes happens today. However, the rate of weight gain usually isn't important for a healthy baby who is fed on an unrestricted basis, latches on well and seems content – as long as he is slowly gaining some weight (or at least not losing any more) and is producing enough wet nappies, and the mother's let-down is working.

Many hospitals have stopped routine test-weighing (weighing before and after a feed to see how much milk was taken) because a low or absent gain can worry people unnecessarily: it worries staff who don't understand that breastfed babies don't need as much milk as bottle-fed babies, and makes some women doubt their ability to breastfeed. Test-weighing is best reserved for the very few babies who aren't thriving in spite of excellent breastfeeding support and advice.

When you've negotiated the earliest days of breastfeeding, you're set to embark on the next stage of feeding your growing baby day by day.

EIGHT

Feeding day by day

Once home with your baby, sit down, have a drink and relax. Don't overdo things, and if possible leave the washing-up, ironing and tidying to someone else for several days at least, as you'll have your hands full with the baby. All too often a woman plunges back into her old routine and quickly becomes exhausted. Then she's surprised and upset when her milk dwindles, which creates a vicious circle. For the next few weeks just take things easy, eat nourishing meals and let the world go by. This is all doubly important if you gave birth at home, have been discharged early from hospital, or have other children.

HELPERS

Hopefully you'll have a relative, friend or paid person to help out for a few weeks, and your partner will hopefully have arranged to have some time off work. Your mother may be the best person to help, but mothers nowadays often don't live nearby. A helper is a very important person. Besides being of practical assistance, the emotional support and on-the-spot reassurance from an empathic helper can be a godsend. Make sure you both understand your roles, though, as there could be a problem if the helper wants to take care of the baby and leave you to run the house and the other children. Your helper should leave you as much time and energy as possible to be with your new baby and to get breastfeeding off to the best possible start. Be sure to get this priority right. Your milk supply may take several weeks to become established and you need time to recover from pregnancy and labour, so make the most of any help available, and don't rush the helper's departure, especially if you have other children.

WHERE TO FEED

You can feed your baby anywhere, but if you are comfortable it'll be more pleasurable and you'll let your milk down better. If you like cushions to support your arm or the baby, for example, make sure they are left in the chair you use. And from time to time try feeding while lying on a bed or sofa.

Keep the room warm if you have a winter baby, as cold air can make the muscle fibres in the areolae and nipples contract, constricting the openings of the ducts at the nipple and delaying the release of milk, which might frustrate your baby early in a feed. The warmth of your baby's mouth will eventually warm your nipple.

Keep your mobile or roving phone to hand, unless you don't want to be interrupted. And if you like something to read while feeding (and you haven't got another young child needing attention), have a book or magazine close by and consider getting a music stand to support it so as to leave your hands free. You may find it relaxing to watch TV or listen to the radio, or just watch your baby feeding, especially if he stares up at you, as many do. A lot depends on how long any one feed takes. If your baby is a quick feeder, you won't get bored. Ideally, feeding is a time to look forward to and enjoy. If you take care of your creature comforts, your baby will get the milk easily and you'll be able to relax and look forward to feed times as oases of peace in the day. Some babies like quiet feed times and refuse to feed well in noisy surroundings. Others, particularly older ones, are easily distracted.

You'll soon find you can breastfeed as you walk around, so you can fetch something you want during a feed or get to the phone without disturbing your baby.

Many women feel very thirsty when feeding, especially in the first few weeks. If you do, get yourself something to drink and put it by you before you start.

WHERE WILL YOUR BABY SLEEP DURING THE DAY?

If you put your baby in a separate room to sleep in the day, you may not hear when he wakes. So try him sleeping in a carrycot near you, or at least well within earshot. Household noise is unlikely to keep him awake if he needs to sleep; if he doesn't, it'll be more interesting for him to watch and listen to what's going on than lie in a quiet room bored, lonely and gazing at the ceiling. Alternatively, cuddle him as he sleeps, or put him in a baby sling or a suitable baby chair. One note of caution though: if he always drops off to sleep in your arms, he'll get so used to it that he'll find it hard to go to sleep in a cot or carrycot.

HOW DO YOU KNOW WHEN TO FEED?

A baby's only way of telling his mother he's hungry is to fidget or cry (unless she carries him by her naked breast so he can feed when he wants, which is what happens in some parts of the world where, as a result, breastfeeding is very successful). In the first few weeks all cries sound much the same to most new mothers (though some swear they can separate them into hungry, wet, dirty and bored cries this soon), so the only way to decide whether it's a hungry cry is to offer the breast. In other words, interpret any cry as a request for food until proven otherwise. Put him to the breast whenever he seems fidgety or restless too, as that may well be his cue to you that he's hungry. This way you'll pre-empt the need for him to cry.

HOW OFTEN TO FEED?

Babies are all different and some want more frequent feeds than others. Early on most babies settle better on frequent feeds, and their mothers find feeds become second nature, rather than occasions to plan for. As they grow older, most babies ask for fewer feeds and some settle into their own individual routines, perhaps of two-, three- or four-hourly feeds, for example. However, not all babies establish a routine, so don't compare your baby with any other. Once you accept your baby may ask for feeds frequently, and erratically, then as long as he's healthy and thriving and latches on well, you're halfway to feeding successfully .

Sometimes your baby may want feeding much more often than usual. He may be extra hungry because he's growing fast; he may need extra fluid and comfort because he's ill or because it's a very hot day; he may need the relief feeding can give to tender or itchy gums if he's teething; or he may need the comfort of being at your breast if he's upset. If he needs more milk, your milk supply will catch up in two or three days if you let him feed as much as he wants.

Women who offer the breast as often as their baby wants usually feed much more often and more successfully than schedule-feeders, and take feeds in their stride. This calls for a different frame of mind compared with bottle-feeding. Bottle-feeding mothers can always say with certainty how many feeds they have given. But breastfeeding is entirely different. The successful breastfeeding woman can't say how many times she has 'fed' in any one day, and early in a baby's life there may even be times of the day when feeds are more or less continuous.

- In a study in Sri Lanka (1994), babies aged four to six weeks breastfed six to twenty times in every twenty-four hours (with five to seventeen feeds by day and one to five at night).
- In a study in North Carolina (1984), successfully breastfed babies

aged five to sixteen months took an average of fifteen feeds every twenty-four hours.

Don't be anxious about conflicting advice from friends, relatives, health workers and books, as some people still promote breastfeeding every four hours (at 2, 6 and 10 a.m., and 2, 6 and 10 p.m.). But this advice is for the birds and bottle-fed babies, not you and your baby! Only a few women produce enough milk using such a routine; most find their milk supply slowly dwindles, because six feeds a day isn't anywhere near enough stimulation for the breasts. Women who *don't* produce enough milk with six feeds a day are the normal ones! And one researcher has found that reducing the number of feeds to five a day causes one in three women to have insufficient milk.

HOW LONG WILL FEEDS LAST?

Let your baby be your guide. Wait for him to come off the first breast spontaneously, then if he's awake change him to the other (perhaps after a short break) and let him carry on as long as he wants. He'll stop when he's had enough, and he'll finish more quickly as he gets older (unless he's tired, bored, ill or upset).

Some babies feed slowly and sporadically, others speedily. And while some babies get most of the milk they need in the first few minutes at each breast, others take longer. The length of a feed depends on how vigorously your baby sucks, how strong your let-down is, how much milk is already in your breasts, how long it takes you to let it down, and whether a baby is simply enjoying being at the breast. There's no reason for you to stop a feed unless you have something else to do, or have sore nipples.

During the first few months there may be times when he wants to feed almost continuously for several hours. This could mean he is using your breast as a dummy to help him sleep, or because he's upset, or he could be having a growth spurt and be trying to increase your milk supply.

ONE BREAST OR TWO?

Many babies drink from only one breast during a feed, which is fine provided you let him go on feeding until he's had enough, you alternate the breast you give at each feed, he is satisfied, and you express when neceesary to prevent your unemptied breast getting lumpy or tense between feeds. If he snoozes after the first breast, wait a while to see if he wakes again and wants the other one. Offer the second breast to see if he is hungry, or if it's full and you want some milk taken off. If he's hungry, he'll feed. Sometimes you may even need to change sides several times during a feed.

YOUR BABY'S FEEDING PATTERN AND BEHAVIOUR

Experienced observers say the behaviour of babies at the breast falls into several categories. Which any one baby falls into depends on his personality, past experience at the breast, how hungry he is, and the way you let your milk down. Some babies always take a long time over feeds. Others regurgitate several times during and after. Many (especially if small or jaundiced) snooze on and off. And some drink in a fast, no-nonsense manner, more like an older baby.

Many babies behave differently at different times of the day and almost all alter their feeding behaviour as they grow older.

NIGHT FEEDS

Night feeds are essential for young babies in particular to get the frequent nourishment they need; they also encourage good milk production and successful breastfeeding. They can be very special quiet times to be together too. Understandably, though, most of us are so used to long sleeps that we can't wait to have unbroken nights again.

Babies wake for many reasons: they may be hungry, thirsty, cold or ill, or be roused from a light level of sleep by noise, light or some other stimulus. There are several practical ways to help your baby to sleep at night as well as his need for milk and level of maturity allow.

Keep things dark

When feeding your baby, don't flood the room with bright light, because this will wake you both up and make you both more likely to stay awake a long time. Put a low-watt bulb in the light you use, or install a dimmer switch. If your baby sleeps in your bed, don't turn the light on unless you have to, to change a nappy for example.

Keep everything quiet, calm and low-key

It's tempting to talk to your baby when you're both awake and everyone else is asleep, but it's better to stay quiet and calm. This way, a feed won't excite the baby so much, and he'll wake less and less often as night feeds become less necessary for adequate nourishment.

Be prepared for nappy changes

Your baby may happily go back to sleep without a nappy change, but it's worth keeping clean nappies to hand so it's easier if you do have to do a change.

Use a more absorbent nappy

Before bedtime put a thick nappy on your baby – perhaps a double cloth nappy, or a nappy pad inside the usual nappy – and if using cloth nappies insert a one-way nappy liner to help keep his skin dry. This means he's less likely to wake from feeling cold or otherwise uncomfortable in a single sodden nappy. He'll also stand a better chance of going through the night without a change.

Cut down on caffeine

Coffee, tea, cola and other caffeinated soft drinks aren't usually a problem, but some babies, particularly preterm ones whose liver can't yet break down caffeine very well, have trouble sleeping if their mothers have a lot of caffeine.

Give up smoking

This might help your baby sleep longer.

Look after yourself

It's easy to believe you need a certain amount of sleep, but most of us experience no ill effects from having less than usual, or having broken nights. However, if you feel tired, get more rest by going to bed earlier yourself, or napping when your baby sleeps by day. If you wake at night feeling hot and sweaty, with full breasts, either wake your baby for a feed, or express some milk, as the longer you leave full breasts unemptied, the more likely they are to become engorged.

Look at the positives

When your baby wakes you, enjoy the feel of his warm, soft body nestling against you. Some busy women enjoy the luxury of undisturbed time during night feeds to think, plan or pray. And if you don't mind having the light on, night feeds can be times for reading or just looking at your baby.

Let your baby sleep in a cot in your room

Many parents of young babies do this, as it makes getting up at night less disruptive and means you are more likely to wake as soon he becomes restless, rather than waiting until he cries. This is less disturbing to everyone and means he's more likely to go back to sleep soon afterwards.

If you put his cot next to your bed, you won't have to get out of bed to lift him out when he needs a feed, though the drop-side of most cots doesn't drop low enough for this to be as easy as it could be. (If you buy the excellent three-sided 'cot-bed' – the Global Bedside Cot, page 418 – your baby will be on the same level as you, so it's easy to put an arm around him to comfort him or to slide him closer to you for a feed, plus he has his own mattress and bedclothes. You can convert it into an ordinary four-sided cot and, when he's older, a bed without sides.)

How long you keep the cot in your bedroom is up to you and your partner. Some mothers move the cot out when their baby sleeps through the night; some prefer to keep close until their baby is a year old, or more; and some like to get the baby used to going off to sleep and waking in a separate room sooner rather than later.

If you can't sleep with your baby in your bedroom, or don't want to, then when he wakes for a feed, either bring him into your bed temporarily, where you'll both be warm and comfy, or make sure you can feed him comfortably in his bedroom.

Let him breastfeed in your bed

This is the easiest way of feeding at night, and means you both stay lying down, which is more restful for you and disturbs your sleep and your baby's much less. Also, there's no crying to wake everyone, because you'll readily sense his restlessness so you can feed him before he cries. You'll also know he's safe and warm.

- One UK study (2003) found that 65 per cent of breastfed babies occasionally slept in the parental bed in the first three months. A recent American study found that over half the babies in the US spent part of the night in bed with their parents. And in some countries most mothers co-sleep with their babies.

After a feed you can leave your sleeping baby by the breast. When you want to feed from the other breast, roll over with him in your arms so he's on your other side. Or just twist your body so he can feed from the other breast. You'll probably find it most comfortable to feed him with your arm crooked round the top of his head, and a hand on his back to keep him in place. When sleeping, most mothers of breastfed babies lie on their side, facing their baby.

Once he's old enough to roll, put a chair-back against the side of the bed to stop him falling out when you're asleep.

You'll probably be able to wind him, if necessary, by sitting him up while you stay lying down.

Don't forget to keep something to drink by your bed – many women feel very thirsty while feeding.

Some women fear suffocating their baby. However, the chances of this are virtually nil in most families. The only parents who shouldn't have their baby in bed are those who are extremely overweight or tired, take sleeping tablets or recreational drugs, or are drunk (all these make suffocation by 'overlaying' more likely), and those who are smokers (there's a link between bed-sharing with smoking parents and sudden infant death syndrome). It's also unwise to 'co-sleep' in bed with a baby if your mattress is very soft, since there's a tiny chance that if he rolls over to his tummy, this could suffocate him. Similarly, he shouldn't lie near a pillow, and you shouldn't co-sleep on a sofa or chair. Put the baby between you and the side of the bed to sleep (rather than between you and your partner), and put the mattress right up against the wall so he can't fall out. Co-sleeping with a baby and partner is more practicable, and safer, with a queen- or king-sized bed, and with a sheet and blankets rather than a duvet. Remove any long ribbons from your nightwear so your baby can't get entangled. Lastly, lie your baby on his back to sleep, and don't let him get too hot.

If you don't want your baby to depend on you lying by him to go to sleep, there's a solution. When you give the last feed before you go to bed, don't let him go to sleep at the breast, but when he seems sleepy lay him in his cot so he gets used to going to sleep in his own bed without you lying by him. When he wakes at night, bring him into your bed for a feed, then take him back to his bed if you want. This means he'll be first in his bed, then yours, then perhaps back in his again. Many families who use this approach go through a transitional phase of 'musical beds' for some months.

Some women feel uneasy about having their baby in bed, perhaps disliking the thought of prolonged contact. Some dads too are antagonistic, though it should be possible to sort this out if you listen lovingly to one another.

Ask your partner to help

If your baby sleeps in another room and you're tired out, ask your partner to get up and bring him to you in bed, then put him back in his cot after the feed.

When will your baby give up night feeds?

This is very much an individual matter. Some breastfeds sleep the night at a few months old, some even earlier, but a great many perfectly normal, healthy babies wake for many months, some even for years. Some wake several times, others just once after their parents have gone to bed, and from time to time a baby might want to breastfeed more or less constantly for a while at night.

Breastfed babies tend to wake more often than bottle-fed ones.

- One study in the UK (2003) found that breastfed babies fed two to three times a night on average in their third month, bottle-feds once or even not at all.
- Another UK study found the most significant factor in the history of three-month-olds who woke for breastfeeds was being breastfed more than eleven times over twenty-four hours in their first week.

However, it certainly isn't worth reducing the number of feeds early on simply to reduce the likelihood of night waking later, because – provided your baby is well latched on – frequent feeds are normal, natural and vital for successful breastfeeding. And it isn't worth stopping breastfeeding just to get unbroken nights, because many bottle-fed babies wake at night anyway, and bottle-feds often take much longer to settle after a night feed.

If your baby gives up night feeds early, make sure you breast-feed often enough in the day to maintain your milk supply and stop your breasts becoming tense. You may also have to express some milk before you go to bed or even during the night to prevent discomfort. If your baby gives up night feeds early and your milk supply dwindles, wake him for a feed before you go to bed.

Sleep patterns change, sometimes with more waking, sometimes less, but young children grow up and night waking doesn't last for ever – though it may seem it will at the time!

Getting your baby off to sleep

Each infant is an individual and has his own sleep requirements which change from day to day according to how he feels and what he's been doing. They also change as he grows older. Young babies tend to sleep as much as they need, unlike some older children, who sometimes get more and more tired yet can't or won't sleep. While some babies go straight to sleep after a feed, others prefer to stare at their mothers, look around, or smile and coo. Don't waste valuable opportunities for getting to know your baby by trying to get him to sleep if he's not ready.

You may be advised to put your baby in his cot after you've fed and winded him, and if he doesn't then go to sleep to let him cry until he does. This advice aims to encourage a baby to develop his own resources for getting off to sleep without needing you there. Such advice may include setting a time limit on the crying, which makes it seem more humane. However, crying suggests your baby is unhappy or uncomfortable, so you may prefer to find another way of helping him get to sleep peacefully and happily.

GOING TO SLEEP AT THE BREAST

The easiest way of helping a sleepy young baby get off to sleep is to let him stay at the breast until he nods off. Some babies do this anyway when they've had enough, while others doze towards the end of a feed, not actually letting go but waking every so often to nibble or lightly suck. If you gently remove your breast, he may drift into a deeper sleep. If you watch him, you'll notice he makes occasional sucking or mouthing movements as if still at the breast and, from time to time, a smile or a frown may flicker across his face as he dreams. (You may see similar expressions just before he wakes.) He may also open his eyes several times as he goes off to sleep as if to check you are still there. Once he's sound asleep and you've finished cuddling him, put him somewhere warm, safe and within earshot to sleep.

However, babies frequently allowed to go to sleep at the breast can easily get into the habit of needing the breast to fall asleep, as if it were a dummy (pacifier). So some women prefer not to let their babies go to sleep at the breast.

What you do depends on whether you enjoy letting him go to sleep at your breast and are happy for him to rely on it; whether you want to be able to leave him with a sitter (many babies settle to sleep easily when their mother isn't there, but some find it more difficult); and whether you are content with the idea of him continuing to need the breast to go to sleep as he grows older.

OTHER WAYS OF GETTING HIM OFF TO SLEEP

Many babies happily go to sleep after a feed if put in a warm, comfortable, familiar place. Rocking your baby in your arms is another time-honoured way of inducing sleep. And some babies regularly nod off in a car, pram or sling, lulled by the motion or noise.

How your baby goes off to sleep may vary with the time of

day, where you are, and what you're doing. Many babies prefer a familiar place, especially when they're older, and if your baby is used to having you there as he drops off to sleep, he'll tend to expect this every time. This is the norm in many families and in many cultures – some of which consider the idea of putting a baby to sleep in another room, apart from his mother, most peculiar.

There's nothing more pleasant than going to sleep yourself with your baby by you if you have the time. You'll wake refreshed and you may find he sleeps extra well when you're there, perhaps because of the familiar and reassuring smell, feel and sound of your body.

HOW LONG WILL YOUR BABY SLEEP?

He may fall into a pattern of sleeping for a certain length of time between some feeds, or he may be an irregular sleeper. Many young babies wake soon after what seemed to be the end of a feed and want to go back to the breast. This is perfectly normal – especially in the evenings or for babies who are very young, preterm or unwell. A few babies fuss and can't get off to sleep because their mother took them off the breast before they'd had enough of the relatively high-fat milk that's available later in a feed at the first breast.

Carry your baby in a sling if he is unsettled when you have to get on with essential jobs. You'll find it's easier to cook, clean, wash up, write and so on with the baby slung on your back than on your front.

LEAKING

The leaking you experience in the first few weeks gradually becomes less of a problem, because your let-down becomes more reliable and the storage capacity of the milk ducts increases so they hold more milk. You'll still leak from the opposite breast during a feed. Frequent changes of cloth or absorbent non-stick paper pads inside your bra will help, and a paper pad with a waterproof outer layer helps prevent milk soaking your clothes; the downside of a waterproof layer is that it can encourage nipple soreness, so such pads are best used only occasionally. Perhaps the best tip is to press firmly over the nipple with the heel of your hand or the ball of your thumb for a short while, as this should quickly stop the leaking.

CRYING BABY

The sound of your baby's cry is designed to alert you to care for him. It's not a sound that's easily ignored, even by a stranger, and a baby who won't stop crying is very disturbing. If a baby cries a lot it's hardly surprising if his mother feels something is wrong with him or his food. Once the doctor reassures her that nothing is medically wrong, some women – and, unfortunately, their helpers – believe they must change the baby's feed. For a breastfeeding woman this means giving formula. But this is almost never necessary (see page 238).

— A crying baby's best interests are only rarely served by stopping breastfeeding and changing to a bottle.

The first thing is to breastfeed as nature intended, which means at least every time he cries. A baby breastfed according to a schedule will almost certainly cry a lot because he will sometimes be hungry before the clock says it's time for a feed and he'll be denied comfort-sucking time. Feeding your baby frequently, whenever he wants, for as long as he wants, will almost certainly reduce or stop his crying.

- One study showed that frequently fed babies cried only about half as much at two months old as those fed less often. By four months the difference was slightly less but still noticeable.

Feeding your baby whenever he cries will also increase your milk supply, which is a good thing if he was crying because he was hungry. Research shows that breastfed babies who are demand-fed cry much less than schedule-breastfed babies. It's difficult to ascertain what the long-term psychological effects of prolonged periods of crying are, but they certainly make the baby and mother unhappy at the time.

Some babies cry because they're bored and need amusement. Others crave company and settle only when held. One way to cope if you're busy is to use a sling. Several types leave your hands free to get on with your work but keep the baby secure and contented as you walk around. One study in the US (1986) found that babies cried only half as much when carried more by a parent. Other babies are pacified by a ride in a buggy, pram or car. Anything is worth trying, but *always try suckling first.* If all else fails, ask a friend, relative or neighbour to look after your baby for a time. If you are constantly worried about the crying, your milk supply will dwindle, which, in turn, will make him cry more. A change of face and scene often quietens a baby miraculously.

HOW YOUR BREASTS FEEL THROUGHOUT THE DAY

Milk-producing cells produce and release milk more or less continuously, so the amount in the breast depends to some extent on the time since the last feed. If your baby doesn't wake and your breasts are uncomfortably full, either express some milk or wake him; you'll sometimes need him to relieve your breasts as much as he sometimes needs you to relieve his hunger.

Hopefully he will have his longest break between feeds at night, in which case your breasts will be especially full first thing in the morning. You may even wake up with your nightclothes and bedclothes drenched with milk. The early morning feed is often the most pleasant simply because it's such a relief to tense breasts.

HOW YOU FEEL THROUGHOUT THE DAY

How much you enjoy feeding depends to some extent on how busy you are. If you slot feeds into a packed day, you may not feel calm, and your baby, sensing your tension, may be unsettled. If you are very stressed you may not let your milk down. If that happens, try to slow down for the rest of the day and cut out a few jobs the next day.

Many women feel most stretched and tired in the early evening. Not only may they have to feed other children and start getting them to bed but they might also want to tidy up, feed the baby and think about the evening meal. The early evening is a physiologically low time for many people anyway.

If it's too much for you and your let-down, be your own time-and-motion expert and aim to organize things so they don't all happen at once. 'Proper' meals can wait as long as you and your family have something to eat to keep you going; older children can be encouraged to help clear up their toys, and you could give them their tea and bath earlier. You could also prepare food for the evening in the afternoon, make full use of your fridge and freezer, and cook dishes such as casseroles well ahead of time.

SOME EVERYDAY CHALLENGES

A woman at home on her own may have practical challenges to consider when breastfeeding. For instance, what do you do if the doorbell rings? You might decide not to answer. You could do up your clothes quickly and go to the door, with your hungry baby either crying in your arms or left safely behind. You could carry on feeding as you answer the door, perhaps with a shawl round you. Or you could stick a notice to the door saying, 'I'm busy with the baby, please ring only if it's important'.

What if passers-by – or the window cleaner – can see in through the window? Just keep a nappy or shawl near so you can cover up if you want. Or draw the curtains.

As for the phone, you could leave it unanswered, though many people don't like doing this. You could take it off the hook. You could sit so you can reach it. Or you could keep the handset of a roving phone by you during a feed, or keep your mobile phone nearby.

Planning how to cope means that when things like this happen you won't worry and your let-down won't be disturbed.

Feeding with other children around

A new baby can be both a joy and a misery to other children, especially if they are very young. The attractions are tempered by their mother having a new and time-consuming interest that is central in her life.

A way round this is to be extra loving and attentive, especially to the next youngest child who will probably be most affected. If he wants to try breastfeeding, let him; he's only trying to compete for your attention and will very soon get bored.

Try to include older children into the intimacy of the breastfeeding circle. For example, you could talk with or read to a toddler and feed the baby at the same time. You could also keep an absorbing toy or game handy for when you're feeding, and remember to spend some time later playing alone with the child who feels left out.

Your children will gain one huge advantage by watching you breastfeed. Simply observing breastfeeding will make a big difference to the likelihood of them breastfeeding (or, in the case of a boy, encouraging his partner to breastfeed) when they eventually have a baby.

Visitors

How you deal with breastfeeding when you have visitors depends on you, your feelings, your feelings about the other people, and their views on breastfeeding.

If you're happy to feed in company, go ahead. You know breastfeeding is natural, normal, healthy and wonderful, and hopefully your visitors will be completely unfazed by it – even delighted. Wear clothes you can pull up enough to feed in a way that doesn't reveal your breast, or use a shawl to cover up. If a visitor is embarrassed, they can go to another room if necessary.

Sometimes you may prefer, or feel it's more appropriate, to feed the baby in another room. If you decide to go this route, try not to hurry the feed, as your baby will be much more likely to be in a good mood afterwards if he's allowed to take his usual time. Some women always choose to feed alone, which is a shame as they miss hours of other people's company.

You may want to think twice about entertaining while you have a young baby, but if you're the sort of person who enjoys looking after people and cooking for them, you'll probably manage fine.

When choosing what to eat, go for something that won't be harmed by being left in a warm oven if you have to feed the baby before you eat. The calmer you are, the calmer he'll be, as babies quickly pick up and react to their mother's feelings. With a little practice it's perfectly possible to feed a baby at the dinner table in a way that doesn't reveal any bare breast, though do be sensitive to your guests' feelings.

GETTING BRIGHT OUTDOOR DAYLIGHT

Aim to take your baby outdoors each day to get some daylight on his skin, especially if he is dark-skinned or you live in northerly parts where sunlight is more oblique and less light gets through the atmosphere. Just getting outdoor daylight on a baby's uncovered cheeks for a few minutes a day in summer provides enough stores of vitamin D to keep his bones strong and protect against the bone-softening disease rickets. And it's good for your bones too. However, don't put a young baby in direct sunlight, and protect an older one from sunburn.

GOING OUT WITH YOUR BABY

Most women prefer to take their baby with them wherever they go, and you can take a breastfed baby almost anywhere. You can easily take your baby with you if you go to a friend's home, even if you have a sitter for the older children in the evening. Tell your hostess in advance that you'd like to bring your breastfeeding baby, as this will give her a chance not to cook anything that might spoil if left in the oven a little longer. Once there, make yourself comfortable when you breastfeed, and ask for a drink, cushions or whatever. You may prefer to feed somewhere private. If not, ask if they mind you breastfeeding with them there – it's better to do that and feed elsewhere if necessary than risk feeling awkward if they are embarrassed.

Attitudes about breastfeeding in public are gradually changing, though some countries are becoming breastfeeding-friendly faster than others. In Scotland at the time of writing, for example, legislation is being planned that will allow women the right to breastfeed anywhere. In Australia women think nothing of breastfeeding when out and about. But in France, apparently, few women breastfeed outside their own homes.

- A study in the UK (2003) found that most people (84 per cent) think it's fine for women to breastfeed discreetly in public.
- Another large survey in the UK (2000) reported that nearly all mothers thought large shops and shopping centres should provide a place for breastfeeding, while four in five thought restaurants should have a mother's room. Only one in three thought there should be feeding facilities in public toilets, which perhaps isn't surprising.
- Over half of new mothers in the UK feel embarrassed to breastfeed when out and about, according to a survey of nearly 7,000 mothers by the National Childbirth Trust (2002), which is a shame.

One particular concern of young women is breastfeeding in front of men (other than their partner). Some even fear that young men will joke about what they're doing or be rude in other ways.

A clever choice of clothing is particularly useful in a public place such as train, bus, park or restaurant. A practice feed in front of a mirror will give you confidence.

If you go to a restaurant it's polite to feed discreetly, if possible, because while you could argue that other people *shouldn't* be upset, the fact is that some may be. You'll do more to persuade them breastfeeding is good if you do it discreetly than if you are careless with their feelings. You may want to choose a corner table where you'll be less conspicuous while breastfeeding and dealing with your baby will be easier. And you may prefer not to go to expensive restaurants if you feel you won't let your milk down so well if concerned about other diners' reactions, or feel they aren't the right environment for breastfeeding.

It's generally better not to take a breastfeeding baby to a cinema, theatre, concert or talk, because gurgles, glugs, goos, cries and so on could rightly be annoying to others who have paid to be there and want to listen without disturbance. However, if you can rely on a young baby to let you know he wants a feed simply by wriggling quietly, and not to slurp or make other feeding noises, you might try sitting at the back of an auditorium, and leave immediately if necessary.

If you go out without your baby, leave a container of expressed milk in the fridge for the sitter to warm when needed and give it from a cup or spoon, or for an older baby who breastfeeds well, a bottle (he won't be confused by a bottle teat and find breastfeeding difficult afterwards, whereas a young baby might). A hungry baby will probably be fine, because the milk is his usual brew and tastes familiar. If you're going to leave expressed milk, though, remember it'll probably take several days of collecting it during and after breastfeeds to collect enough.

CAR JOURNEYS AND HOLIDAYS

Breastfeeding is easy in a car – in fact it really comes into its own – though you must feed only in a parked car, not a moving one.

If you fly, consider flying at night so the baby will be sleepy, the aircraft dark and the chance of privacy increased because more passengers will be asleep. Some airlines have a special seat that can be curtained off for a breastfeeding mother.

If you travel with another adult, ask them to do as much as possible or you could become tense and tired and not let your milk down well.

Holidays are much simpler with a breastfed baby. There's no bottle cleaning or sterilizing to worry about, no boiled water to organize for a feed and the necessary equipment is always to hand.

FEEDING SOMEONE ELSE'S BABY

A few women sometimes breastfeed each other's babies. Historically millions of wet nurses have fed other women's babies. And in developing countries grandmothers sometimes feed their daughters' babies.

The younger a baby is, the more likely he is to accept a feed from someone else. However, no woman should feed someone else's baby unless she has the mother's permission and is healthy. Infection of the nipple with a herpesviruses or thrush (candida) can be transferrred to a breastfeeding baby, for example, and HIV (human immunodeficiency virus) infection can pass to a baby via breast milk.

> Feeding a baby from day to day can be one of the most rewarding things a woman ever does. In the next chapter we'll look at how you can look after yourself while you do this.

NINE

Looking after yourself

There are two especially important reasons for looking after yourself now. Firstly, as a mother you are the kingpin of your home and if you are well and happy the chances are the rest of the family will be too. If you become tired and run down, your state will reflect on those around you.

Secondly, a fit and healthy woman is far more likely to breastfeed successfully than one who is exhausted, not because she produces more milk, or milk of a different quality, but because her let-down is more reliable. An unreliable let-down can frustrate a baby so he takes less and less milk and cries a lot because he feels hungry adding to his mother's exhaustion.

'Mothering the mother' is considered a vital part of successul child-rearing in many cultures. These wise people know a well-cared-for mother stands more chance of looking after her young children adequately. In our culture, it's unlikely you'll have somebody to look after you for much of the time, so it's vital to look after yourself.

Looking after yourself is important whether you're a first-time mum or an old hand. If it's your first baby, you'll have everything to learn, you'll be anxious about doing things right and you'll want all the help you can get to encourage you in your new adventure.

If you've already got a family, you'll need help of a more practical kind as your new addition puts further pressures on your time and energy in an already busy life.

Both situations benefit from loving, sensitive helpers who can mother you and support you in the way you best need. But most people, especially perhaps partners, can't be expected to know what it is you really *do* need. Be assertive and ask for what you want. Helpers can be very well meaning, but tend to do what *they* feel you want or need. So be sure to enlighten them.

REST, RELAXATION AND SLEEP

If you have only one baby, it's comparatively easy to make time for naps during the day when he sleeps. Indeed, if you are waking several times a night, which is highly likely, especially at first, you *must* make time, even if you are the sort of person who turned up her nose at daytime sleeping before you had the baby.

For the mother who comes home after forty-eight hours in hospital, rest isn't a luxury – it's vital. Aim to spend most of your day in and around your bed for the first week after the birth whether you're in hospital or at home. This doesn't mean you should stay in bed all day – you certainly shouldn't. But it's sensible not to busy yourself around the house as if nothing had happened.

The temptation, especially for an efficient woman who held down a busy job before having her baby, is to cram household and other tasks into the baby's sleep time. But you have the rest of your life to be a superwoman – you don't have to be one now. If you are rested, cheerful and content, you'll be a far better mother than if you've cleaned the oven, changed sheets, emailed the office and generally exhausted yourself! Ask someone else to do the housework, or else just do a minimal amount – keep the kitchen and bathroom clean, pick up obvious mess and tidy up so you can sit down and walk around without tripping over. Housework will always be there but you'll probably mother a new baby only a couple of times ever, so make the most of them. To paraphrase the American saying, 'Kissin' don't last – cookery do' – 'Babies don't last – housework does!'.

Relax whenever you can in the day. The secret is not to let

undue muscle tension build up, because this is tiring in itself. Even if you don't sleep, aim to lie down and read, listen to music or put on the radio or TV.

Breastfeeding naturally – on an unrestricted basis and without schedules – will help ensure you sit down for long periods.

At night, accept it'll probably be some time before you return to regular long, unbroken stretches of sleep. If you can't go back to sleep quickly after feeding the baby, make sure you are getting physical rest.

A woman with more than one child needs to be even more certain she gets enough rest. If your elder child still sleeps during the day, try to get the baby to sleep then as well, so you can have a rest at the same time. Otherwise, lie down with your baby, but lie on your bed rather than on a sofa in case you fall asleep, as being in bed is safer for the baby. Sometimes you might ask a neighbour, relative or friend to look after your toddler for an hour or so while you sleep. He'll probably welcome the change too. Or you could arrange with a friend to help each other out this way.

YOUR FOOD

Assuming your usual diet is adequate, well balanced and nutritious, you'll provide your baby with plenty of milk while ensuring your body isn't drained of nutrients. The scent of certain foods in your milk will also help accustom your baby to the taste of your family's food.

If your usual diet isn't so good, aim to improve it, and be sure you don't fill up with empty calories – from foods made with white flour and added sugar, for example. The nutrients most likely to be lacking are iron, calcium and riboflavin (vitamin B_2), so check you eat enough foods containing iron (meat, shellfish, eggs, green leafy vegetables, beans, peas, nuts, seeds and wholegrain foods), calcium (tinned sardines eaten with the bones, shellfish, dairy, eggs, beans, peas, lentils, nuts, seeds and wholegrain foods) and vitamin B (meat, fish, dairy, eggs, beans, peas, green leafy vegetables, mushrooms, nuts, seeds and wholegrains). Be sure, too, to have a good balance of omega-3s and omega-6s (see page 99), remembering that most of us have far too much omega-6 for optimal health.

Do you need to eat more?

Just eat slightly more of everything, since experts believe that the average breastfeeding woman needs only an extra 400–600 calories a day. Things aren't always clear cut, though, because studies show that some successfully breastfeeding women can eat an average of nearly 700 calories a day more than bottle-feeding women, yet still lose the fat they stored in pregnancy. And yet others need no more calories than do bottle-feeding women of the same weight. The digestive system of a breastfeeding woman seems more efficient at getting energy from her food.

Studies suggest a woman's milk supply is more dependable if she spaces her food intake evenly throughout the day, rather than eating the bulk of her daily calories in one meal.

One survey found that stopping breastfeeding because of 'not enough milk' was less likely in mothers who'd been encouraged to eat more. Those who breastfeed longer tend to have larger appetites than before they were pregnant.

Vegetarians

If you are vegetarian, it's wise to check – with a dietitian if necessary – that you have enough sources of vitamin B_{12}. Vegetarian sources include eggs, dairy products and fortified foods (yeast extract, veggieburger mixes, soya milks and some breakfast cereals, for example). Certain seaweeds, and fermented soya products (for example, tempeh and miso), used to be suggested as sources of B_{12}, but we now know their B_{12} is likely to be in a form that can't be used by humans.

Vegans (who eat no foods at all from animal sources) must take particular care to get enough B_{12}; low levels are most likely in first-generation vegans, who haven't the benefit of traditional wisdom in their family on how to prepare nourishing vegan meals. They also need plenty of vegan foods containing calcium (beans, peas, lentils, nuts, seeds and wholegrain foods), iron (peas, beans, nuts, seeds, wholegrain foods, green leafy vegetables, elderberries, molasses, parsley and cocoa), magnesium (beans, peas, nuts, seeds, mushrooms, green leafy vegetables and wholegrain foods), zinc (nuts, peas, beans, wholegrain foods, root vegetables, parsley, garlic and ginger) and riboflavin (vitamin B_2 – found in wholegrain foods and green leafy vegetables).

Is there anything you shouldn't eat?

The vast majority of foods are broken down by your digestive system before they get into your milk, but some small traces do enter the milk. If your baby reacts badly after you've eaten a certain food, simply eat less of it or avoid it until you stop breastfeeding. Some babies are more sensitive than others, and onions, peas, cabbage, cauliflower, broccoli and chocolate seem the most likely to make a baby fuss.

It's wise to avoid too much saturated fat (in dairy food, meat and foods made with butter, lard or hard margarine or other hydrogenated fat).

- A Finnish study (2000) found that breastfed babies of mothers whose diet was rich in saturated fat were more likely to get atopic disorders (allergic asthma, eczema and hay fever).

Avoid any food that looks less than fresh, and avoid foods past their sell-by dates, as they might be mouldy – even if you can't see it. Fungal by-products called aflatoxins can affect health adversely in animals, and the same may apply to human babies.

If your baby is sensitive to something you eat, the speed of his reaction depends on how quickly the food enters your milk and on the type of sensitivity. Some mothers notice symptoms in their babies as soon as after the next breastfeed, while others report a delay of two or three days.

Have no more than two helpings of canned tuna a week (a helping being 140 g or 5 oz of drained tuna) or more than one helping of fresh tuna a week, as babies should be protected from the mercury sometimes found in tuna flesh.

What if you don't eat enough?

Malnourished women can produce very high volumes of good quality milk, and their milk production is extremely robust except in famine or near-famine conditions. Even severely malnourished, starving women can breastfeed their babies for three months before extra food for them is essential if their babies are to continue growing normally. But this is at their own body's expense – they become short of calcium and protein, for example, and the more babies they have and feed, the poorer their physical state becomes. If they eat so little that the level of a protein called albumin in their blood drops below 30 g per litre (1.25 oz per 1.75 pints), their milk supply may fall or even dry up completely.

But this situation is virtually never seen in developed countries, where almost every woman has enough to eat and the only real likelihood of starvation is from the eating disorder anorexia.

SLIMMING

Some women find the fat they put on when pregnant slowly disappears with breastfeeding, but this isn't so for everyone. For your sake and the baby's, you shouldn't go on a crash diet while breastfeeding, but if you want to lose weight, be reassured that a healthy weight-loss diet will neither reduce your milk supply nor be detrimental to the content of your milk or your baby's growth. Nor will slimming release environmental contaminants stored in your body's fat (such as pesticides), as was feared at one time. If you need help, consider going to a slimming club offering a sensible weight-loss diet approved for breastfeeding women, or ask your doctor to refer you to a dietitian for advice on a healthy, weight-reducing diet while breastfeeding. Most importantly, remember that regular exercise can be a huge help in losing weight and keeping it off.

- A Californian study (1994) found that women who breastfed for three to six months lost an average of 2 kg (4.4 lb) more weight than did bottle-feeders; they lost most fat from their tummy, hips and thighs, and the fat stayed off for at least two years. Women who breastfed for longer than six months were more likely still to be losing weight after their pregnancy than non-breastfeeding women. The researchers suggested that the increase in prolactin that occurs while breastfeeding decreases appetite.
- Researchers in Philadephia (1983) suggested three other reasons. The first was that the higher a woman's prolactin level, the lower is her progesterone, which is significant because progesterone encourages fat to be stored. The second was that women who breastfeed frequently have higher prolactin and lose more fat from their fat stores (estimated by measuring their upper arms). The third was that maintaining high prolactin may reduce the activity of an enzyme called lipoprotein lipase, which encourages fat to be stored in fat stores.

WHAT ABOUT DRINKS?

You'll be more thirsty than usual, which isn't surprising considering that the average breastfed baby takes 600–800 ml (more than a pint) of milk a day, depending on their age and weight. Drink as much as you fancy, so you don't become dehydrated, but don't force yourself to drink, because drinking more than you need could actually reduce your milk. If your baby is satisfied and you are producing pale yellow urine, you're almost certainly drinking enough.

Many nursing mothers feel most thirsty while feeding and like to keep a drink close at hand.

Milk?

Milk and other dairy foods are an important part of the traditional diet in dairying countries. However, there's no need to drink more milk than usual, if your diet is well balanced and nutritious. And if you don't like milk there's no need to drink any – you don't need to drink cows' milk to make breast milk. Indeed, most experts consider it unwise for breastfeeding women to eat or drink a large amount of any one food, especially if the baby has a family history of allergy. As cows' milk is so common an allergen, you may want to avoid a large intake while breastfeeding, especially if there's allergy on either side of the baby's family.

Alcohol

Drinking in moderation is acceptable, even though some alcohol passes into breast milk. If you drink larger amounts, correspondingly more gets to the baby. Drinking alcohol raises prolactin in non-lactating women, though no studies have been done to see if this is also true for lactating women. Alcohol flavours breast milk and when a woman drinks it both the intensity of the taste and the alcohol concentration in her milk peak half to one hour later.

However, babies tend to drink less breast milk when their mother has drunk alcohol, and until it's been eliminated from her body, perhaps because the smell in her milk or in her sweat puts them off. The alcohol in the milk may affect a baby's behaviour, making him want smaller feeds. One study (2001) found babies drank about 20 per cent less milk during the four hours after their mother had consumed alcohol.

When babies drink alcoholic milk, they have more frequent short sleeps, though they sleep the same amount in total. Some babies are temporarily uncomfortable and irritable after their mother has a drink. The type of drink may make a difference too.

Drinking enough to make you tipsy may harm your milk supply by affecting your oxytocin output and making your let-down reflex unreliable, or by making you dehydrated, so go easy and aim to have plenty of water or soft drinks along with any alcohol.

Coffee

When a woman has a caffeine-containing drink (tea, coffee, cola or other caffeinated soft drink) the caffeine enters her milk within fifteen minutes and reaches a peak level within an hour. There's still some caffeine in the milk twelve hours later (and even longer in some women). In large enough amounts caffeine is a powerful drug. A young baby's liver breaks down caffeine very slowly and caffeine from a mother who has a moderately high intake (six to eight cups in twenty-four hours) can accumulate and cause abnormal activity and sleeplessness. However, this disappears when she avoids caffeine for a few days. Modest drinking of caffeine-containing drinks (such as one to three cups of average strength coffee a day) is unlikely to cause problems. But if you drink more, aim to have your coffee or other caffeinated drink after you've fed your baby, to give your milk's caffeine level time to fall before you feed again. If you suspect you are drinking too much caffeine, try cutting out tea and coffee for a week to see if this makes any difference to your baby. Smoking increases the effects of caffeine.

VITAMINS

The UK Department of Health recommends that all breastfeeding women take a vitamin supplement to ensure that their milk contains enough vitamins for their baby. However, this is unnecessary if you are healthy, and sure you are eating a nutritious diet, and if you go outside to get some bright daylight on your skin each day (as this is your main source of vitamin D).

Mothers of preterm babies should make sure they have enough

foods rich in vitamin C (especially fresh vegetables and fruits). This is because preterms have relatively low iron stores. The plentiful supplies of vitamin C in breast milk help them absorb iron better.

BREASTFEEDING AND BONES

Breastfeeding may temporarily remove calcium and other minerals from a woman's bones, making them slightly less dense, but as long as you look after yourself (see below) they will soon catch up again.

- Italian research (1999) found bone density decreased for the first six months of breastfeeding, then recovered, and was higher than normal by eighteen months.
- Research in the US (1993) found that the bones of women who breastfed became temporarily less dense, but returned to normal by a year in those who breastfed for up to nine months, and were on their way back to normal in those who breastfed longer.

To help look after your bones while breastfeeding:

- Spend a little time outside each day with bright daylight on your skin (and without sunscreen), to enable it to make vitamin D. This is especially important if you are dark-skinned or tend to wear clothes that cover your arms, legs and, perhaps, neck, or if you live in northerly parts, where the sun's rays are more oblique, or in an urban area where buildings and pollution block light. Outdoor daylight is vital, because window glass filters out a lot of daylight's ultraviolet rays, which are the ones that stimulate the skin to make vitamin D.
- Take regular, moderate weight-bearing exercise (such as walking).
- Eat a healthy diet.
- Avoid crash diets, or otherwise inadequate slimming diets.
- Do not smoke.

There's no point taking a calcium supplement as this makes no difference to a breastfeeder's bone mineral density or to the amount of calcium in her milk.

EXERCISE

Regular, moderate exercise is good for you. It increases your circulation, boosts 'feel-good' hormone-like substances called endorphins, and keeps your muscles strong and flexible and your body fit. So you owe it to yourself and your family to make time for it and to find ways of fitting it into your life. Exercise won't affect your milk volume or quality. However, some babies' feeding behaviour alters after their mother has exercised, and researchers suggest this is because of changes in her sweat.

THE WAY YOU FEEL

Most women have a mixture of heightened feelings after having a baby, and some find the whole of the first year rather like being on a emotional roller coaster. None of this is surprising, because the changes in lifestyle for many women after having a first baby in particular are immense. And becoming a mother means you embark on a role of enormous practical and symbolic importance to your baby, yourself, your partner and society in general.

Memories of being a baby

Simply being with their baby can arouse deep emotions in most mothers. This is a time when memories of her own experiences as a baby are stirred deep in her conscious or unconscious mind. Psychoanalysts believe babies 'split' their impressions of their mother according to their experiences of how she meets their needs. This means they may virtually see her as two different people, a 'good' mother and a 'bad' mother. So when a baby girl grows to womanhood, becomes a mother and observes her own baby's reactions, distant recollections of joy and satisfaction at her hunger being satiated by her own 'good' mother may mingle with long-lost but still imprinted memories of frustration, fear, loneliness, anger, envy and despair over times when she was left alone, hungry and crying, by her 'bad' mother.

Being with her baby can evoke memories of any of these emotions. These echoes from the past are normal and their power in the here and now can be very strong. The astonishingly profound intimacy of breastfeeding can stir a woman's memories even more. And this is one reason behind many women's ambivalence about, or avoidance of, breastfeeding.

Surprised by joy

A woman's delight at having her baby at the breast may stem as much from her own remembered bliss and experience of security at having her own needs met at her mother's breast as from the pleasure of the present experience.

Indeed, breastfeeding is usually a very positive experience. Many women get satisfaction from knowing it's the best and most natural way to feed their baby. They enjoy its convenience and believe it enables them to forge a closer bond with their child. And they realize it's best for them, quite apart from being cheaper than bottle-feeding.

This positive attitude is highlighted by a large British survey which found that the longer a woman breastfeeds, the more likely she is to plan to breastfeed her next baby.

Long-forgotten concerns

On the other side of the coin, a woman's fear that her baby might be underfed, her dismay at being woken yet again by her baby at night, or her anxiety that her crying baby is unhappy, may all echo her own long-forgotten feelings as a hungry baby who feared the breast might never come. Sometimes difficult or painful feelings triggered by our own experiences as babies can be a challenge when we become mothers ourselves.

New motherhood – a challenging time

Psychologists have called new motherhood the 'third childhood', meaning that new mothers enter a sensitive time of far-reaching change – just as they did in childhood itself, or in their 'second childhood', when they were teenagers and met another set of new challenges.

This is a time in which deep feelings, some of them unresolved, are stirred up in every woman, and when most couples find their love life disrupted to some degree.

A woman may find that long-forgotten girlhood fantasies about the sort of mother she would be mingle with remembered and shut-away feelings about the mothering she had as an infant and with her views about mothers in general. As well as this she finds herself having to deal with her feelings about having this baby, with this man, at this time. Her attitude to babies in general and this baby in particular may or may not match those of her partner. Her thoughts about her breasts and the rest of her body, and the family messages she's received about breastfeeding and mothering, join to create a complex mixture of ideas and attitudes through which she has to sift. Some sorting is done consciously and rationally, but a lot goes on unconsciously.

Some women look to motherhood and breastfeeding to answer some of their dilemmas in life; others fear being a bad mother or unsuccessful breastfeeder. A woman may feel pressured into breastfeeding because she wants to please someone or get someone off her back. She may feel the lack of knowing anyone else who is breastfeeding. Or she may be wary about breastfeeding in general and how it may affect her relationship with her partner. She may, of course, not even have a partner, in which case she may worry how she'll cope with breastfeeding, and motherhood in general, on her own. She may have recognized or unrecognized fears about giving up or going back to work, or about not having enough money. And she may feel anxious about having to hand her baby over to someone else when she returns to work. The baby may not have been wanted. Or he may remind his mother of someone in the family she particularly likes or dislikes. Last but not least, some women feel totally unprepared to be a mother, let alone to breastfeed.

Stirred-up emotions represent a challenge that can be seen both as a danger and as an opportunity: a danger if the emotions are unresolved and simply suppressed again; and an opportunity if the emotions are recognized and ways are found to deal with them so that we grow in emotional intelligence.

Personal growth

Personal growth in response to the challenge of being a mother can enrich our lives and make us more sensitive to our own needs and those of our baby and other nearest and dearest.

As babies we may never have learned that our mother was a normally imperfect human being. If it was too difficult and frightening for us to accept our anger or other painful feelings about her as a 'bad' mother who didn't respond to our needs and satisfy them soon enough, we may have suppressed these emotions. This meant we saw her only as a 'good' mother, instead of as a 'good enough' mother who met most of our needs most of the time. In other words, we idealized her.

If this happened to us, we may have internalized the image of the 'perfect' mother and could have trouble adjusting to being an ordinary, 'good enough' mother ourselves. We may set too high a standard, expect to cope easily and then have a shock when reality proves different.

A time of golden opportunity

So how can you help make this time of mothering and breastfeeding a time of golden emotional opportunity?

Here are a few ideas:

Listen to your feelings – Aim to become more sensitive to your emotions by listening to your inner voice. Try recognizing and naming your feelings about breastfeeding first.

When breastfeeding, ask yourself:

1. Am I a 'good enough' mother?
2. Do I know what I'm doing?
3. What will people think of me if I can't breastfeed?
4. Do I like breastfeeding?
5. Will my baby starve?
6. Will it be my fault if my baby starves?
7. Will I feel guilty if I don't breastfeed?
8. Who's really in control if my baby feeds whenever he wants?
9. What will my midwife and doctor (and, in the UK, health visitor) think if I don't breastfeed?
10. Am I comfortable with the sexuality of breastfeeding?
11. Can I bear to care for this demanding baby who never seems to stop feeding?
12. Is my baby the only person who loves me?
13. Does my baby love me?
14. If my baby really loves me, why isn't he happy all the time?

If any of these questions rings bells for you, ask yourself how it makes you feel. For example, questions 1, 2, 3, 5 and 13 make some women afraid; 5 makes some feel helpless too; 6 and 7 make some feel guilty or angry; 8, 11 and 14 make some angry; and 12 give some a sense of desperate longing and neediness.

If these emotions aren't immediately familiar, either they don't apply or they may be suppressed in your unconscious mind. As we've seen, suppressed emotions frequently stem from unresolved experiences in infancy. We aren't aware of them because early on we erected defences to stop them hurting us. But anything that stirs up difficult emotions – particularly being with a baby – can disturb these defences and allow difficult feelings out. Sometimes this creates problems or, rather, challenges.

One relevant challenge for a woman might be a strong feeling that she doesn't want to breastfeed – or doesn't like the idea – without knowing why. Others might include depression, anxiety and compulsive behaviour (such as overeating, a history of promiscuous relationships, dependence on alcohol or drugs, or overwork).

Becoming more self-aware and learning to deal with their feelings helps many women care for their baby more effectively. Otherwise, their own neediness can interfere with their ability to respond to their baby and to be a 'good enough' mother.

Share your feelings – If you'd like to come to terms with any difficult emotions triggered by becoming a mother, brain power and the wish to change may not be enough. You may need to discuss things with your partner, a good and trusted friend or your post-natal class teacher. If this sort of care isn't available, you could seek help from your doctor or health visitor, who may suggest you see a counsellor or therapist.

Get encouragement and support – Dealing with feelings about breastfeeding is one thing, finding ways to give yourself encouragement and support is another. Boosting your self-esteem is a good way of doing this. Remember, you are a valuable person in your own right, and as a mother you are caring for your child at a vitally important time in his life.

So make time to:

- Recognize how valuable you are.
- Focus on things you enjoy and do well (however small they seem). For example, you may love being with your baby (at least some of the time); you may like the change in pace that accompanied leaving work to care for your baby; or you may simply be pleased you've

managed to get out to the shops or cook a meal. Take pride in positive frames of mind and achievements and let them warm you. Increase and spread the glow by telling those close to you.
- Ask your partner, other loved ones, friends or your midwife (and in the UK, health visitor), or breastfeeding counsellor, for encouragement and support. They may not realize you need it unless you ask.

Look after yourself – Take special care to look after yourself as you begin to recognize and adjust to your feelings about being a mother.

Feeling low

In general, whether a woman breastfeeds or bottle-feeds seems to make no difference to her risk of getting post-natal depression. However, one study (1983) found that exclusively breastfeeding women were more likely to get depressed than partial breastfeeders. Another study in Australia (2003) found that women who felt depressed were more likely to stop breastfeeding early.

If you feel low or depressed, several things may help:

- Tell the story of your labour and birth experiences as many times as necessary to make them 'concrete' and 'real'.
- Ask for practical help, being specific about what you'd like done; you may want someone to stay with your baby for a couple of hours a day, for example, so you can sleep or go out.
- Confide in someone you trust and think will be supportive, such as your partner, mother, sister or other relative, or a friend or neighbour. Tell your doctor or midwife (or, in the UK, health visitor) if necessary; they may suggest you see a counsellor, join a group of women in the same situation who are working with a trained facilitator or, if necessary, take antidepressant drugs.
- Check you're eating a healthy diet with plenty of vegetables, beans, peas, wholegrain foods, protein and healthy fats. Supplements of vitamin B complex, magnesium and calcium may help if you're feeling low.
- Get outside every day for at least half an hour in bright daylight to

help prevent winter depression (SAD, or seasonal affective disorder).
- Exercise each day, whether you have a brisk walk, a swim, an exercise class or a workout at home to an exercise video.
- Stay in touch with friends, however tempting it is to shut yourself away.
- Do something you enjoy every day, and do something enjoyable with your baby, such as going for a walk or doing a baby massage.
- Brush up your empathic listening skills and ask a partner or friend to practise with you. Being able to recognize, name and, perhaps, express difficult feelings, brings them into the open and prevents trouble building up.
- Accept that every baby is different. A low-birthweight baby, for example, may spend most of his time feeding, or sleeping, and it may be some time before he matures enough to be alert and responsive and therefore more rewarding for you.

SMOKING

Being a smoker can reduce your milk supply, because nicotine reduces prolactin production. Also, smokers tend to wean their babies from the breast sooner than non-smokers, and very heavy smokers (more than twenty to thirty cigarettes a day) tend to wean earliest of all.

- One study (1992) found that when mothers of preterm babies pumped their milk for several weeks, smokers were already producing less milk by two weeks, and by four weeks only 36 per cent were making enough milk, compared with 72 per cent of non-smokers. Also, the smokers' milk contained on average only four-fifths of the fat of the non-smokers' milk, which would have made their milk less sustaining and satisfying to their babies.

Smoking also increases the effects of caffeine. And large amounts of nicotine in breast milk can have several unpleasant effects in babies, the most common being nausea, vomiting, stomach cramps and diarrhoea.

So cut smoking out or at least down if you can, especially if you're a heavy smoker. Help is available from quit-smoking groups, telephone help-lines and your doctor.

However, if you can't or don't want to stop, at least be reassured that it's generally considered less risky for a smoker's baby to be breastfed than to be bottle-fed.

If you decide to continue smoking, at least consider cutting down, especially with your baby nearby. Inhaling smoke from you or other people smoking increases his risk of respiratory disorders such as pneumonia and bronchitis and puts him at a greater risk of leukaemia. Babies of smokers are also more prone to sudden infant death syndrome.

CONTRACEPTION

Unless you don't mind getting pregnant again soon, you'll need to take precautions after the first eight to ten weeks after childbirth (see also page 84). Choose from the lactational amenorrhoea method (LAM), a diaphragm, a condom, the progestogen-only Pill or, expertly used, the sympto-thermal method. An intrauterine contraceptive device (IUD) is best left till later.

WHEN PERIODS RETURN

Some time after you cut down on breastfeeding or your baby starts on solids, your periods will return (see also page 86). You may need extra reserves of energy and patience a week before and a week after ovulation, as your baby may find it difficult to settle then, probably because your milk tastes different. (Most women ovulate somewhere between the tenth and fourteenth days of their cycle, counting the first day of the period as day one.) You may also find your baby is extra hungry around period time, as your milk supply may temporarily decrease and your let-down become less reliable.

- Australian researchers reported (1983) that the amounts of sugar and potassium in breast milk temporarily fell on the fifth or sixth day before ovulation, and on the sixth or seventh day after, presumably making it less sweet. At the same times, its sodium and chloride increased, possibly making it saltier.

SHOPPING

In the early weeks you'll have relatively little time between feeds to shop. You could do a big weekly shop with your partner, ask someone else to do it for you or find shops that deliver. There's nothing worse than going shopping and having to get a hungry, crying baby home when you're tired and heavy-laden.

SEEING FRIENDS

Some women feel lonely if they leave their jobs, have a baby and don't have many friends in the same position. However, a baby is a very good conversation opener and you'll probably find it easier to make friends now than at any other time. Breastfeeding is no hindrance to seeing people – especially other mothers – during the day. It's best not to arrange set times for meetings because you'll probably end up breaking appointments when your baby wants to spend long, unhurried times at the breast. If you ask friends to your home, remember to make your baby your priority.

BEING A SINGLE MOTHER OR A LONE MOTHER

The number of unmarried and/or unpartnered mothers is increasing in every Western country, and statistics show they are less likely to breastfeed. Each woman has her own reasons for not breastfeeding, and if you decide during pregnancy that you're going to bottle-feed, it's wise to identify your reasons in case this enables you to change your mind. For example, if you believe you won't have enough encouragement and support to breastfeed, you could try talking to a relative, friend, neighbour, health professional, breastfeeding counsellor or leader, or social worker, about the back-up you'll need. You may not know what you'll need until you've had your baby, though, so keep an open mind if your needs change. Mothers who live on their own need to look after themselves especially well.

ASSERTIVENESS SKILLS

Before your baby is born practise being assertive without being aggressive. By doing this you recognize, name and state your needs (as you see them) as a pregnant or breastfeeding woman. At the same time, acknowledge other people's needs and their motives (as you see them) for their behaviour or attitudes. Being assertive means getting your needs met without trampling over others.

You can learn assertiveness ('assertion') skills by copying other people who are pleasant but firm and don't act as doormats. Or you could learn from a book or attend a course.

You'll find such skills useful in many areas of life – including, perhaps, dealing with people who try to put you off breastfeeding or make it difficult for you in some way.

ONE LAST WORD

Having a baby is physically and emotionally challenging, and many women don't feel like their old self for some time – some say at least a year. Remember, too, that having a baby and breastfeeding provide insights and experiences that will change and mature you in ways you could never have predicted.

> Looking after yourself will help you produce plenty of milk and get the best out of mothering. In the next chapter we'll look at the things that affect your milk supply.

TEN

Your milk supply

Many mothers easily supply the amount of milk that matches their babies' needs, others have too much or too little, especially in the early weeks before their milk supply is well established. Too much can be a nuisance but rarely stops a woman breastfeeding. Too little, however, is the commonest reason women stop feeding, or add bottle-feeds, in the first few weeks.

NOT ENOUGH MILK – THE COMMONEST CHALLENGE

You might think that women who stop breastfeeding in the first few months want to do so, but this usually isn't so – at least not at a conscious level. The vast majority don't stop breastfeeding by choice, but because they think they haven't enough milk. This was shown in a large survey (Infant Feeding 2000, published by The Stationery Office) in the UK in 2000, see overleaf.

The message from this study is clear: when a woman stops breastfeeding, by far the most likely reason is believing she doesn't have enough milk. This is more important than sore nipples, far more important than going back to work and beats breastfeeding being 'too tiring' by a long way.

A woman's belief that she has insufficient milk is the main disorder of breastfeeding in the UK; this is also true for other developed countries and, increasingly, for developing countries too.

Yet what most women don't realize is that a poor milk supply is nearly always preventable or treatable. A woman may not have

Reasons mothers gave for stopping breastfeeding	By 6 weeks	By 4 months	By 9 months
	%	%	%
Insufficient milk	53	52	21
Took too long, or tiring	24	17	4
Painful breasts or nipples	23	8	1
Baby rejected breast	13	10	15
Domestic reasons	11	6	1
Mother ill	10	5	8
Baby ill	6	4	2
Baby can't be fed by others	4	8	8
Returned to work or college	2	19	27
Breastfed as long as intended	1	4	5
Didn't like breastfeeding	1	2	1
Time was right to stop	–	–	19
Baby teething or biting	–	–	18

(Percentages don't add up to 100 as some mothers gave more than one reason; the last two questions were introduced only later in the survey.)

enough milk today but the odds of being able to make as much as her baby needs within a few days are stacked high in her favour – if she takes the right steps to increase her milk supply.

Almost every woman can breastfeed if she wants, provided she has enough information and skilled support. Just think how much sadness and disappointment would be spared if only this were understood.

Yet the first advice women with insufficient milk often get is to give top-ups of formula or abandon breastfeeding, which is wrong. *The advice they need is how to increase their milk supply.* The only exception is if a baby is dehydrated or starving, in which case the mother needs to give top-ups of formula or, preferably, donated breast milk, while she increases her milk supply.

Does every woman have enough milk?

Many women think they don't have enough milk – and at any given moment some indeed may not – but the vast majority can make enough if they know how. Indeed, with good breastfeeding techniques most can supply at least twice the volume their baby needs, so most can easily feed twins.

However, just as with dairy cows, some women are naturally capable of making more milk than others. In practice this means some need more breast stimulation, attention to breastfeeding technique and skilled support than others to produce the same amount of milk.

Research also shows that women differ markedly in their breasts' milk-storage capacity, so some have to feed more often than others. As a consequence, a few decide they don't want to devote the time and effort it takes to produce enough milk. This, of course, is their choice.

No one knows how many women are truly incapable of breastfeeding, though in developed countries some studios suggest that up to 4 or 5 per cent are quoted as being unable to breastfeed. But many of these can produce at least some of the milk their baby needs once they know how. The problem rarely lies with these women's breasts but with the fact that they lack good advice and information about successful breastfeeding, and have poor levels of skilled support. The figure of up to one in twenty women being unable to breastfeed is almost certainly an overestimate, as the following studies show:

- Among nearly 4,000 mothers studied in Nigeria and Zaire, including both poor women and the urban elite, *not one* was unable to produce milk.
- Among over 400 babies who survived their first two days in Guatemala, *every one* was successfully breastfed.
- At the Farm Midwifery Center in Tennessee, midwives reported that *only one woman in about 800* had had trouble in producing enough milk.
- *All twenty* babies born in a prisoner-of-war camp in Singapore during the Second World War were satisfactorily breastfed for six months before 'supplementary feeding' was started. All the mothers continued to breastfeed until their babies were over a year old.

However, the fact remains that some babies today in the UK, for example, don't get enough breast milk. It's important to find out which they are, so their mothers can increase their milk supply, or, if they can't, or don't want to, so the baby can be adequately nourished some other way.

One US expert has identified some useful pointers:

- These mothers may have failed to produce enough milk for a previous baby (though this may be because they didn't know how to increase their supply).
- Their close female relatives may have failed to produce enough milk (though this may be because they didn't know how to increase their milk supply).
- They may have noticed little increase in their breast size during pregnancy, and little or no breast fullness a few days after delivery.
- Their breasts may be very different in size (though this may mean very little, as most women have different-sized breasts).

Is your baby getting enough?

This question originates from the years when four-hourly schedules were strictly enforced. Many breastfed babies didn't get enough milk then because the schedules didn't let them feed often enough to stimulate their mothers' breasts as much as was needed to make enough milk.

It's also a loaded question that worries some newly delivered women so much that it hampers their let-down. When this happens, the presence of stagnant milk in the breasts, plus its pressure on her milk-producing cells, and the lack of stimulation from the baby being unable to empty her breasts, combine to reduce her milk production.

Most importantly, it's a question that wouldn't need to be asked at all if women were encouraged to breastfeed as nature intended.

This said, it's a question that must be asked, as breastfeeding is often mismanaged, leading many women to restrict it according to some non-breastfeeding-friendly schedule or routine.

You'll know your baby is getting enough when he:

- Sucks and milks the breast well.
- Feeds often – for example, every one-and-a-half to three hours, meaning eight to twelve feeds or more a day in the first few weeks.
- Is satisfied after a feed.
- Grows – he may lose up to 10 per cent of his birthweight in the first few days. After that your milk will come in and he may gain as much as 113–198 g (4–7 oz) a week, or 445 g (1 lb) every four weeks, during the first month. Work out his weight gain from his lowest weight after birth; rather than from his birthweight.
- Thrives – meaning he has a good colour and firm skin, and is active and alert.
- Has six to eight really wet cloth nappies or five to six really heavy disposables a day from about the fourth day, or whenever your milk comes in. During days one, two and three after birth, a breastfed baby usually has one, two and then three wet nappies a day, respectively, as he needs only small amounts of colostrum.

And when you:

- Are experiencing let-downs.

Knowing what to expect

Many women think that something is wrong if their baby wants frequent feeds day and night or sometimes wants to stay at the breast for ages. If you don't know what to expect it can be worrying when your baby stops feeding, has a short nap, then wants to start again. It's easy to think you don't have enough milk and your baby is dissatisfied, when in fact this is usually perfectly normal behaviour.

Sometimes this unexpected behaviour so disturbs a woman – especially if it's her first baby – that she feels helpless, out of control and hopeless. Her baby wants mothering – and so does she. If this happens to you, be sure to ask health workers, family and friends for whatever help and support you need.

False expectations of how a breastfeeding baby should behave often come about because of comparisons with bottle-feeding babies. When a mother gives her baby a bottle of formula, the only limiting factor is how quickly he can drink it. But breastfeeding is completely different because it's a two-way dynamic process in which both partners give and take and the baby is partly responsible for the amount of milk that's made.

Weighing your baby

Breastfed babies lose substantially more weight than formula-fed babies after birth, and take longer to regain their birthweight. This is normal.

- A Scottish study (2002) of 971 full-term newborns found that breastfeds lost an average of 6.6 per cent of their birthweight, while bottle-feds lost an average of 3.5 per cent. The breastfeds also took longer to regain their birthweight – 8.3 days for breastfeds compared with 6.5 days for bottle-feds.

In the first month, after the initial normal weight loss following delivery, the average baby gains 120–200 g (4–7 oz) a week. From the second to fifth months, he gains 175–225 g (6–8 oz) a week; and from the sixth to twelfth months, 50–75 g (2–3 oz) a week. The average baby tends to double his birthweight by four months and triple it by a year. However, these averages are based largely on formula-fed babies, whereas the average healthy thriving *breastfed* baby puts on less.

You can ignore the change in weight from one week to another, as long as your baby is doing well. A healthy, thriving baby sometimes gains no weight in any one week and may even lose a little occasionally. What's important is that the overall rate of gain is fairly steady over several weeks.

Your doctor or midwife (or, in the UK, health visitor) may suggest regular weighing, as the rate of gain over the weeks is a reasonable guide to growth and health. If your baby isn't thriving because he isn't getting enough milk, they'll spot this early, advise you how to increase your milk supply, and say if your baby needs top-ups while you are doing this. You need extra support if your baby loses more than 10 per cent of his birthweight, doesn't start to gain weight by nine days, or fails to regain his birthweight by two weeks.

Signs your baby may not be getting enough

Your baby may:

- Cry or fuss a lot.
- Often seem hungry after feeds.
- Drink formula if offered after a breastfeed.
- Not soak six to eight nappies a day.
- Not be gaining weight.

And your breasts may:

- Never leak.
- Never feel full.

— Remember that although you may temporarily not have enough milk, you can make more if you know what to do.

Pitfalls

Two things can mislead you into thinking you're not making enough milk, your baby's changing needs – including growth spurts – and the disturbance of coming home from hospital.

Changing needs – It's easy to imagine a baby will take the same amount of milk at each feed. But babies don't necessarily want the same from feed to feed, let alone from day to day. Sometimes he'll want more than you've made, sometimes less. In this sense babies are just like older children and adults. However, when his appetite increases, your milk supply may not immediately match his needs. Don't make the mistake of thinking you can't make enough milk just because he is unsettled for a few days. Be guided by him, take steps to increase your milk supply and marvel at the way your body's demand-and-supply system works. And don't forget, he may be entering a growth spurt.

Growth spurts – If your baby has been satisfied up to now, but becomes edgy and miserable so you think he's still hungry after a feed, he may be starting a growth spurt. Babies can have growth spurts at any age, but they are especially common at around six weeks and three months. US researchers have found that some babies can grow half an inch in length in twenty-four hours! Babies are often restless and cry more before their growth spurt, but settle quietly again after it.

The good news is that when your baby begins a growth spurt he'll automatically ask for more and/or longer feeds, as an instinctive way of increasing the milk supply. However, it'll take two to three days of increased breast stimulation for you to produce significantly more milk, so be prepared for him to be unsettled for this period. Let him feed as long as he wants each time (provided he is well latched on) and give as many feeds as he wants.

If you're already demand-feeding, give at least two extra feeds a day, more if you have time. This way the increased stimulation will soon increase your milk production, though it'll be several days before your supply catches up with his needs.

It's easy for an inexperienced breastfeeder to panic at this stage if her baby seems unsatisfied. But a mismatch between a baby's needs and his mother's supply happens to almost every mother–baby pair from time to time.

Coming home – Another pitfall can occur when you return home from hospital. Your milk supply may well dwindle temporarily, making your baby hungry and unsettled, because of the change in surroundings, the excitement and the extra work you may have to do. Family doctors frequently receive calls from women just home saying their milk has gone. Of course it hasn't gone for good and they can readily increase their supply, but most such mothers, especially first-time ones, don't realize this.

If this happens to you there's no absolutely need to give a bottle or stop breastfeeding. Milk dries up in a well-nourished woman only if her breasts aren't stimulated enough or emptied sufficiently – it's simply a matter of poor technique. All the time in the world spent with a baby who isn't milking the breast as he should won't necessarily produce more milk. But it will tire you both out. When your baby milks you well, you'll let your milk down more efficiently and your breasts will empty more completely. There are many reasons why this may not happen and correspondingly many ways of overcoming the problem.

'Happy-to-starve'

A few seemingly contented breastfed babies are actually starving, and are dubbed 'happy to starve'. The danger is that they risk brain damage or other problems if the problem continues and no one realizes what's happening.

The commonest reason for any breastfed baby to fail to thrive is a restriction in the number and length of breastfeeds by day and night. The three-to-five-hourly, ten-minutes-a-side type of breastfeeding works only for those few women with a very plentiful milk supply. Most of us need to feed our babies much more frequently and for longer to get the breast stimulation and emptying we need to make enough milk.

If you and your professional advisers are concerned because your baby's weight gain is small or non-existent for a few weeks, don't be put off breastfeeding, but do take immediate steps to increase your milk supply (page 230). If complementary feeds with formula are advised, discuss whether it's possible to delay for a few days while you increase your milk supply instead. If your doctor or midwife (or, in the UK, health visitor) agrees it's safe to wait, it's highly likely that your baby won't need formula feeds at all. If he is so undernourished that he needs formula fast, give it by cup after each breastfeed while you spend the next few days increasing your milk supply. Once you are making more milk you'll almost certainly be able to stop giving formula.

If you don't feel confident, ask a breastfeeding counsellor or leader for support. She'll have helped many other women with this problem.

Failure to thrive

If you've taken steps to increase your milk supply, but your baby still isn't growing well, something may be wrong (see page 322).

Never imagine your milk supply is limited to the amount you're currently making – there are many ways of building it up.

TWENTY STEPS TO INCREASING YOUR MILK SUPPLY

1 Position your baby better, if necessary, and check he is well latched on

This allows him to suck and milk more effectively which, in turn, empties your breasts better and stimulates increased milk production (see page 139).

2 Increase suckling time

Breastfeed on an unrestricted basis – meaning frequently and for as long as your baby wants. If he is well positioned and latched on, then the more he's at the breast, the more readily you'll let down your milk, the more he'll take, the more prolactin you'll have, and the more milk you'll make. Breasts respond to the removal of milk by making just as much milk again, and frequent feeds encourage them to make even more. There's no risk of frequent feeds 'using up' your milk.

When you build up the number and length of feeds, your milk supply is likely to take at least two to three days to improve, so don't expect instant results!

While some babies take all the milk they need in ten minutes or so each side, many need much longer. Indeed, many a successfully breastfeeding woman reports that her baby sometimes likes to stay at the breast for up to an hour or even as long as two or three hours, especially in the early evening, feeding, comfort-sucking and having an occasional short nap. An inexperienced breastfeeder may think something is wrong, when in fact her baby is behaving normally. If, on occasion, you haven't the time or inclination to sit with him, no harm will come from curtailing the occasional feed, but as a general rule let your baby decide when to stop. It may help not to think of the time your baby spends at the breast as a 'feed'. Of course, breastfed babies feed from the breast, but they also get comfort and pleasure (and stimulate optimal development of their tongue, cheeks and jaws). It's interesting that women in one African tribe were flummoxed when researchers asked how long their breastfed babies' fed, because they didn't think of the times their babies spent at the breast as 'feeds'. They put their babies to the breast because that made their infants happy.

It's well worth fitting in some extra feeds over and above what your baby asks for – perhaps even twice as many – waking him if necessary.

When you've increased your milk supply and are breastfeeding successfully, your baby may eventually want fewer feeds.

Occasionally a woman's milk supply diminishes because she carries her baby around in a sling or carrier, or on a hip, lulling him so well that he doesn't ask for feeds. If this happens, put your baby to the breast more often than he seems to want.

Remember that giving juice, water or solids may well reduce your baby's requests for the breast. A baby under six months simply doesn't need anything else.

3 Empty both breasts at each feed

Normally it's fine to let your baby feed from one breast, but if you're increasing your milk supply, empty both breasts at each feed. Do this by letting him stay at the first side until he's had enough, then offering the second breast after a short break for a sleep or a nappy change if necessary. When he's had enough at the second breast – or if he doesn't want it – express any remaining milk to encourage greater production. Be guided by your baby as to when he's had enough one side, and don't take him off the breast yourself, because you'll gradually produce less milk if you take your baby off before he has finished.

Emptying both breasts:

- Encourages more let-downs, which encourages a reliable let-down reflex, and boosts the milk supply.
- Prevents pressure within tense breasts reducing the blood supply to the milk glands and thus rendering their milk-producing cells less efficient. Normally, the volume of milk in each breast increases between feeds, but frequent overfilling can counteract this effect.
- Prevents pressure from unemptied milk in tense breasts directly harming milk-producing cells and making them temporarily less able to produce milk.
- Enables tiny muscle fibres around milk glands to contract efficiently so they let down milk well; in contrast, milk glands that are swollen with milk can prevent efficient muscle-fibre contraction.
- Prevents inhibitory factor – a hormone-like substance in breast milk – from slowing milk production.

So whenever your breasts feel full, tense or uncomfortable, put your baby to the breast or express some milk. You can also boost your milk supply by expressing at other times too.

4 Express after and between feeds

Four or five times a day, express the milk remaining in your breasts about half an hour after a feed, and do this for two or three days. This provides extra stimulation to your breasts, which in turn increases your milk supply. Collect it, store it safely, and offer it to your baby in a cup after the next feed if your baby will drink it.

5 Make sure you let down your milk well

You'll need to let down your milk well if your baby is to empty the breast, drink high-calorie, fat-rich hindmilk, and thrive.

Factors such as fatigue, anxiety, fear and pain adversely influence the let-down reflex and may even prevent you letting down your milk at all. During the first few weeks or months a woman's let-down is more vulnerable than later, when her milk supply is established and she is more confident. Confidence from having fed a first baby helps explain why women are more successful earlier on at breastfeeding their subsequent babies.

When people talk of the milk supply becoming well 'established', they mean the let-down reflex has become so well-conditioned through practice that it virtually never fails. They also mean the breasts have adapted their milk supply to match the baby's demands, with no surplus or shortage.

A poor milk supply caused by an unreliable let-down reflex is a common breastfeeding problem, but once you understand what's happening you have every chance of putting it right. Successful breastfeeding depends as much on the efficient emptying of milk – which partly depends on a well-conditioned let-down reflex – as on the amount produced.

Remember that you may let down your milk several times at each breast, especially if your baby stays at the breast for a long time. Stopping him before he's ready may mean he'll miss out on one of these let-downs.

- In one interesting experiment, women who believed they didn't have enough milk were given an injection of oxytocin (the hormone that lets down milk) after a feed, then the researchers measured how much extra milk they let down. Most let down about as much milk again as their babies had already taken. In other words, 50 per cent of the milk potentially available to their baby remained in their breasts after the feed.

If your let-down usually takes two to three minutes to work and you're in the habit of restricting suckling time to, say, ten minutes, your baby is missing out on two to three minutes of what you thought was drinking time. While seven to eight minutes' drinking time is enough for some babies, it leaves others very hungry.

How do you know you're letting down your milk? – You may notice some or all of these signs:

- 'After-pains' in your womb early in a feed in the early days.
- Tingling in your breasts immediately before the milk comes.
- Milk spraying or leaking from your breasts.
- Your breasts feeling warmer than usual.
- Initial nipple pain disappearing as the milk comes down (as this equalizes the negative pressure created by the baby sucking).
- Your baby sucking with rhythmical, one-per-second sucks – the sort which mean he's swallowing milk as it's being let down. You may hear him swallowing too or notice his ear moving in time with his swallowing.

However, some women let their milk down perfectly well yet don't have any of these sensations. The only way they know they're doing it is by:

- Their baby settling at the breast and swallowing in a steady rhythm.
- Their baby thriving and growing.

Making your let-down more reliable – Several things can help:

Condition your let-down reflex

- Try to get into a routine of practical preparations before a feed – a regular chain of events will help condition your let-down into working reliably.
- Don't skip night feeds: you need them to stimulate your milk supply.
- Wake the baby for a feed, or express some milk, when your breasts feel tense and full.
- Aim not to let your baby sleep more than two hours by day, or three to four hours at night (timed from the beginning of one feed to the beginning of the next), as your breasts need regular emptying.
- Wake and feed your baby if you let down your milk unexpectedly.

Be calm, unhurried, and enjoy feeds

- Have everything to hand that you might need during a feed – for you, the baby and any other children.
- Decide in advance what to do about the phone (a roving or mobile phone is ideal), the front-door bell and other people (page 193).
- Cut down on activities that you find stressful but are inessential, such as unnecessary entertaining, emails, working, telephone calls and cooking.
- Cut down on other activities, so you always have time for feeds. This might mean not promising to be anywhere at any set time – simply explain you'll come when you're ready – though you may have to make some exceptions, such as visits to the doctor.

- Relax before and during a feed, and try to clear your mind of any worries.
- Consider listening to some slow music; one study (2001) found that dairy cows produced more milk when listening to slow music!
- Enjoy feeds. Instead of thinking of them as times to get as much milk into your baby as quickly as possible, calm down, stop pressuring yourself and consider them as unique and special times together. Babies grow up very quickly!

Try switch-nursing – 'Nursing' is the American term for breastfeeding. Switch-nursing is a well-tried way of coaxing tired, jaundiced, pethidine-doped, ill or preterm babies, or other weak feeders, into sucking more strongly and milking the breast more efficiently.

It involves swapping your baby from one breast to the other as soon as his sucking slows down and you can hear or see him swallowing less often. So instead of simply giving first one breast, then the other, you carry on by switching back to the first and then perhaps switching to the second again. Try giving him ten minutes each time you switch. If you're feeding two-hourly to stimulate your milk supply, this will mean you'll be feeding for about forty minutes every two hours. Or you could switch from side to side just twice – going, for example, from your left to your right to your left breast again. The time this takes is a small price to pay for increasing your milk supply.

Each time you switch sides, there's milk immediately available in the 'new' breast's reservoirs. So your baby will probably suck and milk the breast more enthusiastically. This is likely to stimulate more let-downs. And more let-downs are good both for your milk supply and for conditioning your let-down reflex.

However, if you usually need several minutes of breast stimulation before you let down your milk, it's worth leaving your baby at the first breast until he comes off spontaneously. Otherwise he may only have time to fill up with relatively low-calorie foremilk. He may then be too tired and full to go on sucking. But he won't be satisfied for long, and your let-down won't get the stimulation it needs.

Keep fit – Take the time and make the effort to find forms of exercise you enjoy and can do at least five times a week. Exercise boosts the body's endorphins (natural feel-good chemicals) and having a fit body helps you to relax. So it helps you let down your milk and also increases the blood flow through the breasts – which stimulates milk production.

Look after yourself

- Avoid getting over-tired. Aim to have at least one nap in the day; put your feet up whenever you sit down; avoid unnecessary domestic chores; organize shopping to make it as easy as possible; and cut down on outside commitments. If you feel exhausted, you may let your milk down less reliably.
- Make sure you're comfortable when feeding because things like aching shoulders or a draught around your feet won't help.
- If you have sore nipples, aim to trigger your let-down before your baby starts feeding. Remember, the pain will eventually go and is unlikely to last throughout a feed anyway (page 256).
- Have a small alcoholic drink just before a feed. This will relax you and help your let-down (though see page 206), though it's unwise to to this more than once a day.
- See if a hot shower encourages your let-down, though this obviously isn't practical before every feed. Sometimes you might like to feed in the bath, as its warmth will help you relax and encourage your let-down. Your baby will probably like it too.

6 Encourage your baby to keep alert and awake

Help your baby stay awake enough to feed well (see page 280) by talking, stroking and switch-nursing. This should mean he sucks and milks your breasts more strongly and avoids getting into the habit of snoozing for long periods at the breast.

7 Help your baby suck and milk more effectively

(See numbers 1, 5 and 6 above, and page 315).

8 Get help

Ask for help from your midwife, (and, in the UK, health visitor), doctor or breastfeeding counsellor if your baby isn't gaining weight well, or is losing weight. They can help you increase your milk supply by improving your breastfeeding technique. They can also check that your baby's underlying health is good.

9 Avoid formula if at all possible

Giving formula will probably diminish your milk supply, because if your baby no longer has to rely on your milk, he's unlikely to want to feed often or for long enough to stimulate your breasts well. However, be reassured that if your breast-fed baby had 'top-ups' of formula in hospital, you're highly likely to be able to breastfeed fully once you get home.

If your baby is already taking some formula, reduce its amount by 15 ml (about ½ fl oz) at each feed, so he wants more breast milk. Give the formula not by bottle but with a cup or spoon (or, if necessary, a supplementer, page 302), or he may get so used to a bottle that he'll be loath to breastfeed.

Take steps to increase your milk supply. For example, feed him more often and let him stay at the breast as much as he wants – even just for comfort at an empty breast. Your milk supply will begin to increase after two or three days. Be prepared for long and frequent feeds – perhaps forty minutes every two hours, and remember that he might sometimes want to stay at the breast and nap on and off for several hours. Look after yourself by doing as few other things as possible – just rest and cuddle the baby. You *can* build up your milk supply. All you need is information, confidence and patience.

Check that your baby is wetting his nappies as he should (page 225) and stay in contact with your health-care professionals or breastfeeding counsellor or leader.

- Experts recommend that women should give nothing but breast milk for the first six months.

10 Avoid a dummy

It's better not to give your baby a dummy (pacifier) if you think you may not have enough milk, because it will satisfy some of his need to suck and may stop him asking for as many feeds as you need to stimulate your milk supply. One study (2001) in New Zealand reported that mothers who gave a dummy were more likely to think they didn't have enough milk and to stop breastfeeeding early.

Some babies diminish their mother's milk supply by sucking their thumb or fingers. They may have got into the habit because they haven't been allowed enough comfort-sucking time at the breast.

11 Eat an enjoyable and healthy diet

Your diet should make no difference to your milk supply provided you eat well and drink according to your thirst – bearing in mind that you may need to eat slightly more than when you weren't pregnant or breastfeeding.

12 Exercise to increase the circulation in your breasts

Regular whole-body exercise encourages a reliable let-down reflex and also increases the amount of milk you make by boosting the circulation to your whole body, including your breasts and the hormone-producing glands in your brain. Over any given period of time the volume of the blood flow through the breasts is 400–500 times the volume of milk produced, and the greater the blood flow the more milk you'll make.

13 Wear a comfortable bra

A breastfeeding woman who wears too tight a bra may find her milk supply decreases, because constricting the breasts may reduce or even stop milk production. If you have small or medium-sized breasts, consider not wearing a bra at all.

14 Be positive

Women who really want to breastfeed produce more milk. One study found that those women who said at first that they preferred bottle-feeding were three times more likely to find their baby refused the breast and twice as likely to say their baby was a bad feeder compared with women who intended from the beginning to breastfeed. This indicates that positive attitudes are very helpful. Interestingly, in the same survey, women who wanted to breastfeed reported that their babies refused the bottle.

But the fact remains that many women who really want to breastfeed fail because they believe they haven't enough milk. Indeed, many a woman's greatest single concern before embarking on breastfeeding is that she won't be able to produce enough milk. This concern seems ingrained in many modern women, and it's tempting to wonder whether it's symbolic of a deep-seated albeit unconscious feeling of not being good enough or having enough to give.

15 Get plenty of rest and relaxation

Looking after yourself in this way is essential while you are putting so much concentration and energy into building up your milk supply.

16 Come off the combined Pill

The contraceptive pill, unless of the progestogen-only type, usually reduces the milk supply. (See page 217 for alternative contraceptive methods.)

17 Stop smoking – or at least cut right down

Smoking can decrease the milk supply by lowering prolactin levels. It can also hinder the let-down.

18 Drink more fluid?

Lots of people will tell you to drink plenty, but be careful to drink only what you want, because drinking any more usually isn't helpful. You'll know you're getting enough fluid if your urine is pale yellow.

19 Consider traditional milk-boosters

Throughout the centuries women around the world have used amulets, potions, herbal skin rubs and other remedies, special foods and drinks, chants and prayers to ensure they produce enough milk. There's no harm in trying milk boosters (galactogogues), provided you also use proven methods (above) for increasing your milk supply.

Let's look at them:

- Alcohol, especially heavy beers and stouts. These increase prolactin, but babies tend not to drink as much milk when it tastes of alcohol, so they don't stimulate the breasts as well as usual. Having small amounts of alcoholic drinks may help but only by making you relaxed and therefore encouraging your let-down reflex. Drinking too much may interfere with your let-down.
- Vitamin B. This could improve your sense of well-being, which might help if you've been feeling tense and haven't been letting down your milk well.
- Cows' milk. It used to be said that this helped breastfeeding women make milk but we now know this isn't true. If you're eating a healthy diet there's no need to drink any cows' milk unless you like it.
- Dark green leafy vegetables are traditional milk boosters.
- Corn, peas, beans, lentils, chickpeas, oats, barley and brown (wholegrain) rice are traditionally said to boost the milk supply, but there's no scientific evidence to back these claims.
- Walnuts and almonds are said to be good for milk production, as are fenugreek, sunflower, sesame and celery seeds. You can add these to your meals, or take a fenugreek capsule. Animal studies show that fenugreek seeds have oxytocin-like activity.
- Caraway seeds, dill and fennel – made into tea or used in your diet – are traditionally considered 'warming'. This means they could ease tense muscles, which may aid the let-down. Fennel in particular is a traditional milk booster.
- Borage leaves and seeds, ginger root, coriander and cumin seeds, nettle leaves, and alfalfa sprouts – made into tea or added to meals – have been used for centuries to increase the milk supply. You can also take both nettle and alfalfa leaf in capsule form, and nettle as a tincture.
- Vitex agnus castus (chaste tree) seeds stimulate the pituitary gland and enhance a low prolactin level. One study found it increased milk production in four out of five women; after

twenty days the average milk production was three times as high in the women taking chaste tree as in those not taking it. You can use these seeds to make a tea.

- Saw palmetto berries are reputed to help the breasts function properly and can be made into a tea.
- Herbal teas made from raspberry leaves, cinnamon or blessed thistle can help if you're feeling stressed, which may in turn help you let your milk down better. However, beware of drinking too much of certain herbal teas: in one report, mothers who drank two litres (nearly four and a half pints) a day of a tea said to stimulate milk production and containing liquorice, fennel, anise and *Galega officinalis* found their babies reacted badly, with restlessness, vomiting, floppiness, tiredness and a weak cry, as well as poor growth. The symptoms disappeared when their mothers stopped drinking the tea.
- Vervain tea is said to boost milk flow.
- Geranium and fennel oils can be added to a carrier oil (such as sweet almond) and used for a whole-body massage to boost your milk supply. Add about ten drops of essential oil to one tablespoonful of carrier, but remember to wash the oil off your nipples and areolae before feeding your baby.
- The homeopathic remedy Agnus castus is said to help.

Note that peppermint, sage, parsley, sorrel and carrot juice are reputed to reduce the milk supply.

20 Consider taking prescribed drugs

Chlorpromazine, other phenothiazine drugs and the rauwolfia group of drugs can increase the milk supply, but can also have side effects, such as restlessness, tremors, involuntary movements, changes in breathing and heart rate and extreme tiredness.

Metoclopramide can increase the milk supply by boosting prolactin, and only small amounts enter breast milk. Small trials in which mothers of preterm babies took 10 mg three or four times a day for a week, then tapered it off over a week, show it usually increases the milk supply within two to four days. However, it can have side effects, including depression.

Domperidone also stimulates prolactin, but because it doesn't enter the brain, it can't cause depression.

Age

Women who have their first baby in their forties tend to produce less milk than do younger women, though only at first.

Does the number of children you've had matter?

Women breastfeeding their first baby tend to produce less milk at first than those who've already breastfed one baby or more.

- A study in the UK (2001) found that women breastfeeding their second child produced about 31 per cent more milk in week one and slightly more by week four. Those with the lowest milk production when feeding their first baby had the greatest increase when feeding the second.

Remember, you can readily increase your milk supply however many babies you've had.

WHAT IF I CAN'T BREASTFEED?

Even with the very best motivation and the very best help, a tiny percentage of women are unable to breastfeed.

If you are one of these, there are several things you can do:

- Be grateful you have an alternative.
- Focus on the positive aspects of your experience and recognize them as successes. An example might be the enjoyment you and your baby have had during some of the feeds you've done together. Remember that the breastfeeding you have done is better than none.

And your baby is lucky to have a mother who has tried her best. No one can expect straight A's for everything in life.

- Forgive yourself. And if later you discover you might have been able to breastfeed had you known more, received more support and done it differently, don't blame yourself or other people but work out what to do if there's a next time.
- Allow yourself time to recognize, name and come to terms with your feelings about being unable to breastfeed. You may experience a whole mass of conflicting emotions, with sadness and disappointment, perhaps, mingling uneasily with anger, frustration and helplessness. You might also be delighted yet feel a twinge of guilt because deep down you know breast is best.
- It may help to talk to someone who's prepared and able to listen, or you might find you want to write about what's happened or about your feelings, or paint or do something else creative. This could help you move on and enjoy your baby as he grows without dwelling unproductively on what might have been.
- Don't transfer your disappointment, anger or guilt to your baby. It isn't his fault and it isn't yours either. Your love for your child is more important than your milk, so don't allow difficult feelings to harm your unique relationship.
- When you bottle-feed your baby, hold him as you did when breastfeeding, not like a doll held at arm's length.
- Consider giving the occasional breastfeed – perhaps in the early morning – if you still have some milk. With the relief of your anxiety over not having enough milk, you might even start letting your milk down better and, as a result, produce more than you thought you could.
- Try using a nursing supplementer (page 302) to supply your baby with some formula while he is breastfeeding. This gadget enables a baby at the breast to get what breast milk there is, and at the same time receive formula through a fine tube that enters the baby's mouth along with the nipple. It also allows his sucking and milking to stimulate the milk supply, and gives both woman and baby the pleasure of breastfeeding, while at the same time assuring adequate nutrition.

Try again next time

If you have another baby, try breastfeeding again. Many women breastfeed second or later babies successfully even though they failed before. You'll be more confident and experienced as a mother next time, which should help. Remember that failing to breastfeed for as long as you wanted the first time may mean you'll need more encouragement, practical back-up and skilled support next time. It's up to you to make sure you get it.

IF YOU WANT TO STOP

It's usually easy to make your milk dry up. Simply reduce the length of time your baby spends at the breast by gradually cutting down the number and length of feeds, over several weeks, if possible. Too rapid weaning can cause problems such as engorgement and blocked ducts. As your baby receives less breast milk, give more formula by bottle.

A woman who finds breastfeeding a gruelling or annoying chore may want to reconsider what she's doing. It's better for a baby to have a happy mother who bottle-feeds than to have an unhappy breastfeeding one, who may even become depressed or bear a grudge against her baby. However, practical help may be all you need if you are finding breastfeeding unacceptably time-consuming and tiring, so don't to be too proud to ask.

Drying up your milk after childbirth

If you choose to bottle-feed, your milk will still come in and your breasts may feel very full, especially between the third and fifth days. Whenever they start feeling this way, express or pump enough milk to make them comfortable. Neither restricting drinks nor taking diuretics (drugs to remove water from the body) works, and Epsom salts are best avoided because they can cause diarrhoea. Neither heat, ice nor a tight bra seem useful, but some women find putting cabbage leaves inside their bra makes their breasts feel better. Herbalists suggest eating plenty of garden mint, sorrel and sage to help dry up milk and French women sometimes eat a parsley omelette when they want to stop breastfeeding. (See also page 254 for suggestions for herbal remedies to reduce engorgement.)

Doctors once used oestrogen (stilboestrol) to dry up milk. However, this sometimes had potentially serious side effects, such as a blood clot in a vein (venous thrombosis), and stopping it often caused a rebound increase of milk production. A synthetic form of oestrogen called chlorotriansene may be safer. A newer drug, bromocriptine, is effective but unnecessary and expensive and can produce side effects (headache, nausea, heartburn, dizziness and, rarely, high blood pressure, a temporary stroke-like illness and even a heart attack). Drugs, when used, are taken for fourteen days, starting from the day of birth.

In south India women traditionally put strings of jasmine flowers on their breasts to dry up their milk. Research shows these are as effective as bromocriptine!

— An advantage of not using drugs to dry up your milk is that if, like many women, you change your mind and decide after all to breastfeed, you'll find it much easier to build up your milk supply if you haven't suppressed it artificially.

TOO MUCH MILK

In the early days, before your milk supply matches your baby's demands, you may have too much milk. Over a few days your supply will gradually adjust, but the abundance can cause problems, especially towards the end of the first week. A newborn baby can be bewildered and almost choked by an over-exuberant flow of milk. He'll turn his head away, cough, splutter and be reluctant to go on feeding. He may also swallow too much air as he tries to drink from this 'fire hydrant', and then suffer from colic.

Cope with an over-abundant milk supply by expressing some

milk before a feed, either by hand or by allowing the milk to leak away if you start letting down your milk before your baby goes to the breast.

A similar problem can arise if you allow your breasts to overfill by letting your baby sleep too long between feeds. Instead, wake him when your breasts feel full and tense, or express enough milk between feeds to soften them.

Many women overcome the problem of too much milk by feeding from one breast only at each feed. The presence of milk in the unemptied breast, together with its pressure as it builds up, stops the milk-producing cells making so much. If you feed from only one breast in a feed, though, ensure you don't allow the unemptied breast to become overfull before the next feed. Express just enough milk to remove any lumpiness or tension. And, if necessary, express a little milk just before the next feed so your baby can easily take the breast into his mouth.

It may also be a good idea to stop your baby comfort-sucking and snoozing at the breast and allow only 'nutritive' sucking (the sort when he actually swallows milk). You can recognize this sort of sucking by its rhythm of one suck per second.

You may find your baby prefers to feed in an 'uphill' position if your milk flow is fast and furious, as this position prevents a strong spray of milk tickling the back of his throat. Hold him facing you on your lap and offer your breast, holding your nipple if necessary.

As your baby grows, he'll be better able to cope with an efficient, fast let-down reflex without choking.

If you still have too much milk, think about donating the extra to a milk bank, where it would be used for preterm or sick babies whose mothers don't want to or can't breastfeed. Ask your doctor or midwife (or, in the UK, health visitor) for details.

> Knowing what affects your milk supply will stand you in good stead if you are faced with one of the challenges commonly experienced by breastfeeding women. We'll look at these in the next chapter.

ELEVEN

Other common challenges

Each mother–baby pair with a breastfeeding concern needs an individual plan of action, since what works for one may not always be best for another. The baby's age, health and birth history are important factors, as are the mother's and baby's personalities, their home environment, any other advice they've had, the parents' expectations, and the amount of encouragement and support they get.

If you can't work out what to do yourself, seek help from a breastfeeding counsellor or leader, or an experienced health professional. And be reassured that breastfeeding problems nearly all pass in time, given good information and support – so hang on in there!

PAINFUL BREASTS OR NIPPLES – AN OVERVIEW

Breast pain can be caused by engorgement, mastitis (due to a blocked duct or, less often, a breast infection) or thrush.

Some breastfeeding women experience burning or shooting pains in one or both breasts after a feed. Possible triggers for this poorly understood plight include thrush, a badly fitting bra, muscle tension from an uncomfortable feeding position and trouble from old scars or other problems in the breast. It's been suggested that such pain can result either from a particularly forceful let-down temporarily making milk ducts collapse or become unduly sensitive, or from the breasts refilling particularly rapidly after a feed.

Painful nipples can be due to soreness, or to a cracked or blanched (whitened) nipple.

These conditions often make women stop breastfeeding, so let's take a good look at how to prevent or treat them.

ENGORGEMENT

There are two types: physiological and pathological.

Physiological engorgement

In the first few days after birth, the breasts swell as mature milk comes in. This swelling results from three things – increased milk volume, more blood flowing through the breasts, and congestion in the breasts due to pressure from swollen milk glands making fluid leak from lymph and blood vessels into the surrounding tissues.

This is common and should lessen in a day or two as your milk production adjusts to meet your baby's needs. But it could occur again at any time if you don't feed (or express) frequently enough.

Help prevent or treat it by breastfeeding on an unrestricted basis, checking your baby is well positioned, and expressing a little milk between feeds if necessary. Give your baby the expressed milk by cup or spoon after a breastfeed if he needs it.

Pathological engorgement

In some women congestion builds up so much that the breasts become pathologically engorged – extremely swollen, as well as lumpy, hard, tense, oversensitive, painful, inflamed, hot, red and shiny, with the skin pitted like orange peel and easily bruised. Swollen ducts and reservoirs sometimes stand out as lumps and cords under the skin, leading some people to describe the breasts as 'stringy'. You'll probably feel hot all over and shivery, you may indeed have a low fever and you may sweat profusely. You'll also be thirsty. Drink as much as you want. *Don't* limit fluids, as some people used to suggest. Some women feel weepy, either because of the discomfort or because it coincides with the 'baby blues' or actual post-natal depression.

Breast swelling tends to flatten the nipples, making it difficult for a baby to get a good enough mouthful of breast to latch on and feed well. High pressure in the breasts also squashes and flattens milk-producing cells, making them unable to produce much milk. While this may be good in the short term, in that reduced milk production reduces any further build-up of pressure, it's bad in the long term because the cells' ability to produce milk can be damaged. Indeed, allowing engorgement to continue is one method of drying up milk. Also, milk contains a factor that can inhibit milk production if the breast is left unemptied for long. So while you might imagine you have plenty of milk, you may in fact be on the way to having too little. If you were to limit the number of feeds, you'd eventually relieve engorgement because your milk production would diminish, but the problem is that it might never again regain its former potential and would eventually dry up.

> — Unfortunately, poor management of engorgement is one of the commonest reasons for a woman's milk supply to fail in the early days, yet such failure is preventable.

Women whose milk dwindles after a week because of engorgement could almost all have breastfed successfully had they only known what to do.

Another problem with engorgement this bad is that it encourages mastitis, infection and blocked ducts.

Dealing with engorgement

If you've had poor advice (and one leading American specialist believes engorgement is a problem caused by doctors!) you can take steps to deal with the resulting engorgement and lay the foundations for successful breastfeeding in the months ahead.

TEN STEPS FOR TREATING PAINFUL ENGORGEMENT

1 **Breastfeed frequently, day and night**, offering feeds every one and a half to two hours by day and every two to three hours at night. Breastfeed or express whenever your breasts feel full, even if your baby hasn't asked for a feed or is asleep. He should have no bottles and shouldn't use a dummy (pacifier).

2 **Encourage your milk to let down before you feed (or express or pump).** Do whatever helps you relax, and swing your arms vigorously, first in one direction twenty times, then in the other twenty times. While warmth encourages the let-down, it can also encourage congestion, so most women find it's better not to have a hot bath or put hot flannels on your breasts.

3 **Express or pump before a feed if you need to soften your breast** to make it easier for your baby to feed. A baby who tries to take a tense areola into his mouth is unlikely to latch on properly; instead he'll chew the nipple, which will make it sore, and he'll also get very little milk. This is because he simply can't take a big enough mouthful of the swollen, tense areola to drain the milk reservoirs, and because the pain he causes by chewing your nipples may prevent you letting down your milk. If you're badly engorged, you'll find an electric pump more comfortable than hand expression or a hand pump.

4 **Make sure your baby is well positioned** so he can suck and milk effectively. You'll know he's taking milk well if you see him swallowing regularly and purposefully, he's satisfied by feeds, and your breasts are softer after a feed. Use breast shells for half an hour before a feed if you need to make your nipples stand out better.

5 Feed your baby at least for long enough to remove fullness and lumpiness.

6 Gently massage your breast when your baby pauses between bouts of swallowing.

7 Express or pump after a feed to remove any remaining lumpiness. Such lumpiness is most likely if your baby is too tired, apathetic or unwell to suck and milk the breasts effectively for long. There's no need to empty your breasts fully.

8 Express or pump between feeds if your breasts ever feel full, tight or tender and you don't want to wake your baby.

9 Relieve tenderness and pain – see below. This is *as well as* doing numbers 1–8 above.

10 Give yourself a pat on the back. You're doing a grand job by breastfeeding and taking steps to overcome this temporary problem. Keep going.

Relieving tenderness and pain

There are many ways of doing this.

Wear a supportive bra, checking that its fabric band or underwire beneath the breasts doesn't cut into them.

See whether cooling your breasts for about twenty minutes makes them more comfortable by decreasing congestion, though don't do this in the half-hour before you're likely to feed, as it might hinder your let-down.

Try:

- An ice pack – for example, a packet of frozen peas, a plastic bag filled with ice (crushed ice is more comfortable than cubes) or a chilled gel-filled cool-pack. Wrap any of these in a piece of cloth to protect your skin.
- A chilled cabbage leaf.

- A cold flannel – wrung out in ice-cold water.
- A cold-water splash.

Some women find that warming the breasts before a feed – with a warm, not hot, shower or a wrapped hot-water bottle, for example – is, on balance, worthwhile because it helps the milk to flow, though it might make the breasts temporarily more uncomfortable.

Aromatherapists suggest *very* gently massaging or smoothing in a little oil or cream containing two to three drops of rose or peppermint oil in a tablespoonful of carrier oil (for example, sweet almond), but don't get this on your areolae or nipples as its taste could put your baby off feeding, or be dangerous for him. You could also apply an aromatherapy compress. Put a few drops of rose, lavender, geranium or fennel oil in a bowl of hot water. Cut a round hole in the centre of a large hanky, then lay the hanky on the surface of the water so it picks up the film of oil. Now apply the hanky to your breast, with the hole over your areola and nipple. Cover it with a towel and wait five minutes Repeat every few hours. The hole in the hanky prevents oil getting on your areolae and nipples, as your baby might not like the taste.

Medical herbalists have suggestions too, and you can buy the herbs suggested below from a medical herbalist or a herbal supplier:

- Mke cleavers tea by pouring 600 ml (1 pint) of boiling water over 30 g (about 1 oz) of dried cleavers (*Galium aparine*) leaves, stems and flowers. Cover and steep for ten minutes, then strain. Wring out two flannels in the tea, and apply to the breasts. Repeat frequently. Cleavers is traditionally used as it's said to be cooling and to relieve congestion.
- Make a poke-root decoction by grinding 30 g (about 1 oz) of dried root with a pestle and mortar, covering with 600 ml (1 pint) of water in a pan, simmering for ten minutes, then straining and using as for cleavers tea. This is a traditional remedy for engorgement.

If you are engorged in summertime, and lucky enough to have jasmine flowers in your garden – or know someone who has – try copying women in southern India who relieve swollen breasts by covering them with jasmine flowers.

Painkillers aren't much help for the pain, but if you want to take something, paracetamol is considered safe.

SORE NIPPLES

Up to nine in ten breastfeeding women have sore nipples at some time, especially early on, and particularly in the first week. About a quarter have severe pain or a crack. While it isn't always possible to prevent soreness, several things can help, and it nearly always improves with time.

Some sore nipples appear undamaged; more often the skin is roughened and there's reddening and swelling of the small projections (papillae) on top. There may also be a crescent-shaped stripe across each nipple, composed of tiny blood spots in the skin (petechiae). This occurs on the part of the nipple that's been exposed to maximum suction, with the baby's palate above the stripe and his tongue below. Women with no visible damage may have tougher skin that resists suction better. If the skin is broken it may be crusted too.

A sore nipple hurts most when the baby starts feeding, but this pain generally lasts only a minute or two, provided the skin isn't too damaged, because the baby no longer needs to suck so strongly when the milk lets down. In women breastfeeding on demand, soreness is usually worst on the third day and starts decreasing on the fourth day, whereas in women breastfeeding on a four-hourly schedule it's worst on the fourth day. Schedule-fed babies may damage nipple skin more as they tend to get more hungry and therefore suck more strongly. Large babies may cause more soreness for the same reason.

The pain from a sore nipple is usually described as feeling as if the baby were biting. It usually goes as soon as the milk lets down, so it's nearly always less in the second breast.

There are several possible explanations for soreness. The most likely is that your nipples are unaccustomed to being sucked, and the good news is that their skin toughens as the days go by. Or your baby may have been feeding with the breast poorly positioned (perhaps because you've been holding him awkwardly, or you have poorly protractile nipples or engorged breasts, or he's been snoozing at the breast and letting it half slip out) – in which case he has to suck particularly hard to try to get milk and/or keep the breast in his mouth. Or you may be feeling stressed and therefore taking a long time to let down your milk, which could be a problem as a baby sucks especially strongly before milk lets down. Or your baby could be sucking and milking the breast very strongly at the beginning of a feed out of frustration because so little milk is available. After your milk comes in, this shouldn't be a problem, as there should always be some foremilk in the reservoirs when he starts to feed. If not, it could be because your milk ducts are constricted and not allowing milk through because you're cold, in which case have a warm shower or bath before feeding, put on some more clothes, heat the room or bathe your breasts with warm water.

Here are some useful tips for overcoming soreness.

TWENTY STEPS FOR TREATING SORE NIPPLES

Steps 1–10 are for everyone, but you can pick and choose from the rest.

The cardinal rule is, *don't stop feeding*.

1 **Change your feeding position several times a day** so no one part of the nipple takes the full force of the baby's suction every time. For example, in the morning sit up and hold your baby on your lap; in the afternoon and evening sit up and use the 'football' hold; and at night lie on your side, with your baby lying facing you; by adjusting your position you can feed from your lower or upper breast.

2 **Make sure your baby is well positioned.** If your nipples

look sore, with stripes across them, your baby is highly likely to be sucking very strongly simply to hold on to the breast. He's unlikely to have enough breast in his mouth, so the nipple endures all the force of his sucking and milking. This draws the nipple in and out of his mouth, which soon makes it sore. Also, and most important, a poorly positioned baby doesn't stimulate the breasts well, so milk production and flow are poor and milk doesn't flow into his mouth quickly enough to fill the vacuum and reduce the high suction pressure on the nipple. Some experts believe nearly all nipple soreness results from poor positioning!

3 **Feed your baby frequently.** This encourages mature milk to come in sooner and makes your let-down reflex more reliable. You may get sore nipples sooner than a schedule-feeding woman, but your soreness will disappear before hers, your breastfeeding will almost certainly be more successful and you'll be less likely to have a blocked duct or breast infection.

4 **Don't limit drinking time but limit total sucking time.** Taking your baby off the breast (see number 10) when he's finished drinking may help by limiting his total sucking time but not his actual drinking time. It isn't always easy to know when babies have finished drinking, because they have breaks between bouts of sucking. But if your baby spends long at the breast without swallowing regularly and sucking purposefully at a rate of one suck per minute – even though you are trying to keep him alert and interested by encouraging your let-down – then it's time to stop.

As soreness eases over the next day or two, go back to letting your baby suck for as long as he wants or your milk supply may diminish.

5 **Encourage your milk to let down before putting your baby to the breast** by going through a routine of preparing

for a feed by keeping warm and perhaps by gently massaging your breast; your baby then won't have to suck and milk your breasts so strongly and for so long to stimulate the let-down. This is also wise because both fear of pain, and actual pain, can delay the let-down.

6 **Always offer the less sore nipple first.** By the time you offer the other one, your milk should be flowing well and you may have little or no pain.

7 **Distract yourself** to take your mind off the pain during the first part of a feed when your nipples feel most sore. Try reading, watching TV, or doing breathing exercises or other relaxation techniques.

8 **Care for your nipple skin as advised on page 157.**

9 **Express some milk after each feed, rub it on your nipples and let it dry.** This is a successful, simple and traditional tip for helping sore nipples heal. Breast milk contains various factors that are soothing and anti-infective and encourage cells to grow.

10 **If you have to take your baby off the breast, break the suction by putting a fingertip into the corner of his mouth and pushing the nipple to one side.** Pulling him off may increase soreness.

11 **Treat any engorgement,** as a baby finds it difficult to get a good mouthful of an engorged breast, so is more likely to chew the nipple.

12 **If your nipples don't stand out well, try using breast shells for half an hour before a feed.** This lets your baby take a bigger mouthful of breast and thereby avoid sucking on the nipple alone.

Be sure to keep the shells clean, so they can't infect damaged skin.

13 Apply lanolin cream. This encourages 'moist healing', which has been shown to be better for sore nipples than keeping them dry. Cream containing lanolin (extracted from sheep wool) is useful, but choose a brand (see page 259) free from residues of pesticides used on sheep to prevent blow-fly infestation.

14 Apply a warm moist compress to soothe any soreness lasting between feeds.

15 Consider applying hydrogel dressings (page 416) to encourage 'moist healing', though not if you suspect any infection.

16 Cool your nipples immediately before feeding your baby. Do this by splashing them with cold water, or applying a cloth-wrapped cool-pack (from the fridge) or a polythene bag of crushed ice or ice cubes. It's best to encourage your let-down to start working first since coldness can hinder the let-down.

17 Have a small alcoholic drink twenty minutes before a feed if you think pain is likely to hinder your let-down, though don't repeat this if you think it makes your baby less keen to drink your milk. Obviously don't overdo your alcohol intake by having such a drink before every feed!

18 Consider whether you could have a skin sensitivity. If your nipples feel sore throughout a feed, you could have contact dermatitis from sensitivity to washing powder, fabric softener, a toiletry (for example, soap, shampoo or deodorant), a cream or other remedy for sore nipples, food particles in your baby's mouth, or the plastic of a breast shell or pump. Either stop using each suspect one by one, for a week at a time each, so you discover what's to blame, then avoid it in future, or avoid all suspects at once, reintroducing them one by one when your soreness is healed.

Sometimes a teething baby's saliva triggers soreness. And some women with continuing soreness need treatment for thrush, eczema, psoriasis or seborrhoeic dermatitis. If your doctor prescribes any topical treatment, wash it off before your baby feeds.

19 Avoid antiseptic sprays. Some women spray their nipples with the antiseptic chlorhexidine, thinking it will prevent sore nipples, nipple cracks and mastitis. However, there's no evidence that this is useful for preventing or treating soreness.

20 If all else fails, try a very thin rubber nipple shield. This has a teat for the baby to suck, but it's recommended only as a very last resort, as it has so many potential drawbacks. First, it may not help. Second, if not properly cleaned after each use it can harbour bacteria or fungi and infect damaged skin. Third, it can reduce the milk supply, because milk production and the establishment of a reliable let-down depend on the baby stimulating nerve endings in the skin of the nipple and areola, and a shield reduces such stimulation. Fourth, it can prevent a baby getting all the milk; the thinnest shield keeps back 22 per cent, while thicker ones keep back up to 65 per cent! Fifth, some babies get so used to a shield that they won't take the breast without one.

It's best not to use a shield unless you absolutely have to. If you do, stop as soon as possible. If your baby is reluctant to breastfeed without a shield, cut away a little more of the rubber before each feed so he gradually becomes used to the feel and taste of your skin again. Or try slipping it out once he's sucking well.

Rarely, a sore nipple bleeds and the baby swallows tiny amounts of blood. This can look horrifying if regurgitated in a mouthful of milk, but your blood won't harm your baby, so just treat the soreness and carry on feeding.

THRUSH

This infection with the yeast-like fungus *Candida albicans* (also known as Monilia) can make the nipples and areolae sore. Some affected women report sharp burning pains that shoot deep into their breast during a feed and worsen immediately afterwards. Sometimes they continue between feeds.

You may also have itchy nipples, with flaky pink, red or purple areas. There may be fine cracks around the nipple, perhaps with white matter inside. The areola may be shiny and slightly swollen, and have a bright red ring around it. Very occasionally thrush shows up as adherent white spots on the nipples.

Candida is a normal inhabitant of our skin and bowels but in certain circumstances it can multiply and cause infection. If a mother or baby has a thrush infection (for example, in the mother's vagina or the baby's mouth or nappy area), they can pass it backwards and forwards to each other. Thrush in a baby's mouth may show up as white spots inside the cheeks or on the tongue or gums; a nappy rash infected with thrush may look shiny or have a bright pink raised edge.

Candida thrives in warm, moist situations and likes milk, so a baby's mouth and a mother's nipples and areolae (particularly if she wears a bra and uses breast pads) make very suitable breeding grounds. You are more likely to get thrush if you have recently taken antibiotics, have sore or cracked nipples, or are on the Pill.

Both mother and baby need simultaneous, prompt and vigorous treatment of any infected areas. This is best carried out for two weeks, even if the infected area seems better earlier. There is no need to stop breastfeeding. See also page 272.

Anti-thrush medication

A pharmacist or doctor can recommend suitable anti-fungal medications (such as nystatin, miconazole or clotrimazole) for you and your baby; nystatin is usually used for a baby's mouth, while miconazole seems more effective on the nipples. Certain medications are available only on prescription. If you have vaginal thrush, your partner may need to be treated too.

Rinse your baby's mouth carefully with water after each feed and put a little (1 ml) nystatin suspension into his mouth. Wash your nipples and areolae after each feed, dry well, then apply anti-fungal cream. Continue the therapy until the symptoms have been gone for at least ten days. If you have deep shooting pains, you may need to take tablets of anti-fungal medication for at least two weeks as well.

Ideally, avoid using breast pads as they can encourage thrush, but if you do use them, change them after each treatment. Have a clean bath towel each day, and when laundering towels and bras use water that's as hot as is safe for the fabric and put a cup of vinegar in the rinse water.

If thrush still doesn't clear, your doctor may prescribe 1 per cent aqueous gentian violet solution for use on your nipples and in your baby's mouth. Apply it once a day and for no longer than three days. The stain will make your nipples and your baby's mouth look dramatically purple.

Other measures

A baby can become reinfected from anything that has previously been in his mouth, so if he uses a dummy (pacifier), for example, boil it daily for twenty minutes. If you have repeated vaginal thrush, cut down on added sugar and other refined carbohydrates in your diet, as well as yeast-containing foods and drinks, including alcohol.

Home remedies

Research shows that treating thrush on the nipples by applying a vinegar solution (made with a teaspoon of vinegar in one cup of water) after each feed, and treating thrush in a baby's mouth with a bicarbonate of soda solution (made by mixing a teaspoon of bicarbonate of soda in a cup of water) may help stop itching, but doesn't cure the thrush.

Sunshine, or UV light from a sunlamp may also help get rid of thrush on your nipples, but take care not to get burnt, and protect your eyes with suitable goggles if you use a sunlamp. Expose your breasts for half a minute on day one, one minute on days two and three, two on days four and five, and three on day six. Reduce the exposure time if the skin reddens at all.

BLANCHED NIPPLE AND AREOLA

In a few women, nipple pain is sometimes followed by the nipples and areolae turning white and going numb, presumably because the blood supply suddenly reduces. The pain is like a cramp; it begins during a feed and continues afterwards; and the blanching and numbness begin either during the feed or soon after. It can persist for half an hour or even much longer until the blood supply returns, when the nipples may turn blue or red before returning to their usual colour. The symptoms are a type of Raynaud's phenomenon (which more usually affects the fingers).

Avoid sudden temperature changes. Warmth (for example, from a covered hot-water bottle) may ease the pain. Keeping warm, checking your baby is well latched on, eating foods rich in calcium and magnesium (meat, fish – including sardines eaten with the bones, shellfish, dairy, eggs, beans, peas, lentils, green leafy vegetables, mushrooms, nuts, seeds and wholegrain foods), or even taking these nutrients in supplement form, may help. If the problem is serious you could discuss with your doctor whether to take a prescription drug called nifedipine (a calcium-channel blocker) that encourages blood vessels to widen.

NIPPLE CRACK

A crack usually follows poor treatment of nipple soreness and is very painful. It usually develops along a line representing the baby's maximum suction pressure while feeding. Indeed, if when you have sore nipples you see a red or white stripe across your nipple during or after a feed, you need to adjust your breastfeeding technique to prevent it cracking open. Some cracks become infected by thrush. Cracks are the commonest cause of bleeding from the nipple (other causes include a benign tumour called an intraduct papilloma, so unless you are sure blood is coming from a crack, it's wise to consult your doctor).

- A Turkish study (2000) comparing three groups of women for ten days after childbirth found that those who kept their nipples dry and clean were less likely to get cracks than those who applied breast milk after feeds, or used warm moist compresses four times a day.

Do everything you can to heal a crack and prevent it happening again. There is no need to stop your baby feeding. When the crack heals, prevent it reopening by varying your baby's feeding position regularly.

What to do

The best treatment is as for sore nipples. Changing your feeding position, limiting time spent at the breast without drinking, making sure your baby is well latched on, and applying breast milk after a feed are particularly useful for speeding up healing if you get a crack.

Dermatologists say that elsewhere in the body skin is more likely to crack if it contains insufficient internal moisture, and cracked skin heals better if it contains sufficient internal moisture.

They see no reason why this shouldn't apply to cracked nipple skin too. Applying cream, ointment, oil, hydrogel or a non-adherent burns dressing can increase the internal moisture content of nipple skin, allowing slower, more gentle drying. This gives the outer layer of skin time to return to normal and prevents rapid drying and scabbing creating tension either side of the crack, drawing its edges apart and delaying healing.

However, dermatologists also recommend removing surface moisture from nipples after a feed, or after leaking, since moisture on the skin doesn't have the same benefits as moisture in the skin, but can make the surface of the skin soggy and more prone to infection.

If a crack doesn't heal within a few days you may, temporarily, need to take your baby off the breast because of the pain, in which case either express your milk or use a pump for a while – perhaps as long as four or five days, but most likely only one or two. Give the expressed or pumped milk to your baby from a cup.

It isn't wise to use a nipple shield so you can carry on breastfeeding, as this reduces breast stimulation, so could reduce your milk supply. Anyway, an Australian study showed that women preferred to express or pump. As the crack heals, gradually resume breastfeeding, starting twice a day and continue to express or pump regularly between feeds.

BLOCKED DUCT

This causes a red, tender lump that may progress to a local area of inflammation (mastitis) that makes you feel flu-like and achy.

A duct becomes blocked (or 'plugged') either because of pressure from a badly fitting bra, or from engorgement with inadequate emptying of one particular duct. Milk builds up in the duct behind the blockage, causing a lump. Letting down your milk makes the pressure build up more.

If you treat a blocked duct early, the lump should subside with no further problem. If you do nothing, the surrounding breast tissue will probably become inflamed. This inflammation results from fluid and certain constituents of dammed-up milk escaping, making the overlying skin redden and increasing your body temperature. Inflammation from a blocked duct alone has been known to make a woman's temperature rise as high as 40°C (104°F)!

Treatment is urgent because stagnant milk – in the blocked duct and the glands supplying that duct, and in the surrounding breast tissue – can easily become infected. However, simple measures started at the first suspicion of anything wrong put things right almost every time.

TEN STEPS FOR TREATING A BLOCKED DUCT

1 **Empty your breast thoroughly each time your baby feeds,** since the lower the pressure of milk in the breast, the better your chance of clearing the blockage. Check your baby is well positioned, let him feed as long as he wants and express any milk remaining after a feed.

2 **Vary your feeding position** at each feed. This simple tip is one of the most helpful. If possible, position your baby with his chin over the block; the milking action of his tongue and lower jaw then have a better chance of clearing it.

3 **Feed your baby more often** if your breasts – or part of a breast – feel lumpy after a feed. This ensures frequent drainage of the ducts. Fit in as many extra feeds as you can, even if you're already feeding on demand.

4 **Offer the affected breast first**, to ensure best possible emptying, and either return to it later in the feed, or express it afterwards.

5 ***Gently* but firmly massage the lump towards the nipple**

during a feed (and after if it's still there) in an attempt to release the block and its dammed-up milk.

6 **Check your bra isn't pressing anywhere** and causing the block, especially if you wear one that leaves a band across the top of the breast when its flap is open, or you pull the cup of an ordinary bra down to feed, or your bra has an underwire that presses on your breast because it doesn't fit well.

7 **Relieve pain** by applying a hot wet compress every hour, or putting a covered hot-water bottle over the area. Immersing the breast in a basin or bath of hot water for five to ten minutes before a feed may help too.

8 **Take antibiotics if the lump persists after twenty-four hours in spite of these measures**. This will prevent infection, and your doctor can prescribe ones suitable for a breastfeeding woman. *Don't stop feeding.* Eating a little live yoghurt twice a day, or taking probiotic capsules (from health-food stores) may help prevent the antibiotics causing diarrhoea and, perhaps, thrush.

9 **Get plenty of rest and relaxation.** Go to bed – even just one day in bed will make you feel better and may boost your resistance. This will help prevent any local inflammation spreading. (It's possible that stress encourages a blocked duct by boosting adrenalin; this increases blood fats, enabling more fat to enter milk; extra fatty milk is thick and may encourage blockages by forming an adherent coating on the lining of the milk ducts – much as fatty blood encourages fat to coat the lining of the arteries, making blood clots more likely.)

10 **Take more exercise**, as this may help dislodge the block. Do whole body exercise to boost your general circulation, plus shoulder, arm and upper-body stretching exercises.

One extremely unusual – and unproven – therapy for lumpy breasts and mastitis comes from the field of kinesiology and is said to reduce congestion by increasing lymph drainage. There seems to be no medical explanation, but it's included here as it can do no harm and some women have found it helps. You can do it yourself or ask someone to do it for you. Put one hand very lightly on the lumpy area of your breast. With three fingers of the other hand, massage the outside of the same-side leg along a line from just below the knee to the hip (think of the side-seam of a trouser leg). Use a firm circular motion for about ten seconds, and gradually move your fingers up the line. Repeat if necessary with your other hand on another lumpy area of the breast.

Expressing a 'plug'

Some women who persevere with gently trying to express milk from a blocked duct, eventually express a very small firm 'plug' of white or yellow, cheesy or granular matter from the opening of that duct at the nipple. This is made of milk that dried out (due to its water being absorbed) while dammed up behind the blockage. The milk they then express from that duct is often unusually thick and may flow slowly of its own accord for a while. Once all the dammed-up milk has come out, the milk looks normal.

If a plug is near the nipple, you may see a swollen milk reservoir bulging in the areola – rather like a varicose vein.

Repeated blocked ducts

In women plagued with repeated blocks, various factors may be making their milk unusually 'sticky', or encouraging certain constituents (such as fat globules) to adhere to the lining of their milk ducts, so reducing their diameter and encouraging blockages.

Several measures are worth trying:

Adjust your diet – Check your diet is healthy, with at least five daily helpings of vegetables and fruit.

Avoid too much saturated fat (in meat, dairy food, margarine, and white cooking fat and other commercially made products containing hydrogenated or partially hydrogenated fats), as it makes blood more sticky and could possibly have the same effect on breast milk.

The best way of doing this is to change the balance of the fats in your diet so you eat relatively more polyunsaturated ones and less saturated fat. Do this by including nuts, seeds and wholegrain foods in your diet.

It may also help to eat more foods rich in omega-3s (green leafy vegetables, walnuts, oily fish, walnut oil and linseeds). Include onions, garlic (about three cloves a day), pineapple, ginger, avocados and foods rich in vitamins B_1 and B_6 (meat, fish, egg yolk, wholegrain foods, green leafy vegetables, peas, beans, lentils, avocados, bananas, nuts and seeds), vitamin C (green vegetables, potatoes and most fruits), vitamin E (nuts, seeds, soya, lettuce and vegetable oil), flavonoid plant pigments (vegetables and fruits) and salicylates (vegetables, fruits and seeds). All these emulsify blood fats (disperse them into smaller globules) so it's reasonable to suppose they may do the same with milk fats.

Consider a supplement of omega-3s or lecithin from health stores or pharmacies. Omega-3s can help reduce inflammation. And both omega-3s and lecithin may make milk less sticky and likely to dam up.

Manage stress effectively – Your reaction to stress could interfere with your body's production and balance of omega-3 and omega-6 essential fatty acids. You can't avoid stress – indeed, stressors are a normal and necessary part of life – but you may need to learn better ways of dealing with it so it doesn't get to you.

Smoking – If milk behaves at all like blood, which is likely, then smoking (and passive smoking) will make it stickier. Smoking is already known to encourage one type of breast inflammation (periductal mastitis).

Check your sleeping position – Some women find that sleeping on their front can lead to a blocked duct.

Homeopathy – The homeopathic remedy Phytolacca is said to help. The dose is 30c or 12c tablet two or three times a day. Avoid food, drink and brushing your teeth for fifteen minutes before and after taking a homeopathic remedy.

Herbal remedies – Medical herbalists recommend drinking dandelion-root tea (no more than a cupful three times a day) and smoothing linseed oil combined with a few drops of geranium or rose oil into inflamed breasts, but remember to wash the oil off before feeding your baby.

MASTITIS

This means the breast is inflamed. Many people assume every inflamed breast is infected, but studies show that of every two women with mastitis, only one has an infection, while the other has engorgement or a blocked duct.

It's important to recognize a breast infection because this is potentially serious and needs antibiotics. Fortunately, lab tests (see opposite) help resolve any doubt.

Mastitis is most likely to begin in the upper part of the breast, in the side nearest the arm. If left untreated, local inflammation can spread.

Breast infection (mastitis with infection)

Breast inflammation due to infection can be called mastitis with infection, infected mastitis, or simply breast infection. It happens to around one in forty breastfeeding women, most often between two and five weeks after childbirth.

Infection may affect just one part of the breast or the whole of it. The infected area is red, swollen, hot, painful and tender, the overlying skin is shiny, and the woman feels shivery, ill and achy, as if she has flu, with a fever of 38°C (100.4°F) or higher. She may feel nauseated and might vomit, and sometimes it's possible to squeeze pus from the nipple.

If only a part of the breast is involved, the symptoms are like those of a blocked duct, but worse.

If the infection involves the whole breast, it may look as if it's badly engorged, but unlike severe engorgement, which nearly always affects both breasts, mastitis due to breast infection usually affects only one.

Diagnosing infection – It can be difficult to distinguish inflammation caused by infection from inflammation caused by severe engorgement or a blocked duct. However, the woman's description of how it started usually helps to identify the underlying cause of mastitis.

It's best to have a sample of your milk sent to the pathology laboratory before starting to take an antibiotic. If immediate checks show that your milk's white-cell and bacteria-colony counts are high, this suggests you need antibiotics. The lab will inform your doctor and begin culture and sensitivity tests to see which bacteria are responsible, and which antibiotic is best; such tests take several days.

If you have obvious signs of infection, and initial tests suggest you need an antibiotic, your doctor will prescribe the one that's most likely to help. If the culture and sensitivity test results show another one is more appropriate, it's worth changing, because the wrong antibiotic encourages continued or recurrent infection.

The tests will suggest:

- *Engorgement*, if your milk has a normal white-cell count (less than 10^6 per ml) and a normal bacteria-colony count (less than 10^3 per ml), indicating it's either sterile or contains normal amounts of skin bacteria.

- *A blocked duct* if your milk has an increased white-cell count (more than 10^6 per ml) and a normal bacteria count (less than 10^3 per ml), indicating it's either sterile or contains normal amounts of skin bacteria.
- *A breast infection requiring antibiotics* if your milk has an increased white-cell count (more than 10^6 per ml) and an increased bacteria count (more than 10^3 per ml).

Test for thrush – Ideally the pathology lab should test your milk for fungal infection with thrush (*Candida albicans*) as well. One survey showed that one in two women with mastitis had candida, though this doesn't necessarily mean it was causing the inflammation, as candida is often a normal inhabitant of the skin. However, if candida seems to be the culprit, you need anti-fungal treatment rather than antibiotics.

What to do if you have an infection

- Take antibiotics early. Flucloxacillin (500 mg four times a day) is best to start with, as long as you aren't allergic to penicillin. (If you are, you can take 500 mg of erythromycin twice a day). Neither will harm your baby. (Tetracycline, ciprofloxacin and chloramphenicol are unsuitable, as they can harm a breastfed baby).
- Check your feeding technique and in particular keep your breasts well and frequently emptied by your baby and/or by expression or pumping. This maintains your milk supply and helps healing. If you let your breasts remain too full – or try to let your milk dry up – you run the serious risk of getting an abscess.
- If you've had a blocked duct, turn to page 266).
- If you've been engorged, turn to page 252.
- If you've had a cracked nipple, turn to page 264.
- Rest more. One study showed that women with mastitis due to a breast infection had had fewer hours of sleep at night than other women and were less likely to be taking daytime naps. Take special care of yourself when life is busy, for example, around Christmas or other holidays.
- Treat the pain with hot flannels.
- If you smoke, cut down or give up. If you can't, eat more foods

rich in vitamin C and take a vitamin-C supplement (at least 100 mg), as smoking reduces your levels of this infection-fighting vitamin.

- If you're in hospital, ask for a disinfectant hand-wash solution. German researchers reported that if breastfeeding women – and the staff who touched them – carefully and regularly washed their hands with such a solution, there was very much less chance of mastitis.
- Find effective ways of managing stress, as high stress levels can lower your resistance to infection.
- Check you are eating a healthy diet with plenty of fresh fruit and vegetables, and consider taking supplements of vitamins C (at least 100 mg a day) and E (10 mg of tocopherol acetate daily).
- Try gently smoothing in some vitamin E cream, or a simple cream scented with three drops of geranium oil to each tablespoon, but remember to wash the oil off before feeding your baby.

Causes of breast infection

Breast infection can occur at any time in breastfeeding women. But what makes a woman vulnerable to infection with bacteria that are usually normal residents of her skin is often unclear. The organism involved is nearly always *Staphylococcus aureus*, though *Staphylococcus epidermidis* or streptococci are occasionally responsible. Infection can begin in the tissue surrounding the milk glands and ducts, or in the milk ducts themselves.

Some affected women have been breastfeeding successfully for several weeks or months. However, certain breast infections follow poor or delayed treatment of engorgement, a blocked duct or a cracked nipple. Other infections are thought to enter the breast via the nipple from the baby, who is likely to have picked them up in hospital and been carrying them in his nose without symptoms. When several mothers and babies at once have a breast infection in hospital, or soon after they leave, their mastitis is called 'epidemic' mastitis.

Can your baby still have your milk?

Generally, yes. It's almost always better to go on breastfeeding: better for the baby and better for you.

However, if – and only if – initial lab tests of your milk show it contains particularly large counts of bacteria (dead or alive), there's a very small possibility of gastro-enteritis or even septicaemia, so your baby shouldn't drink it even if it's sterilized. In this case, either feed only from your unaffected breast, or give your baby donated breast milk, or formula. Pump or express your infected breast and discard the milk. When the bacteria count drops you can breastfeed again. Remember, it's perfectly possible to breastfeed successfully from one breast, so don't panic.

What if it doesn't get better?

If, despite excellent treatment, your breast remains inflamed and infected, yet there's no abscess, your doctor should change the antibiotic to co-amoxiclav (taking care to monitor your baby carefully for jaundice).

If this doesn't help, you should have a cancer check.

BREAST ABSCESS

This usually follows the poor or delayed treatment of mastitis. One survey showed that *abscesses occurred only in women who stopped breastfeeding when they got mastitis*. A lump caused by an abscess isn't tender.

Treatment is as for breast infection. If the abscess doesn't resolve, either repeated aspiration (drawing off pus through a needle) or, as a last resort, surgical incision and drainage (nearly always done under local anaesthetic) are necessary.

You can feed your baby from the affected breast if you and your doctor are reasonably sure the infection is contained within the abscess (which is usually the case). Otherwise, carry on feeding entirely from the other side and expressing and discarding the milk from the one with the abscess.

LUMP IN THE BREAST

Women of all ages and at all stages of their reproductive lives can develop a breast lump, so it's important to be 'breast aware' – familiar with the day by day feel and appearance of your breasts, so you can report anything unusual to your doctor without delay. It's more difficult to feel a lump if your breasts are large and firm, but if you do, take it seriously. Having said this, the lactating breast is often lumpy, though such lumps are usually 'here today and gone tomorrow', whereas a significant breast lump stays.

The causes of a lump during breastfeeding are much as at any other time but, not surprisingly, those related to milk production come highest on the list.

A blocked duct causes a lump that with suitable treatment should disappear in a few days.

An abscess has usually been preceded by mastitis.

A galactocele (milk-retention cyst) is a non-tender, smooth, rounded swelling filled with milk. Such a cyst is thought to be caused by a blocked duct that never re-opened. If you ignore it, the milk inside will gradually thicken and become creamy, cheesy or oily, or even form an abscess if it becomes infected. Sometimes gentle expression can empty the milk via the nipple; if not, try the various other ways of dealing with a blocked duct (page 265). If a cyst that doesn't respond to these measures is aspirated (emptied using a hollow needle), it simply refills with milk, but if necessary it can be surgically removed under local anaesthetic and you can carry on breastfeeding.

A lump called a fibroadenomas is commonly found in the breast, lactating or not, and may appear for the first time during lactation. It contains fibrous and glandular tissue, and if necessary can simply be removed (preferably under local anaesthetic) and breastfeeding continued.

A breastfeeding woman who develops breast cancer will probably be advised to wean because the drugs used for chemotherapy will enter her milk and harm her baby. The type of breast cancer that develops during pregnancy or breastfeeding is sometimes particularly aggressive, so never delay seeking advice about a breast lump unless you are sure of the cause.

CHALLENGING FEEDERS

Some babies take to the breast within a few minutes of being born and never give their mothers any trouble. Others, however, seem completely disinterested, perhaps feeding briefly, then letting go and crying, while others seem to battle with the breast. There's nearly always a reason for such behaviour; the challenge is deciding how to manage.

Whatever the cause of the difficulty with feeding, keep your milk supply going. Though a few babies never feed enthusiastically, virtually all do feed eventually, given the right help. An unenthusiastic baby may not stimulate your milk supply well enough, so you'll need to express or pump after each feed, and you may need to keep this up for some weeks.

Before you even think of labelling your baby as a difficult feeder, deal with any engorgement and check he is well positioned. Some women have to take special care at first because they have poorly protractile nipples.

Poorly protractile nipples

Some babies have difficulty latching on because their mothers' nipples don't stand out well enough for them to draw them well back into their mouth. This situation tends to improve after several weeks of breastfeeding. However, it may help to wear breast shells for a few minutes before a feed, as this makes the nipples stand out just long enough for the baby to take a good mouthful of breast. Using a breast pump for a short while before a feed has a similar effect. Once your baby latches on, your nipple should stay out for the duration of the feed. When he stops feeding, it'll probably go back in.

You can also help your baby latch on by taking your nipple and areola between your finger and thumb and gently making a flat 'biscuit' for him to take into his mouth. Hold it so it's parallel with the line of your baby's lips, not at right angles, and release your grip as soon as he's feeding well because otherwise you could obstruct the reservoirs and ducts and stop the milk flowing.

Baby kept from you after birth

The best time to start suckling is in the first half-hour after birth. After this the baby's urge to feed gradually falls off for some time, and you may need more patience to get him interested.

Baby affected by drugs you've had in labour

The painkiller pethidine (also known as meperidine) is a common offender, while in the US many babies are also affected by barbiturates. These babies may be drowsy and apathetic about feeding for up to five days, though the effects usually wear off more quickly. You might not be able to get your sedated baby to feed well but you can avoid giving a bottle, and you can keep your milk supply going by expressing or pumping after each feed. You can also give him expressed milk from a cup or spoon when he's finished at the breast, and offer him the chance to go back to the breast if he wishes. Wake him often for a feed – every two or three hours at least – as the sooner he learns how to breastfeed, the better. While you or a nurse may be able to get him to bottle-feed even if he won't feed from you, this isn't a good idea as he'll then be less likely to take to the breast once the sedation wears off.

Another culprit is syntocinon – synthetic oxytocin – given as an intravenous drip to stimulate labour contractions. The problem is that this temporarily suppresses the production by a woman's pituitary gland of her own, natural, oxytocin, so it may take longer than usual for her to establish a reliable let-down reflex.

Jaundiced baby

A jaundiced baby (page 308) is often sleepy and difficult to interest in feeding. Frequent small feeds are best. As the jaundice clears, he'll become more interested, so be patient and keep your milk supply going by expressing after each feed.

Baby has been given a bottle

A baby who learns to bottle-suck will try to breastfeed using the same technique. Unfortunately, this often doesn't work and he has to learn how to breastfeed. With patience, you'll be able to get him to feed from you, but it's far better to avoid giving a bottle in the first place. Once a baby has fed from the breast for many weeks, the occasional experience of bottle-feeding shouldn't matter, though some older babies quickly learn that milk comes from a bottle more easily and are then reluctant to take the breast if there's the slightest chance of a bottle!

The technique a baby uses for bottle-feeding is easier than the one he uses for breastfeeding. When bottle-feeding, a baby applies a little suction, lets the milk pour into his mouth, and then swallows. There isn't much up-and-down or in-and-out movement of his tongue, and little jaw movement either.

If a baby bottle-sucks at the breast, he gets very little milk. There's much more work involved in breastfeeding, so it's hardly surprising to find that the muscular effort expended is good for the development of a baby's jaws.

If you're teaching your baby to breastfeed once he's been given a bottle, it's no help if you constantly muddle him by giving both breast and bottle. If you want to breastfeed, never give a young baby a bottle. If for some reason he isn't getting all his nourishment direct from the breast, give him complements of expressed breast milk (or formula if you must) by cup or spoon or from a supplementer (page 302).

You can tell whether your baby is trying to bottle-suck during a breastfeed because you'll occasionally see him sucking his cheeks in (caused by him sucking his tongue – if you pull his lower lip down you'll see his tongue is above the nipple instead of below it). He may also stick his tongue out (which is known as tongue-thrusting, and makes him come off the breast) and do a lot of fast fluttery sucking at a rate of two or three sucks per second, rather than the slower sucking at a rate of about one suck per second that accompanies drinking. Your baby won't swallow very often (check by listening, and by watching for the ear movement that accompanies swallowing), and there'll be long intervals between bouts of sucking. Feeds take a long time because his poor milking action doesn't encourage you to let your milk down.

In the rare event of a mother being so ill that she can't feed her baby, he should have her milk (or donated breast milk, or, if unavoidable, formula) from a cup or spoon, not from a bottle.

Full baby

If your baby has had some formula since you last fed him, he may not be hungry when you next expect to breastfeed him. This is because formula stays in the stomach much longer than breast milk. Rather than give a hungry baby formula, it's better to breastfeed him (or, if you aren't there, for the carer to give him expressed breast milk). Remember, you need your baby to breastfeed so you produce plenty of milk. A baby full of formula is no help to your breasts as he simply won't feed.

Exhausted baby

If you feed your baby according to a schedule in hospital he may cry from hunger for some time – perhaps as long as an hour – before it's time for the next scheduled feed. This is especially likely to happen at visiting times and at night. By the time you get him he's exhausted and goes to sleep after feeding for a very short time, sometimes even before your milk lets down.

This is obviously ridiculous. You must insist on feeding your baby as soon as he cries. Remember that the smaller the baby, the more often he'll need feeding and the quicker his crying will exhaust him.

Sleepy baby

A sleepy baby may be suffering from you having had a long labour or from the effects of painkillers you had in labour, he may be jaundiced, he may be tired out from crying between feeds, or he may simply need a lot of sleep.

You'll find it helps if he is alert (but not crying) when you start to feed him. You may be able to wake him up more by taking his clothes off (though don't let him get chilled!), rocking him gently or stroking his back firmly. Watch for any of the signs that show he may be ready to feed even though he isn't asking for a feed. These include eyes darting around beneath closed eyelids, sucking movements, putting his hand to his mouth, moving in general and making small sounds.

Encourage him to continue sucking by gently expressing a little milk into his mouth while he's at the breast, or by gently stroking his cheek low down towards his jaw. If he's too sleepy to get enough milk, however much you try to keep him awake and interested in feeding, make sure he gets some of your higher-calorie fat-rich hindmilk. Do this by expressing after he's finished a feed. Collect the milk and give it to him by cup or, even better, by a supplementer (see page 302) halfway through the next feed.

Baby overwhelmed by milk supply

If your let-down is so powerful that the milk gushes into your baby's mouth and nearly chokes him, collect this early milk and allow him to feed only when the milk stops flowing so exuberantly. Give him the collected milk by cup or spoon afterwards.

Babies who try to swallow quickly enough to cope with an exuberant milk supply often swallow a lot of extra air and get colic or regurgitate more than usual after a feed. Some babies bring up almost a whole feed because of this. Expressing or simply collecting the initial milk you let down should get over the problem. If you were to allow the baby to bring up a whole feed and then feed him again, he should keep the milk down because the flow would be much slower and he wouldn't swallow as much air, but your milk supply would increase because of the law of demand and supply and your let-down would subsequently work even better, making the problem worse at the next feed.

One way to overcome the problem of too much milk is to give one breast per feed. This allows him to suck for comfort without getting two breasts full of milk at each feed. Express some milk from the unused breast if necessary to keep yourself comfortable. See also pages 247–8.

Crying baby

(See pages 166 and 191.)

Baby wants feeding very often

How often a baby wants to feed depends on his personality, how hungry and thirsty he is, how tired he is, and whether or not he is well and happy. In other words, there may be some specific reason why your baby sometimes or always wants frequent feeds, or he may just be asking for what is perfectly normal and desirable for him.

Check whether you're making enough milk and, if not, increase your milk supply (page 233). If he feeds very frequently at one particular time of the day (which is most likely to be in the evening), and cries if you don't feed him, see page 168. If he is healthy, thriving and gaining weight, he may simply have got into the habit of feeding frequently. If you are not happy to go along with this, you may be able gradually to lengthen the gaps between feeds by distracting him with various activities or by asking someone else to look after him when he might otherwise be likely to want a feed. A good tip is to get him used to larger feeds. Try expressing some milk in the morning (which is when most women have most milk). Keep this milk in the fridge and when your baby starts wanting frequent feeds – perhaps in the evening – give it to him from a cup after a feed. This may fill him up and allow you to have a longer break.

Excited baby

A baby who is so excited by the idea of feeding that he 'bounces' at the breast as he searches and lunges for the nipple, and at the same time waves his arms around, may be too active to settle down to a feed. He disturbs himself so much that he becomes overwrought and ends up frustrated and crying. Try wrapping him firmly but not too tightly in a shawl or cloth to keep his arms by his sides. Encourage your milk to let down before he goes to the breast, so there's milk there for him as soon as he starts to feed. Rub a little milk over your areola to see if its smell helps him focus and concentrate. If his behaviour puts you off so you find it difficult to let your milk down, you could try using a supplementer (page 302). This provides a stream of your expressed milk from a tube that he takes into his mouth along with your nipple.

Baby fights at the breast

A baby who fights at the breast may have had the experience of being smothered by a full breast while feeding, and therefore have learned that getting milk means not being able to breathe through his nose. Make sure your breast isn't obstructing his nose. You may find it helps to lift your breast gently with your fingers from underneath. With patience on your part he'll forget his early unpleasant experiences.

Don't confuse fighting at the breast with the common fussing or playing and butting some babies do while waiting for milk to let down. These babies are happy once the milk is flowing, whereas true fighters carry on thrashing around and never seem to feed properly.

If your baby is still reluctant to take the breast, try the trick of popping a rubber teat, perhaps filled with expressed milk, into his mouth. Once he latches on, withdraw it and substitute your nipple.

Baby refuses a feed

If your baby uncharacteristically refuses to feed, it could be that you smell different from usual, perhaps because you are wearing perfume, or a different perfume, or you've used a new soap, cream or other toiletry.

Your baby may also notice a change in your body's natural scent, and in the taste of your milk, at different times in your menstrual cycle. There are changes in the composition of milk, for example, five to six days before ovulation (for thirty to forty hours) and again six to seven days after ovulation.

Babies can also sense when their mother is upset, and a few then become reluctant to feed. Sometimes a baby takes a dislike to the flavour of something his mother has eaten, so it's worth thinking back over your last two meals to see if you've had something unusual.

Some babies stop feeding for no apparent reason. They go on a 'nursing strike' and all you can do is keep offering your breast and give your expressed milk by cup.

Baby refuses the breast

Occasionally a baby takes a liking to one breast and refuses to feed from the other. He may be more comfortable on one side or the milk may come more easily from that breast. Unusual causes include the baby being blind in one eye or being deaf or having an ear infection in one ear.

Try beginning a feed from the side he prefers, so the milk starts flowing from the other side. Then transfer him to the other breast without turning him round, letting him feed in the 'football' hold. This may do the trick. If not, express milk from the unused breast to maintain its milk supply and keep trying at each feed time. He'll almost certainly come round to the idea of feeding from both sides again. Many babies (and, come to that, many mothers) prefer one side to the other. It's quite possible to end up rather lopsided if you feed your baby more from one side. The side that isn't stimulated as much will, in time, respond by producing less milk. Most women have breasts that are unequal in size before they become pregnant. This doesn't matter at all, though they may always have more milk on one side.

Baby throws his head back

This behaviour is most often seen in preterm babies and generally disappears by eight weeks. Try gently bending your baby forwards, so his back curls up, to see if this more relaxed position helps him settle at the breast. Wrapping him firmly in a small blanket can help keep him in a curled position. You may find that he relaxes as soon as he sucks.

If your baby arches his back at the same time, feeding him as you hold him firmly in the 'football' hold may help. Try to arrange yourselves with his bottom against the back of your chair and his legs bent upwards, so his body bends forwards at the hips.

Floppy baby

If your baby is floppy, he probably has very relaxed muscles and may not feed very effectively. As a result, feeds are extremely time-consuming. You may find expressing your milk after and between feeds and using it in a supplementer (page 302) helps you continue breastfeeding.

LOW BIRTHWEIGHT

About 7 per cent of newborn babies have a low birthweight, defined as less than 2,500 g (5 lb 8 oz). Two-thirds of these are born early, after less than thirty-seven weeks of pregnancy, and are called preterm. The others have a weight that is not appropriate for their gestational age (length of pregnancy) and are described as small for dates. Worldwide, 22 million low-birthweight babies are born each year.

Breast is best

Both preterm and small-for-dates babies do best on breast milk (if they are mature and well enough to receive milk at all).

This is because:

- The composition of a preterm baby's own mother's milk is designed to meet his needs at his level of maturity. It contains relatively more protein, ionized calcium, chloride and immunoglobulin A, and less lactose than milk from a full-term baby's mother. It also has more lactoferrin and lysozyme. As a baby grows, the composition of his mother's milk gradually adjusts to meet his changing needs.
- Preterms may not have had enough time in the womb to build up big enough stores of iron in their liver, as such stores increase most rapidly in the last few weeks of a full-term pregnancy. However, preterm breastfeds are less likely to become anaemic than preterm bottle-feds, because although there's more iron in formula, the iron in breast milk is better absorbed. (Some breastfed preterms do eventually become anaemic, though, and your doctor will recommend iron supplements if necessary.)
- Preterm babies digest breast milk earlier and better than formula (including preterm formula) and are less likely to bring it up.
- Breast milk enables a good growth rate, of around the rate a baby would have grown had he stayed in the womb, or a little slower. Experience in the US shows that preterms who receive sugar-water and formula top-ups lose more weight than those who are breastfed

frequently and given nothing else. Also, small-for-dates breastfed babies grow faster in the first year than those that are formula-fed. Their heads also grow faster in the first three months, probably reflecting better brain growth.

- It's particularly important for preterms to get plenty of the Omega 3 fatty acid docosahexanoic acid (DHA – needed for the brain to grow rapidly in the first three months after birth), as they miss out on the large amounts of DHA that pass across the placenta in the last weeks of a full-term pregnancy.
- A preterm baby particularly needs the protection against infection and allergy that only breast milk can provide.
- A breastfeeding mother may feel closer to her baby. This is important because enjoying your baby can be difficult amid the paraphernalia of a special care baby unit.
- A breastfed preterm whose mother cuddles him close (when he can leave the incubator) is greatly advantaged by the pleasure and stimulation of being near her, hearing her voice, heartbeat, breathing and tummy rumbles, sensing her delight and interest in him, smelling her unique natural body scent and – when he's able – tasting the sweetness of her milk.
- Studies in Chicago (1999) showed that preterm babies breathed better if they were breastfed than if they were bottle-fed, and were less likely to have episodes when they were short of oxygen. Some preterms are already short of oxygen (from respiratory distress syndrome or a heart defect), so this is especially bad for them. Preterm bottle-fed babies also have a slower heart rate than breastfeds.

Some mothers of very low-birthweight babies (up to 1,500 g or 3 lb 5 oz) find it difficult to produce enough milk, possibly because their short pregnancy didn't allow their breasts' glandular tissue enough time to mature. (Others choose not breastfeed, in which case a breast milk bank will hopefully provide donated breast milk.) Be with your baby as much as you can and cuddle him a lot when he is able to leave the incubator for short periods. You'll let your milk down better when you're near him and he'll benefit from being near you.

- A UK study (1988) found that very low-birthweight babies who had plenty of cuddling next to their mother's naked skin cried less at six months old. Their mothers also breastfed them for longer than mothers who hadn't had this skin-to-skin contact.

What about formula?

While preterm formula is better than standard formula for preterm babies younger than thirty-four weeks post-conception age, breast milk is generally superior to both, though it needs to be fortified for some babies. (The post-conception age is the number of weeks from conception to birth, plus the number of weeks of life since birth, and it gives an idea of a preterm's maturity compared with that of a baby that stays in the womb for the normal time. Note that the usual way in which women calculate their unborn baby's age is from the first day of the last period, but conception is generally around two weeks later than this.)

Manufacturers continue to try to copy preterm breast milk, which is why they've recently added docosahexanoic acid (DHA), but they can't add such things as live cells and antibodies. Breast milk is best for all babies, preterm or full-term.

Your baby doesn't need formula unless you can't provide enough milk – in which case he can have top-ups of formula or, perhaps, milk donated from another mother.

Babies fed breast milk and preterm formula grow faster than those given breast milk and donated milk, possibly because donated milk is usually drip milk, and because the pasteurization (heat treatment) of donated milk destroys the fat-releasing enzyme lipase.

Providing breast milk for your preterm baby

With patience, perseverance and support you can provide breast milk for your baby and at the same time build up your milk supply. At first he may need to be tube-fed with your expressed or pumped breast milk; later this can be given by cup. A baby mature enough to suck can practise taking milk from the breast.

Have confidence that you'll be able to provide enough milk. If you want to increase your milk supply, plan an intensive campaign of more frequent feeds for two or three days at least, and read chapter 10.

With enough support from the nurses and doctors, and knowing you couldn't do better for your preterm baby than give him your milk, you'll probably succeed. Try to relax and enjoy this time as you mother your baby in such a special way. Talk, if you can, to other mothers breastfeeding preterm babies; some hospitals have regular group support meetings.

Collecting your milk

For the first few days it's best to collect milk by expressing it. Learn how to express as soon after delivery as possible, because it's easier to learn before your breasts fill up.

- A study reported in the journal *Pediatrics* (2001) found that pumping didn't help milk come in more quickly, and the researchers concluded it should be strongly discouraged until the milk comes in.

When your milk comes in, perhaps on the third or fourth day, you may want to pump it instead or as well as expressing it. Expressing takes longer at first but some women prefer it.

Start collecting milk as soon after delivery as you can. It won't take long in the first two or three days because colostrum is produced only in small amounts. But this early milk is particularly valuable for your baby, so treat it like liquid gold.

Empty your breasts as well as possible every two to three hours by day, and aim for at least eight milk-collecting sessions in twenty-four hours – six or seven sessions would be too few to stimulate optimal milk production and to help your let-down reflex develop reliably. Although some women can go six or seven hours at night without being woken by full breasts, and still manage to fit in enough times to express during the day, it's best at first not to let more than four or five hours pass at night without expressing or pumping. In addition, express or pump any time, day or night, if your breasts feel uncomfortably full. Collecting milk frequently builds up your milk supply, though your baby won't need large volumes yet. It's just as important to start expressing or pumping your milk soon after birth as it would have been to breastfeed very soon after birth had you had a baby of normal size. It also helps prevent engorgement.

Wash your hands before expressing or pumping, using disinfectant solution if you are in hospital. Encourage your milk to let down by keeping warm and gently massaging or stroking each breast towards the nipple. Pump for ten minutes each side and switch from side to side every two or three minutes if necessary to encourage the milk to flow.

Store any milk your baby doesn't need straight away, as a reserve for later. Liaise with the nurses so you know how much he takes down the tube at each feed. Amounts as small as 10–15 ml (two to three teaspoonfuls) are normal for a baby weighing 1,000 g (2 lb 3 oz). Put the amount necessary for a feed in a bag or other container, fill as many containers as your baby needs, then close them securely and label them with your name and the date.

If you have plenty of milk, you may be advised to discard the milk you collect early in a pumping or expressing session and give your baby the higher-calorie, higher-fat milk collected later in the session.

IV feeding

The smallest (under 1,000 g or 2 lb 3 oz) and most unwell babies, including those on a ventilator, can be fed only with liquid feed given via a drip into a vein. At first this contains glucose and salts and later, perhaps, amino acids, vitamins, minerals and fats as well.

Tube-feeding

Breast milk can be given directly into the stomach via a fine tube (gavage or nasogastric) to any baby who:

- Weighs less than 1,500 g (3 lb 5 oz).
- Is less than thirty-two weeks post-conception age.
- Isn't well enough to suck.
- Breathes faster than seventy-five breaths a minute.
- Can't yet coordinate sucking, swallowing, breathing and gagging.

A doctor or nurse passes the tube down his nose and via the back of his throat into his gullet and stomach, where it usually stays between feeds. You or a nurse then give tiny and frequent – perhaps hourly – feeds of your milk down the tube.

Tube-feeds are small. A 900 g (2 lb) baby, for example, might need an average of 10–15 ml (two to three teaspoons) of milk an hour. The milk may be propelled down the tube at frequent intervals (perhaps one to three hourly, depending on size and need) using a syringe, or propelled continuously by an electric pump. Most babies don't seem to mind the tube remaining in place between feeds, but if your baby objects, a new one can be inserted for each feed.

Feeding by mouth

A preterm baby who is able to feed by mouth may use several methods as he matures, for example:

- Breast (practice-sucking at first) and cup.
- Cup alone.
- Breast, cup and supplementer (page 302).
- Breast plus supplementer.
- Breast alone.

Once low-birthweight babies (even the heaviest) start breastfeeding, it's often some time before they feed effectively, so they may need to continue for some time with tube- or cup-feeding.

If a baby needs more breast milk than you can supply, he can have formula (preterm if necessary) by cup or supplementer as well, but it's best not to give it by bottle.

Being able to drink from the breast requires a baby to be able to swallow and to have gag, rooting and sucking reflexes, though they can practise being at the breast before they have these skills. Babies can *swallow* early (possibly from eleven weeks post-conception age). The *gag reflex*, which stops milk going down the wrong way, develops from twenty-six to twenty-seven weeks post-conception age. The *rooting reflex* appears from twenty-eight weeks post-conception age. A strong *sucking reflex* appears from thirty-two to thirty-four (sometimes thirty-six) weeks post-conception age, though many younger babies are able to suck. Jaundice or other health problems, or pethidine given in labour, sometimes temporarily dampen effective sucking. The older the baby, the more strongly he'll suck.

Preterm babies can practise breastfeeding – be at the breast without drinking – at any age if they are out of the incubator.

They can drink from the breast or from a cup once they can coordinate breathing, sucking and swallowing without choking. Some babies manage this from thirty to thirty-one weeks, when they weigh 1,300 g (2 lb 14 oz); others don't manage it until they are thirty-two to thirty-four weeks post-conception age, and weigh over 1,500 g (3 lb 5 oz).

Most preterms can manage full breastfeeding at about thirty-six weeks.

Studies show that babies can coordinate sucking and swallowing earlier at the breast than at the bottle.

Practice-sucking at the breast for tube-fed babies – If your baby can come out of the incubator, give him lots of opportunities to be at your breast even if he isn't yet able to suck. It's preferable to be somewhere quiet and comfortable. Hold him at your naked breast several times a day to get him used to the warmth, smell and feel of being there. It's a good idea to put him by your breast while he's actually receiving milk down the tube. Express a few drops on to your nipple every so often, and bring him close enough to smell it. One day, when he's mature and interested enough, he'll start licking the milk and, eventually, start doing some practice-sucking. Be guided by your intuition and keep trying. He should show increasing interest once he first tastes your milk and experiments with sucking.

Persevere with practice-sucking for days or even weeks if necessary, keeping your milk supply going meanwhile by frequent expression or pumping. *Don't be surprised if your baby just licks your breast, or seems to sleep for up to twenty minutes between bouts of one, two or three proper sucks.* He's regaining his strength and he'll be all right as long as he's warmly wrapped up next to your warm body. Coordinating sucking and swallowing is challenging at first, but every day makes a difference, and practice makes perfect.

Eventually he'll take three, four or five sucks, then, if you listen hard, one day you'll hear him swallow. All he's taking at this stage is a little of the milk that drips or flows during a let-down, or leaks from your nipple if your breast is full.

Practice-sucking boosts your milk supply. And babies allowed to practice-suck have higher oxygen levels, are more alert between feeds, gain weight better, develop earlier coordination of breathing, sucking and swallowing (allowing them to cup-feed or breastfeed sooner), and go home earlier. One explanation for the last three benefits is that practice-sucking during a tube-feed enhances digestion, perhaps by stimulating the vagus nerve, which then decreases the level of the hormone somatostatin so milk stays in the stomach longer; it also boosts insulin, which helps a baby use glucose; and it increases gastrin, which releases stomach acid, boosts stomach movements and encourages gut lining cells to grow. Another explanation is that a baby who practice-sucks spends more time being calm, which frees energy for growth.

Time spent encouraging your baby gives you the opportunity to hold him and get to know him. The physical contact also helps him deal with the stress of living in an incubator in a special care baby unit.

Part tube-, part cup-, part breastfeeding (thirty to thirty-two weeks post-conception age) – Your baby can start drinking from a cup and breast when he is mature enough to coordinate breathing, sucking and swallowing without choking.

Cup-feeding small babies is better than feeding them with a spoon or dropper. Start teaching a tube-fed baby to cup-feed with the tube in place. He'll like cup-feeding because he'll be able to taste the sweetness of your milk.

Put about 5–10 ml (one or two teaspoonfuls) of expressed milk into a sterilized baby cup, perhaps the one known as a 'Baby Beak' (see the Appendix, page 415). Hold your baby on your lap, sitting half upright, preferably by your naked breast so he can smell you and your milk. Put a drop of milk on to his tongue with your finger, so he can taste it. Gently tilt the cup so it touches his lower lip and allows a little milk to enter his mouth. Take great care not to swamp him. Within a few days or weeks he'll start lapping it up like a kitten. Don't worry how much he takes; the nurses will work out whether he needs a top-up by tube. Make this time as peaceful and relaxed as possible, so he associates cup-feeds with pleasure and tranquillity.

Continue until he takes all he needs from a cup and the breast, then the tube can be removed. This will be a red-letter day.

Part cup-feeding, part breastfeeding with gradually more breastfeeding and less cup-feeding – your baby will probably be able to suck and swallow efficiently from your breast when he's about thirty-two to thirty-four weeks post-conception age, when he'll probably weigh more than 1,500 g (3 lb 5 oz).

Encourage your milk to let down before he starts sucking. The nurses will offer skilled advice on positioning him so he gets as good a mouthful of breast as possible and he can feed most effectively. Move him from one side to the other every so often during a feed and let him feed as long as he wants. He'll need frequent breaks because he'll get tired. When he seems to have finished, express or pump the rest of your milk. You can then give this to him by cup.

It's important that you and your baby between you empty your breasts frequently, as it's the stimulation from frequent feeding/expression/pumping that builds up your milk supply. So as he gets used to the breast, aim to fit in *at least* eight to ten breastfeeds a day. A full-term baby would have this number and a preterm, who takes smaller amounts, needs at least the same number and ideally more in order to take enough milk.

If you prefer, give your expressed milk via a supplementer (page 302). This device enables your baby to have expressed milk via a tube taped to your nipple while he is breastfeeding. An advantage of a supplementer is that a baby can get more milk more quickly, which is useful if feeding tires him a lot. A disadvantage might be that he gets it so much more quickly that he doesn't give your breasts the stimulation they need to make plenty of milk. Get over this by allowing your baby to comfort suck as much as he wants, and by making sure you empty your breasts well after each feed. Store this expressed milk to put in the supplementer for his next feed.

Transition to full breastfeeding (thirty-two to thirty-six weeks post-conception age) – Eventually your baby will become so good at breastfeeding that he can give up the cup completely. Most low-birthweight babies are thirty-six weeks post-conception age before they can suck well enough to take adequate nourishment from the breast alone. You may have to wake your baby to feed, and give him plenty of encouragement to keep at it during a feed, because preterms often don't 'ask' for feeds until their post-conception age is near the equivalent of full-term.

Your preterm baby will never need a bottle; indeed, if he were to become used to bottle-feeding he might have problems learning to breastfeed effectively.

What if you go home ahead of your baby?

During the transition from full tube-feeding to full breastfeeding, you'll find it much easier if you live in the hospital as near your baby as possible. Ideally, stay alongside your preterm baby until he comes home. One of the many advantages of this is that you are there every time he needs a feed. He'll also benefit from the anti-infective properties of fresh breast milk.

If you go home without your baby, borrow an electric pump so you can take your milk to hospital each time you visit and the nurses can give it to your baby by cup when you aren't there. It's also a good idea to have an insulated cooler bag, plus ice packs, for transporting your little containers of breast milk to the hospital.

Mothering your preterm baby

Preterms are nursed in incubators in special care baby units (SCBUs) to keep them warm and protect them from infection. Unfortunately, few SCBUs have beds for mothers. However, physical contact is very important both for your baby and for the development of your mothering instinct. So, if possible, hold him as often as you can. If he has to stay in his incubator, stroke him gently through the armholes.

You may like to consider sleeping with your baby too. In Pithiviers, in France, preterms that slept in their mother's bed gained weight faster than the others.

It's easy to take cues about how to handle your baby from the nurses. However, nurses are expert at nursing and may not have time to give their charges the cuddling, stroking, holding, attention and talking they need. It's up to you to mother your baby as warmly and intimately as possible, even if this feels awkward at first.

Perhaps a lack of physical contact and mothering is partly why babies born preterm tend to cry twice as much as full-term ones. No one will laugh if you talk to your preterm baby, spend time looking at him or ask to do as many routine jobs, such as nappy changing, as possible. And when you take him home, take all the time in the world to get to know each other and enjoy one another's company.

- Canadian researchers (2004) reported that baby rats whose mothers spent a lot of time licking and grooming them grew up to be less fearful and better adjusted adults, who in turn gave their own babies the same kind of care. They believe this 'physical mothering' causes long-term changes in one of the genes that influence how well the brain controls stress hormone levels.

Kangaroo care

Researchers have found that preterm babies can go home sooner if their mothers have spent a lot of time with them next to their bodies, safely tucked into their clothing between their breasts, like a young joey kangaroo in his mother's pouch. According to South American researchers, most babies weighing 1,200 g (2 lb 10 oz) or more can be cared for like this. Researchers at the Hammersmith Hospital in London also found that babies over 1,500 g (3 lb 5 oz) did better if cared for like young kangaroos! Your partner can carry the baby next to his naked chest in the same way if he likes.

Looking after yourself

You'll have a lot to deal with if you have a preterm baby, and it's very important to look after yourself and ask for all the help and support you need from family, friends and hospital staff. This is especially important if you have other children or live on your own. The more people you have supporting you the better, and the longer you're likely to breastfeed.

Take every opportunity to relax and enjoy yourself, and make sure you are as comfortable as possible in hospital. For example, you could take in a CD/tape-cassette/radio player with headphones, and ask relatives and friends to bring in favourite foods and drinks or take you out for a meal. Your partner could give you a shoulder or back massage as you feed the baby and all three of you could have a cuddle together. As the breastfeeding mother of a preterm baby you are a very special person and need high maintenance.

Confidence, support and encouragement

Although preterm babies do so well on breast milk, nurses and doctors sometimes seem reluctant to encourage mothers to provide it. This may be partly because they perceive it as difficult and time-consuming for the mothers and themselves. It may be because the SCBU simply has a bottle-feeding ethos. Or it may be because they don't want to make women who don't breastfeed feel guilty (though see page 403).

— Hold on to the fact that if you know what to do and have enough skilled advice, encouragement and support, you are very likely to be able to breastfeed your pre-term baby.

- Research in the US (1995) found that most mothers who continued breastfeeding when they took their preterm babies home reported a turning point after two weeks. Their babies stayed awake at the breast longer (which is much more rewarding for the mother) and breastfed more effectively. Many preterm babies start to suck really strongly at the breast only at about the time they were originally expected to be born.
- A North Staffordshire study (1994) found that encouraging mothers of preterm babies to breastfeed raised the proportion who left hospital exclusively breastfeeding from 1 per cent to 58 per cent!
- Researchers in a special care unit in Bombay (1985) found that 95 per cent of mothers could breastfeed their preterm babies successfully when encouraged to do so. A big bonus was that the babies were very much less likely to develop infections and die from them. The cost of running the unit also fell as more babies received breast milk.

Small-for-dates babies

Occasionally a baby is smaller than expected from the duration of the pregnancy, in which case he is called 'small for gestational age' or small for dates. This is almost certainly because he has been poorly nourished in the womb. At first some small-for-dates babies suck poorly and have a poorly coordinated swallowing reflex. They also tend to produce a lot of mucus, which can make them gag and regurgitate.

Your small-for-dates baby may have a sucking reflex in spite of weighing very little, so it's worth giving him the opportunity to suck every so often, whatever his weight, unless he's also very premature. He'll need frequent feeding, and this will help keep his blood sugar level within normal limits. He'll also need to be kept warm.

Fortifying/enriching breast milk

Although most preterm babies of over thirty-two weeks do well on breast milk alone, the very smallest ones tend to grow slowly and have a higher risk of the bone-softening disease rickets, so expressed or pumped milk may need to be fortified (enriched) with 'human milk fortifier' containing protein, vitamins (such as E) and minerals such as calcium, copper, iron, phosphorus and zinc. After about two weeks such a baby may benefit from an iron supplement too.

If your baby is receiving donated breast milk, it'll almost certainly need to be enriched with fortifier or combined with preterm formula, to provide extra protein, calories and minerals. This is because donated milk, being mature milk, differs in composition from preterm breast milk; it's also likely to contain a high proportion of relatively low-calorie, low-fat milk from early in a feed, as it's likely to have been collected while dripping from the breast.

A tube-fed baby may need extra calories to replace those lost when milk fat sticks to the lining of the feeding tube.

Once a baby weighs 2 kg (just over 4 lb), or is discharged from hospital, it's usually no longer necessary to add fortifier to breast milk.

BREAST PUMPS

Most women never need a pump. And however good a pump, it's never as effective as a healthy baby at milking the breast and stimulating the milk supply.

If a baby is unlikely to be able to feed directly from the breast for some weeks, electric pumping can be less tiring than either hand expression or hand pumping. However, it's wise to hand express as well as often as possible, as this stimulates the milk supply better than an electric pump.

You might need a pump

If your baby:

- Is too immature or unwell to get any milk directly from the breast, or to get enough.
- Has to stay in hospital without you (or vice versa); he can then have pumped milk by cup or spoon or tube (but preferably not by bottle).

Or if you:

- Have inverted nipples; using a pump for a minute or so before a feed helps bring the nipple out.
- Want to collect milk to leave for your baby if you are going to be apart for a while.
- Are taking essential medications that might pass into your milk and harm your baby. Throw away the pumped milk but keep your milk supply going by frequent, regular pumping and hand expression, until you are off the drugs and can breastfeed again.
- Have a serious infection that temporarily precludes your baby having your milk. Throw away the pumped milk but keep your milk supply going by frequent, regular pumping and hand expression, until your infection is under control and you can breastfeed again.
- Are building up your milk supply after giving your baby bottles of formula.
- Have let your milk dry up after delivery, or later, but have now decided you'd like to breastfeed.

- Work away from home and want to pump and/or hand-express while away so you can take milk home and/or keep your milk supply going.
- Are building up your milk supply in order to feed an adopted baby.

Using a pump

Before using an electric pump, you must sterilize all the parts that come into contact with milk. This protects your baby and your nipples from infected milk residues.

Position the flange (the pump's funnel-shaped receiving end) so your nipple rests at the inside of its upper part. Pumping draws your nipple in and out, and contact with the flange encourages let-downs. Spread the first few drops of milk over the skin in contact with the flange so it slides over the skin easily. Don't press the flange too tightly against your breast as this could obstruct the underlying milk ducts or reservoirs. Aim to start your milk letting down before you begin using the pump, by gently and rhythmically massaging your breast and by hand-expressing. Massaging your breast while pumping aids milk flow and encourages further let-downs.

Change to the other breast when the milk flow diminishes or stops. You can change from one breast to the other several times during a pumping session, just as you would when hand-expressing, or with your baby at the breast. At first you may collect only very small amounts of milk – perhaps only 7–8 ml (¼ fl oz, or one and a half teaspoonfuls). It's a good idea to finish a pumping session by hand-expressing the last little bit of milk, as this will produce the richest milk, especially in the first breast.

You'll need to use the pump at least as often as a baby this age would generally want a feed, because pumping isn't as effective as a baby at stimulating your milk supply. Four-hourly is rarely enough – it's better to aim for a minimum of eight to ten sessions a day (meaning two-to-three-hourly). As long as your nipples don't become sore, you should be able to increase your milk supply by pumping more often and for longer each time, as the increased stimulation will boost your prolactin.

Ideally, pump both breasts at the same time, as this saves time and produces more milk.

Women often use pumps unnecessarily, especially in hospital. This is because the pumps are there, because intervention in nature's process is attractive to those who don't understand how breastfeeding works, and because many women have learned a poor breastfeeding technique. If your baby can breastfeed, this is far better for both of you.

Many babies given bottles of formula soon refuse to breastfeed because they've learn to bottle-suck, which is easier than taking milk from the breast. If a mother then pumps her milk and gives it by bottle, it makes the situation worse. If your baby finds it hard to take milk from the breast, but is mature enough and well enough to swallow, give it from a cup and keep trying the breast as well, or use a supplementer (page 302) as you breastfeed.

Only rarely is it necessary to stop breastfeeding temporarily because of nipple soreness or cracking but, if you have to, it's less painful to hand-express milk than use a pump.

Hand pumps

The cheapest and simplest of these are also known as 'breast relievers' and consist of a plastic or glass container with a rubber bulb that produces suction. The milk you collect is likely to contain large amounts of bacteria because a rubber bulb inevitably retains some milk and is difficult to clean; bacteria thrive on the milk residue and contaminate the next milk collected. Such pumps are also not particularly effective, compared with hand expression, at removing milk from the breast. You can buy hand pumps of varying efficiency from pharmacies and by mail order.

Electric pumps

In general, the larger the pump, the quicker it builds up suction (vacuum). The price reflects a pump's sturdiness and quality of engineering. Some women find that pumping with a large pump is the fastest way of obtaining milk.

Electric pumps are available for hire or loan from some hospital maternity and special care baby units, and some breastfeeding self-help groups. You can also buy them from medical supply houses and some pharmacies, and by mail order.

USING A SUPPLEMENTER

This device can be very useful but is plagued by having several names, as it's also known as a nursing supplementer, a nursing trainer, a supplemental supply line and a nursing system.

It enables a breastfeeding baby to get milk directly from the breast, plus, at the same time, either expressed breast milk, donated milk (from a milk bank) or formula, from a bag or a bottle. The Lact-Aid Nursing Trainer bag has a fine flexible plastic tube coming from it. You fill the bag with milk, hang it around your neck, then tape a tube to your breast so its free end protrudes just a little beyond the nipple and enters your baby's mouth when he breastfeeds. When he's finished that side, you tape the tube to your other breast. With the Medela supplementary nursing system, you hang the bottle around your neck and tape one tube to each breast.

It's useful for:

- Teaching a baby who's used to bottle-feeding to suck effectively at the breast.
- Giving a larger feed to a preterm baby who hasn't the energy to suck for long; you express your milk between and after feeds and put this in the bottle.
- Supplementing your adopted baby's breastfeeds with formula.
- Avoiding the need for a bottle so the baby doesn't learn to 'bottle-suck'.

You can buy a supplementer (see page 417), but some women who need to use one for only a short time make one of their own. If you'd like to try, you need some very thin, flexible plastic tubing (as used for naso-gastric tubes in special care baby units); number 5 French size tubing is fine for full-term babies, number 8 for babies with a cleft palate, and number 3 for preterm babies. Take a bottle and teat, make a hole in the teat and push the tubing through. Put some of your milk in the bottle, hang it upside down around your neck and tape the free end of the tube to your breast so the end is at your nipple.

Be sure to sterilize everything thoroughly after a feed.

MILK BANKS

Women with milk to spare can supply it to a breast milk bank. Donated milk can be transported from milk banks by road or rail to preterm or sick babies in other hospitals.

Babies whose own mothers aren't feeding them and who may particularly benefit from donated milk include very low-birthweight preterms in their first week of life (as they tolerate donated milk better than preterm formula), babies who aren't growing and thriving, those who've had bowel surgery, those who have a poorly functioning immune system, and certain older babies with diarrhoea and other bowel symptoms from severe food intolerance.

Donor mothers are carefully screened by asking about their medical history and drug intake, and doing blood tests. A donor should not have a current medical condition requiring medication, nor a family history of tuberculosis (TB) or Creutzfeldt-Jakob disease (CJD). She shouldn't ever have taken growth hormone. And she shouldn't have been vaccinated recently. If a woman is taking any drugs – including aspirin, herbal remedies and the Pill – her milk may be unacceptable (though certain drugs, for example insulin, or those in asthma inhalers, are all right). And she shouldn't be a smoker, drink more than a small amount of alcohol, or drink an excessive number of caffeine-containing drinks each day. She'll be tested for HIV 1 and 2, hepatitis B and C, human T-cell leukaemia viruses (HTLV 1 and 2), and syphilis.

If screening is satisfactory, the woman receives detailed instructions about how to collect, store and transport her milk; this is then cultured to make sure its bacteria count is low enough, heat-treated/sterilized/pasteurized at 62.5°C (144.5°F) for thirty minutes (if following UK milk banking guidelines) to kill as many disease-causing bacteria and viruses as possible (including cytomegaloviruses and HIV that hasn't shown up in blood tests), and then frozen for up to six months.

Ideally, breast milk should not be heat-treated (pasteurized) at all, as this destroys live cells. However, heating it to temperatures lower than 62.5°C (144.5°F) may not kill certain bacteria, for example, those that cause tuberculosis. It also destroys lipase; babies fed heat-treated breast milk gain less weight than those given raw milk, as lipase acts to help absorb fat.

Another problem is that donated milk is often 'drip' milk – milk that drips from one breast while the donor's baby feeds from the other. And drip milk is low in fat anyway, containing only two-thirds of the calories of expressed milk. However, donated breast milk has helped save the lives of many sick or tiny babies whose own mothers could not or would not feed them themselves.

If you have milk to spare and want to donate it, your doctor or midwife (or, in the UK, health visitor), or the staff at the nearest hospital that has a special care baby unit, will advise you what to do.

The addresses for more information about milk banks can be found on page 417.

In some countries women are paid to donate spare breast milk to milk banks. One woman in Norway was recently reported to be providing up to 11 litres (over 19 pints) of milk a week (whereas a typical donor might provide up to 2 litres – 3½ pints), and being paid £11 per litre.

THE BABY WITH TEETH

Some babies are born with one or two teeth, though most don't get their first tooth until six months. There's no reason why teeth should interfere with breastfeeding, as the gums aren't used for feeding – the pressure comes from the tongue below and the palate above.

Whether or not your baby has any teeth, he may try the odd bite when he's around six months or older, and he will be very interested if you make a big fuss. Say 'no' firmly and gently take him off the breast. If you smile, he may think you like it and do it again! A few babies think it's a good game.

Some babies bite only towards the end of a feed. You'll get to know when he's about to bite, so take him off the breast before he starts.

Some babies bite from frustration if the breast is too full or there isn't enough milk, in which case just deal with the underlying problem.

> Managing common problems with breastfeeding can be both challenging and rewarding. The same applies when managing the special situations discussed in the next chapter.

TWELVE

Some special situations

If you find yourself having to manage mothering and breastfeeding a newborn while facing a special situation, you'll need good information and practical support, not to mention plenty of tender loving care. Remember, you're doing a very important job.

TWINS OR MORE

Two babies stimulate the breasts twice as much as one, so you'll automatically make more milk. Many mothers breastfeed twins successfully for as long as they want, without giving either of them formula feeds or top-ups. It may help to bear in mind that the average healthy woman with a normal milk supply can completely nourish her baby from one breast only.

At first it's easiest to feed each twin separately, but to save time later it's worth learning the knack of feeding them both at once. This said, there'll always be times when you'll enjoy the luxury of feeding them individually.

You can feed them together in one of several positions. The easiest is probably to hold each one in the 'football' hold. Or you could hold one in the conventional position, while the other lies facing the same way at the other breast, parallel to him, with you supporting his head with your hand. Another idea is to have both babies in the conventional position, with one lying across the other.

Position each baby carefully and check they are well latched on, as your nipples are more likely to become sore if they drag on the breast. Once you get used to feeding them both, you'll find it works well.

Should you wake the second baby for a feed every time the first one wakes? The answer is 'yes' if you want to save time, and 'no' if you'd like the occasional chance to suckle one at a time. If you're at all unhappy about the adequacy of your milk supply, always wake the second baby and feed them both.

How about alternating the breast each twin feeds from? The usual advice is that this is advisable, so the twin that sucks more strongly stimulates each breast alternately. However, each new-born animal in a litter usually chooses a nipple and keeps to it, so it's possible that human babies might prefer to do the same. Certainly in the first few weeks, if you always feed one baby from one breast and the other from the other, and if one sucks more strongly and so drinks more each time, you'll find your breasts became rather lopsided. Almost all women say their breasts become more equal in size once their milk supply is established.

Many mothers have successfully breastfed triplets, though sometimes formula is necessary as well, especially early on. However many babies you have, it's good if you can provide at least some milk for each one.

Mothers of 'multiples' say that the more support and encouragement they have while breastfeeding, the better. So don't be shy to ask for as much as you need, and to be clear about exactly what you'd like done to help.

The Twins and Multiple Births Association (TAMBA) in the UK, telephone (in the UK) 0870 770 3305, or visit www.tamba.org.uk, offers information about breastfeeding, details of support groups, and telephone support for mothers of twins or more.

Last but by no means least, take as much care of yourself as you can. For example, you'll need plenty of good food to eat and plenty of rest.

- Research in the Gambia (1986) found that all the women studied were able to feed their twins successfully.

BABY ILL OR IN HOSPITAL

A sick baby needs the very best nutrition available. He also needs the comfort of being at his mother's breast. Unless your baby is so ill or immature that he can't have milk at all, he'll do better with your milk than with any other. He'll also recover more quickly after an illness such as gastro-enteritis if he doesn't have to cope with the stress of digesting formula. If your baby has a respiratory illness, with difficulty in breathing, breastfeeding is easier than bottle-feeding (a bottle-fed baby tends to breathe in a more gasping fashion between swallows).

If your baby has to go into hospital, it's best if you go too so you can comfort and feed him. If you can spend only the day with him, leave expressed or pumped milk for the nurses to give from a cup at night.

If you can visit only infrequently, you may need to bring enough milk to last for several days. It calls for real patience to express or pump your breasts frequently (more often than your baby usually feeds) day after day. However, it can be done and is easiest if you hire or buy an electric breast pump.

BABY JAUNDICED

In the first few weeks of life there are many causes of jaundice (a yellow skin colour caused by high levels of bilirubin). These range from the normal 'physiological' jaundice seen in many babies, both breast- and bottle-fed, to abnormal jaundice from conditions such as bowel obstruction, infection, a congenital defect, drugs, an underactive thyroid, maternal diabetes and blood group (ABO or rhesus) incompatibility. Abnormal jaundice can be serious if not treated properly. The diagnosis depends on the time of onset of the jaundice and on blood tests.

Only a few full-term jaundiced babies need treatment; whether this is necessary depends on the type of jaundice and the bilirubin level.

Babies with a moderately raised bilirubin level for whatever reason are often treated with phototherapy (light therapy). They are placed naked for short times in a cot 41 cm (16 inches) beneath a strong blue light, with their eyes covered with a mask or coloured perspex shade. Some hospitals place babies on special blankets that emit blue light. The light changes the shape of the bilirubin molecules in the blood, allowing the body to eliminate them. Light therapy may hinder frequent and unrestricted breast-feeding, but if the nurses agree, you can take your baby from under the light when you want to feed him.

If your baby is otherwise well, the paediatrician may agree to your taking him home and giving him daylight phototherapy. Do this by placing him naked in a cot or somewhere else safe by a window in strong daylight. Ask how long he should be exposed; beware of sunburn and don't let him get too cold or too hot. You'll have to take him to hospital for blood tests to monitor the bilirubin level. The advantage of being at home is that you can breastfeed much more easily.

Preterm babies are affected adversely by lower raised levels of bilirubin than are full-term babies, so any treatment must be started sooner.

Physiological jaundice

This follows the normal breakdown of red blood cells in a newborn baby, appears on the second to fourth day of life, and usually disappears by about a week. It's more common in breastfed babies and there's no evidence that it causes long-term problems.

This early-onset jaundice is less likely in babies breastfed soon after birth and on a frequent and unrestricted basis, but the fewer feeds a baby has, the more likely he is to have jaundice. All that many physiologically jaundiced babies need is more breast milk. You can arrange this by feeding more often and for longer so as to increase your milk supply. One expert says ten to twelve breastfeeds a day is the minimum number for reducing the risk of jaundice.

Colostrum helps a baby's bowel get rid of meconium – the first bowel motions, which contain a lot of bilirubin. If meconium isn't excreted quickly it can be reabsorbed into the bloodstream. Frequent breastfeeds help get rid of it more quickly.

Studies show that giving an infant water isn't helpful and may interfere with his mother's milk supply. This is because he'll want fewer breastfeeds if his tummy is full with water.

Breast-milk jaundice

Some healthy breastfeds become jaundiced a little later, towards the end of the first week of life. One or two in every hundred breastfed babies develop this 'breast-milk jaundice'. It is worst during the second to third week and lasts from four to sixteen weeks.

Most paediatricians aren't too concerned about bilirubin levels below 20 mg per decilitre of blood (mg/dl). And although higher levels from other sorts of jaundice can damage a baby's brain, such damage has never yet been attributed to breast-milk jaundice. Indeed, there's considerable evidence that breast-milk jaundice has no serious long-term effects.

However if, as occasionally happens, the bilirubin level rises to 20 mg/dl or above, many paediatricans prefer to be cautious and suggest a woman does one of two things:

1 Stop breastfeeding for a while (the time recommended varies between twelve and forty-eight hours, but you may like to start off with twelve and extend the time if necessary). If this happens to you and your baby, keep your milk supply going by expressing or pumping more frequently than you would have fed the baby, and discard the milk until you can breastfeed again. Meanwhile, your baby can have donated breast milk or formula from a cup, rather than a bottle. This works because something in your milk must have

made him jaundiced, but another woman's milk won't have the same effect. His bilirubin level will fall significantly and you can then resume breastfeeding. The bilirubin then usually rises slightly before falling slowly and steadily. If it were to rise significantly again, interrupt breastfeeding once more. If it doesn't fall significantly after a short break, extend the break by six to twelve hours; the hospital staff will measure the bilirubin every four to six hours. If the level rises during the breaks from breastfeeding, the jaundice isn't due to breast milk.

2. Carry on breastfeeding but at the same time dilute your milk by giving donated milk (from a milk bank) or formula via a supplementer (page 302). If you do this, be sure to empty your breasts after each feed by expressing, because your baby may feed for a shorter time as he'll also be getting milk from the supplementer. The bilirubin will fall more slowly than if you'd interrupted breastfeeding, but it'll be more comfortable for you and will allow your baby to go on getting some of your milk.

The cause of breast-milk jaundice isn't clear. One theory is that it's due to a chemical in milk which interferes with bilirubin metabolism. Another is that it is caused by high levels of fat-splitting enzymes (lipases) in milk which break down fat and release fatty acids which then inhibit the normal breakdown of bilirubin.

Abnormal jaundice

Babies with abnormal jaundice look yellow at birth or within twenty-four hours. Whatever treatment is necessary, they need early, frequent and unrestricted breastfeeds for the reasons outlined above.

DIARRHOEA

Breastfed babies are very much less likely than bottle-feds to get a bowel infection, but if they do, studies show it's better and safer to carry on breastfeeding. Babies who stop are five times more likely to become dehydrated than those who continue. If your baby is severely ill he may need to drink a solution containing oral rehydration salts from a cup, as well as to go on breastfeeding. Even if a baby becomes so dehydrated that he needs intravenous fluids, he can continue to breastfeed. Only extremely rarely must such a baby stop breastfeeding.

BABY WITH LOW BLOOD SUGAR (HYPOGLYCAEMIA)

Breastfeed your baby as soon as possible after birth, then on an unrestricted basis – with frequent feeds to help keep the level of sugar (glucose) in his blood within normal limits. Blood sugar provides his cells with energy, and your milk is a good source of sugar and of the nutrients from which your baby can make sugar.

Quite a few preterm newborns develop low blood sugar as they adapt to having intermittent feeds instead of the continuous supply of nutrients, including sugar, that they received before birth via the umbilical cord. Very immature preterms can have difficulty in digesting any type of milk, but especially formula. This means the milk stays in the stomach for a long time, which delays the release of glucose and allows the blood-sugar level to fall.

Signs of low blood sugar include sweating, weakness, limpness, floppiness, disinterest in feeding, tiredness, a high-pitched or weak cry, blue lips, a rapid pulse, irritability and frequent juddering or shaking movements (jitteriness) – particularly when disturbed. Some babies have seizures (fits). And at worst the baby may go into a coma or his circulation may fail. If the blood sugar dips repeatedly or stays low for a long time (days rather than hours), his brain may be damaged. This is why doctors do blood-sugar tests on any baby who shows signs of low blood sugar or is likely to have a low level. Such a baby may also need other tests to find out whether an underlying condition (such as an infection) is responsible.

Definitions of low blood sugar vary; one definition is a level below 35 mg per decilitre (mg/dl) – 1.9 millimoles per litre (mmol/l) – of whole blood; however, some doctors are unconcerned if a full-term baby's level drops to 30 mg/dl (1.6 mmol/l), or a preterm or small-for-dates baby's to 20 mg/dl (1.1 mmol/l), as long as there are no symptoms. In one study of newborns with a level below 20 mg/dl but no symptoms, other than jitteriness, who continued breastfeeding, neurological tests some years later showed they had no problems.

Low blood sugar is unusual in healthy full-term normal-weight babies who feed frequently. Many experts consider that these babies need blood-sugar tests only if they have symptoms suggesting low blood sugar.

- A Danish study (2000) of 223 healthy breastfed full-term babies found that very few developed low blood sugar. The researchers said there is no reason for such babies to have routine blood-sugar tests.

Certain babies are more likely to have low blood sugar. They include those who are preterm or small for dates, have an infection, were short of oxygen during labour, have become chilled, had a delayed first breastfeed, are breastfed infrequently, or have been given sugar water (which causes a sudden rise in blood sugar followed by a sudden dip); and those whose mothers had pre-eclampsia, have diabetes, had an intravenous glucose drip in labour, or have taken certain drugs. Such babies need routine blood-sugar tests.

All these babies, including those preterms who are mature and well enough to have milk, should ideally have undiluted breast milk (preferably from their own mother), by tube, breast or cup, as soon as possible after birth. They need the milk frequently and on an unrestricted basis. If a mother isn't producing enough milk, then while she takes steps to increase her milk supply, her milk can be topped up with formula or donated breast milk. If she doesn't want to breastfeed, her baby can have formula. If necessary, sugar solution can be dripped into a baby's vein.

RHESUS ANTIBODIES

Some mothers who have rhesus antibodies in their blood and have a rhesus-positive baby worry that breastfeeding may pass the antibodies to the baby. Certainly a woman with rhesus antibodies in her blood has them in her milk too. However, they won't affect her baby because they are inactivated by his gut. So it's perfectly safe to breastfeed. Indeed, it's the best way to feed such babies, according to several studies. It's also safe to breastfeed after having an injection of anti-D immunoglobulin.

SUCKING AND MILKING PROBLEMS

A baby may be tired, jaundiced or full. There may be practical problems such as poor positioning at the breast, poorly protractile nipples or engorgement. Giving a breastfed baby one or more bottles of formula can play havoc with breastfeeding because he very easily learns to bottle-suck – which involves a different technique from breastfeeding – and may then find it difficult to breastfeed. Other reasons for poor sucking and milking include the effects of drugs given to the mother in labour, the after-effects of a poor oxygen supply in labour, and being born preterm.

Mechanical factors that can affect a baby's sucking and milking action include a large tongue, cleft lip, certain congenital abnormalities of the gums and jaws and severe tongue tie. A baby may have difficulty with swallowing for a variety of reasons, including cleft palate, inflammation following intubation for breathing difficulties at birth, and a small lower jaw. If swallowing is difficult, a baby milks the breast poorly too. Less common medical reasons for difficulty with breastfeeding include certain neurological and neuromuscular problems, and hypothyroidism.

Some of these conditions are relatively easy to treat, and the baby's sucking and milking action improves after treatment. Others improve spontaneously. But a baby with an untreatable or less easily treatable condition may need a lot of help to breastfeed.

The usual story of a baby with a poor sucking, milking or swallowing action, who fails to gain enough weight in spite of unrestricted breastfeeding, is that he wants the breast very frequently, sometimes hourly, or even more or less non-stop day and night. The mother may be tired out and desperate for help. Some babies aren't interested in feeding and sleep a great deal; they may even be 'happy to starve'.

Such a baby probably gets only the relatively low-calorie milk produced early in a feed from the first breast, because poor sucking and milking don't stimulate the breast to let down the later, higher-calorie milk. This means that although he has frequent feeds, he doesn't put on much weight. The lack of stimulation to let down milk eventually decreases milk production.

If there's no apparent reason for poor sucking and milking, if the cause is untreatable, or if it's been treated successfully yet your baby still has problems, try these ten steps to help him get your milk.

TEN STEPS TO HELP A BABY WHO BREASTFEEDS INEFFECTIVELY

1 Check your feeding position

2 Offer your nipple and areola 'attractively' – Soften your breast first if it's very full, by expressing a little milk; encourage your nipple to erect; put some of your milk on your nipple so your baby can smell it and taste it straight away; encourage your milk to let down before he feeds; consider using a supplementer so milk flows immediately when he's at the breast; and either hold your breast as if on a shelf, with your opposite hand supporting it from below, or use a cigarette hold to make a 'biscuit' of the nipple and areola in such a way that it's parallel with the baby's mouth. Some experienced counsellors say that 'shelf support' works best for babies with sucking and milking difficulties. Try gently touching your baby's lower lip with the nipple, and when he opens his mouth, draw him closer to the breast.

3 **Change sides as soon as he stops swallowing** during a feed (called switch-nursing, or the 'burp and switch technique'). This encourages him to suck better and stimulates the let-down. As you change him over, encourage him to wake, if he's sleepy, by burping him (bending him at the waist is a good way).

4 **Feed somewhere quiet** or try talking or singing to rouse him. Praise him after a good sucking session: even a very young baby may respond by doing it again.

5 **Experiment with his clothes** – See if he feeds better when firmly wrapped and warm, or when unwrapped and not too warm.

6 **Try feeding with you and him both naked** to see if the skin contact stimulates him to suck better.

7 **Rock or jiggle** him to arouse him, if necessary.

8 **Feed more frequently** – As your baby's sucking and milking improve by using the above steps, don't forget to wake him for feeds if he's in the habit of sleeping for long periods. Your milk supply needs stimulating, and it's no good getting him to suck properly if there's little milk for him because you haven't been feeding (or expressing or pumping) often

enough. While his improved sucking will in itself increase your milk supply, it needs to be combined with reasonably frequent, unrestricted feeds, with no long gaps. Aim at first for no more than two hours from the start of one to the start of the next during the day, and three hours at night, though if your baby wants more put him to the breast sooner. If your breasts feel tense between times, either express a little milk to soften them or wake your baby for a feed.

9 **Aim for realistic goals** – If your baby has been putting on no weight, then a gain of 60 g (2 oz) in the next week is very good. If he's been losing, then staying the same is excellent.

10 **Try a supplementer** (page 302) if you can't improve your baby's sucking and milking actions. Fill the container with milk you expressed or pumped after a previous feed. Your baby gets your milk both directly from your breast and from the supplementer. However, he'll get more of it, and he'll get it more quickly and easily. A supplementer is also useful if he needs extra milk immediately. If you can't produce enough to put in the supplementer, use formula or donated breast milk. At the same time you can increase your milk within a few days by expressing or pumping regularly and frequently. As a last resort, bottle-feed your baby with your expressed or pumped milk.

Tongue tie

The frenulum is the little central sheet of tissue between the root of the tongue and the floor of the mouth. In a few babies it is shorter (from top to bottom, with the baby upright), longer (from back to front), and thicker or tougher than usual. This can tether the tongue to the floor of the mouth so it's said to be 'tied'. You or your advisers may see that the tip of the baby's tongue can reach neither the upper nor the lower gums. The back of the tongue may roll forward over the gums because its tip is held back by the frenulum. This can make the leading edge appear notched, puckered or heart-shaped.

The problem, insofar as breastfeeding is concerned, is that the baby may not be able to push his tongue far enough forward to feed effectively. This means he holds the breast in his mouth between his upper and lower gums, instead of between his upper gums and his tongue. He may not be able to hold the breast in his mouth very well, and milk may dribble from the side of his mouth. He may also make a clucking noise as he tries to milk the breast. His mother is also more likely than other women to have sore or cracked nipples. And the ineffective sucking can lead to a poor milk supply and blocked ducts.

The best way of dealing with minor degrees of tongue tie is to be particularly careful over your breastfeeding technique. The odds are that your baby will manage, and the more practised he becomes at feeding, and the older he gets, the easier breastfeeding should be.

Tongue tie that causes continuing breastfeeding problems responds very well to minor surgery to cut the frenulum.

- A US study (2002) found that 127 of 3,036 breastfeeding babies (just over 4 per cent) had significant tongue tie. Seventy of these babies weren't latching on to the breast well, and fifty-three of the mothers had nipple pain. The mothers of 123 of the affected babies agreed to surgery. The poor latch improved in all cases, as did the nipple pain.

Cleft lip and/or palate

The initial shock and disappointment of discovering that your baby has a cleft lip, with or without a cleft palate, may make you reluctant to breastfeed. Once you get over this initial feeling, you may want to bear in mind that you virtually never see older children or adults walking around with a noticeable deformity of their lips. Plastic surgery is so good today that the defect can be almost perfectly repaired.

A cleft lip in itself needn't interfere with breastfeeding. Some milk may leak around the cleft but you'll soon learn how to mould your breast around the cleft. This way you can make a seal around the baby's lip (which you couldn't do with a bottle teat). Your baby will be able to suck (unless the cleft is exceptionally severe) and milk your breast. Prevent engorgement, and try not to let your breasts become too full, as both these conditions make it more difficult to form a seal around the baby's lip. If your breast is very full before a feed, soften it by expressing.

Many hospitals now repair cleft lips within two days of birth, though others wait the traditional three months or so. Early surgery is by far the best from the point of view of feeding. Not only does it make feeding easier for the baby but it also makes the mother more inclined to breastfeed.

Different surgeons advise waiting for different lengths of time before letting a baby suck after a cleft-lip repair. Because of the danger of the scar splitting some suggest waiting three to four weeks, others allow sucking at ten days, and some allow it immediately after surgery. From the breastfeeding mother's point of view, the sooner her baby starts feeding the better, though obviously the healing of the scar must take priority.

- Sixty out of one hundred babies resumed breastfeeding immediately after their operation in a survey reported in 1987. There were no complications and breastfed babies gained weight faster than those fed from a cup.

While you wait to resume breastfeeding after surgery, keep your milk supply going by frequent and regular expression or pumping. You can give your milk to your baby in a cup.

If the operation is postponed for several months, you'll need a lot of patience while breastfeeding, as babies with a cleft lip tend to take a long time over their feeds.

If your baby has a severely cleft lip and you find it impossible to breastfeed, give him your milk from a cup, a specially shaped spoon, or a bottle with an adapted teat. Ask your paediatrician about these.

A baby with a cleft *palate* can't suck well because he draws in air from his nose when he tries. Make up for the loss of suction by holding your nipple and areola in his mouth while he feeds. With practice he'll be able to suck and milk your breasts satisfactorily. You may find a supplementer useful while he's learning to milk your breast.

Milk can enter the nose of a baby with a cleft palate, but breast milk won't irritate the nasal lining, whereas formula might. Most mothers prefer to breastfeed in a relatively upright position to minimize the chance of milk going into their baby's nose.

Breastfeeding is associated with less otitis media than is bottle-feeding. This is good because babies with a cleft palate are particularly prone to ear infections.

- In 1994 researchers recommended breastfeeding cleft-palate babies for as much of the first year as possible.

An affected baby can use a plastic dental plate (feeding plate) until the cleft is repaired, usually after he's a year old. The plate is made with the help of impressions taken of his palate. It can be inserted as early as three days after birth (sometimes not until ten days) and not only helps him feed satisfactorily but also improves the shape of the dental arches. Some hospitals make plates routinely, others only for severe clefts.

LEARNING DIFFICULTY

There's every reason to breastfeed a baby with a learning difficulty. He'll gain the same benefits as any other baby and it will help your relationship to develop.

Many mothers feel such babies deserve every possible chance in life and consider, rightly, that breastfeeding gives the best start.

Like your baby, you will need plenty of encouragement and

support as you learn to breastfeed, so ask the hospital staff and your family and friends for as much as you need.

Down's syndrome

One mother of a baby with Down's syndrome commented, 'I'm sure that breastfeeding and the closeness that came with it helped me to love and accept him just as he was.'

These special babies are particularly prone to infections, especially respiratory infections, so the protection provided by breast milk is very valuable.

Some feed slowly, weakly or with little interest, because of muscle weakness, a poor sucking reflex or sleepiness. However, bottle-feeding would be just as time-consuming. With patience you're highly likely to succeed with breastfeeding and you'll be sure you're doing the best for your baby. Just as with any baby, avoid using a bottle, because learning to bottle-suck interferes with learning to breastfeed. If your baby is too tired to suck for long, express some milk and give it from a cup. You may need to encourage him to suck by giving him lots of skin contact, encouraging your milk to let down before you put him to the breast, and expressing a few drops of milk into his mouth. Feed him before he has to cry, to avoid tiring him. If he's so sleepy that he doesn't wake very often, wake him for a feed every two hours or so if necessary during the day, and every three hours at night.

NEUROLOGICAL OR NEUROMUSCULAR CONDITIONS

These babies include those with cerebral palsy, infantile spinal muscular atrophy, congenital muscular dystrophy, neonatal myasthenia gravis and infections of the central nervous system. Each causes feeding problems.

For example, a baby with cerebral palsy may sometimes arch

his back while feeding. Because of their condition, other babies may be apathetic during feeds or have problems with sucking (a poor sucking reflex, uncoordinated sucking, or poor sucking due to muscle weakness).

See page 315 for information on how to encourage such a baby to suck, milk and swallow more effectively, and while feeding remember to pay attention to the position of his whole body as well as his tongue, jaw and lips. It's well worth persevering because most such babies can breastfeed with enough help, and most become much better at it as time goes by.

BABY ISN'T THRIVING

The terms 'failure to thrive' or 'weight faltering' simply mean a baby isn't growing as he should. Each baby has to be assessed as an individual, but for practical purposes something may be wrong if a baby continues to lose weight after ten days of life, hasn't regained his birthweight by three weeks, gains at a very slow rate after the first month, or gains at an increasingly slow rate. There's particular reason for concern if he is also unhealthy.

There are many reasons why a breastfed baby may not grow as he should. He may not drink enough milk (most likely because of poor positioning at the breast, infrequent short feeds or poor sucking or swallowing). His mother may currently not be producing enough milk (because of poor technique, an unhealthy diet, illness or exhaustion). Or she may not be letting her milk down well (because her baby isn't positioned well, for psychosocial reasons, or because she's a heavy smoker or drinker or takes certain drugs). An unreliable let-down reflex eventually leads to poor milk production. It's vital to check whether you need to correct poor positioning, improve your breastfeeding technique or increase your milk supply.

The baby may be losing nutrients (because of malabsorption, diarrhoea or vomiting), may have an infection (for example in his urine), or may have high energy needs (for example, a baby who is small for dates or who has a congenital heart disease) that aren't being met. Several of these problems may be combined, which is why a doctor needs to take a careful and complete medical, social and dietary history, examine the baby thoroughly, look at the mother's breasts, watch a feed and arrange lab tests.

BABY NEEDS AN ANAESTHETIC

If a baby needs an anaesthetic before an operation, US research (1994) concluded that breastfeeding could safely continue until up to three hours before.

RARE ILLNESSES WITH IMPLICATIONS FOR BREASTFEEDING

Galactosaemia is an inborn condition, caused by an enzyme deficiency, that can sometimes be fatal if the baby is not put on a diet free from lactose (milk sugar). There is no alternative but to wean your baby from the breast at once and give him a special lactose-free formula.

Certain other 'inborn errors of metabolism' can be diagnosed soon after birth. Phenylketonuria, for example, causes high blood level of phenylalanine, which can lead to brain damage and learning difficulties. Breast milk contains lower levels of this amino acid than does formula. Such a baby can be breastfed. Monitoring phenylalanine levels means that if they were to rise dangerously high, the baby could have a combination of breast milk and a special low-phenylalanine formula or, if necessary, this formula alone.

IMMUNIZATIONS

Just after your baby has his immunizations he may go off his milk and be more fussy than usual for about twenty-four hours. If your breasts are very full because he isn't sucking well, express a little milk every so often.

The five-in-one vaccine (diphtheria, pertussis/whooping cough, tetanus, polio and HiB – Haemophilus influenzae B) isn't affected by breastfeeding, and a breastfed baby can have it at the normal recommended times. The same applies to rubella, mumps, measles, yellow fever, cholera and typhoid vaccines.

MOTHER IS ILL

If you are acutely ill at home, and too unwell to have your baby by your bed, you'll need someone to look after you both and to bring the baby to you when he needs a feed. If you have to be in hospital, you may be able to take him with you, but this will depend on what's wrong with you and on the hospital's facilities. If you can't have your baby with you in hospital, see if someone can bring him to you for feeds. This entails a lot of work and commitment, and means you'll need to be in a hospital close to your home.

Another way of continuing to breastfeed if you're in hospital is to express or pump milk and send it home for your baby. It should be stored in a fridge and collected by a friend or relative for the baby to have from a cup.

A few illnesses rule out breastfeeding. Others do so temporarily because of the drugs needed. If you have a long-standing illness such as severe asthma or kidney disease, you may feel so tired and run down that you won't be able to face breastfeeding. However, some mothers find that breastfeeding makes them rest and tires them less than bottle-feeding would.

DIABETES

Diabetes affects about 3 per cent of the population and can run in families. Breastfeeding for at least nine to twelve months reduces the risk of a baby with a family history of diabetes getting it himself one day.

- In one US study of seventeen breastfeeding mothers with type 1 diabetes, all breastfed successfully, and fourteen breastfed for more than nine months. Several tips came out of their experiences, particularly that high motivation and support from family, friends and health professionals were important.

A mother with diabetes whose baby goes into a special care unit after delivery needs to be particularly sure to breastfeed, or express or pump her milk frequently, since establishing her milk supply early on will help her to balance her dietary needs and her insulin dose. After about five to seven hours – whether or not she breastfeeds – she'll have an increased risk of a low blood-sugar level (since the loss of placental lactogen hormone is associated with temporarily increased sensitivity to insulin), but balancing diet, insulin dosage and, when she's up and about again, exercise, stabilizes her blood sugar.

Most women need less insulin in the first four to six weeks after childbirth than before they were pregnant. Some, however, need more insulin in the first three months, probably because they eat more and exercise less.

If their blood sugar falls because they've used too much insulin, this releases adrenalin, which decreases the blood flow in their breasts and can also inhibit the let-down reflex. Traces of insulin and adrenalin pass into milk but are largely inactivated by digestive enzymes in the baby's stomach. Any minute amounts of insulin that enter the baby's bloodstream simply mean he temporarily produces a little less of his own.

Infections are more common in women with diabetes, and any

antibiotics taken must be safe for the baby. Women who have diabetes should particularly watch out for thrush.

Any breastfed baby may sometimes want more or less milk, perhaps because they are having a growth spurt. A change in the amount of milk a mother with diabetes needs to make can make her blood sugar unexpectedly dip or rise, in which case she must compensate by adjusting her diet, exercise and insulin.

Some women find their diabetes is more stable when they are breastfeeding than it was before.

- One study (1993) found that if a woman had pregnancy diabetes, breastfeeding helped reduce or delay her risk of developing type 2 diabetes in the future.

INFECTIONS

Several infections can produce temporary breastfeeding problems, but in no case is it necessary to dry up your milk.

If it's advisable for your baby not to breastfeed or to have your expressed or pumped milk, keep your supply going by frequent expression or pumping, and discard the milk. This prevents engorgement. Once your baby is allowed breast milk again, you'll then have plenty of milk.

Herpes simplex

This viral infection can cause 'cold sores' (usually on the lips but sometimes in the mouth or on the breasts) or a genital infection in mothers. It can be very serious for newborn babies. No one with a cold sore or a sore mouth from a herpes infection should kiss a baby.

Women with herpes sores on the breast should not breastfeed and should discard their milk until the sores have healed and therefore aren't shedding viruses.

If there are no sores on the breast, experts simply recommend strict hygiene precautions, treating the infection and continuing to breastfeed. It's *extremely* unusual for breast milk to contain herpesviruses.

A few experts, however, advise a woman with a *first* herpes attack, especially of the genital area, not to breastfeed. This is because of the danger of a newborn baby becoming infected with viruses that are potentially very dangerous to him, as his immune system is vulnerable and breast milk hasn't yet had a chance to develop much anti-herpes protective activity. These experts also say there's more chance of developing a sore on the breast during a first attack.

A woman advised not to breastfeed can keep her milk supply going by frequent expression or pumping, but should discard the milk. Once the infection has cleared and she's no longer shedding viruses, she'll then have plenty of milk and can start to breastfeed. The anti–viral drug acyclovir has considerably brightened the outlook for treatment.

Hepatitis

Women who are carriers of hepatitis B viruses can breastfeed, as there is no evidence that this increases their baby's risk of the infection, especially if they receive hepatitis B vaccine and hepatitis B immune globulin soon after giving birth.

- Research (1995) reported in the *Lancet* suggested that on currently available evidence, it's safe for women who test positive for hepatitis C to breastfeed.

Tuberculosis

If you've had lung tuberculosis (TB) and have been free from the disease for two years, you can safely feed your baby.

If you've had active lung TB in pregnancy, with a positive tuberculin test, a positive chest X-ray and positive sputum or gastric washings, and if your treatment (with triple therapy: three drugs) was begun *at least a week before your baby was born*, you needn't be separated from him and can safely breastfeed *provided he is also treated with isoniazid*.

If you are bacteriologically negative, you can breastfeed even if you've only just begun treatment, provided he too is treated with isoniazid (in a smaller dose than for a baby whose mother is bacteriologically positive). It's important that your baby doesn't have too much isoniazid because he'll get some in your milk as well, and an overdose can cause nerve damage (peripheral neuritis). Some experts suggest monitoring a baby's liver function to make sure this doesn't happen. Because one of the commonly used drugs (para-aminosalicylic acid) isn't recommended for babies (as no one is sure how much gets into milk), a breastfeeding mother should have streptomycin or kanamycin instead. If other drugs are used, special precautions may be advisable.

If a breastfeeding mother contracts active, bacteriologically positive TB, separation from her baby may be recommended for safety while treatment begins and until cultures of her sputum and gastric washings are negative. If her milk isn't infected, it's reasonable for the baby to have expressed or pumped milk from a cup. Treatment usually makes a woman non-infectious in a very short time.

It could be argued that if a mother and baby have been together before the mother's TB was diagnosed, there's no point in separating them. However, because the complications of TB are more hazardous in newborn babies, it's worth taking every precaution to reduce a baby's risk of catching it.

In certain developing countries, and among certain other economically disadvantaged people, it's virtually always safer to leave a mother and her baby together, because breastfeeding is so much safer than bottle-feeding, given the lack of money for formula, the lack of clean water, fuel and other bottle-sterilizing necessities, and the high risk of infections. In such circumstances the risk of drug toxicity is relatively unimportant. These breastfed babies should be carefully treated with isoniazid, however, and vaccinated with a special type of BCG vaccine (isoniazid-resistant). The mother's active TB needs thorough treatment at the same time.

Gonorrhoea

If this is diagnosed at delivery, your baby shouldn't have your milk, or be with you, until twenty-four hours after treatment has begun.

HIV infection

Up to one in two of the 1.5 million HIV-positive children in the world acquired their infection from breastfeeding from an HIV-positive mother. However, the vast majority (85 per cent) of children breastfed by an HIV-positive mother do not become infected, possibly because breast milk contains anti-infective factors that protect the baby, the baby's gut isn't damaged by allergenic foreign proteins, and a hormone called erythropoietin may strengthen the lining of the breasts' blood vessels and milk glands and ducts, and so make the viruses less likely to enter her milk.

If a woman is HIV-positive, her decision whether to breastfeed needs to be based on the risks and benefits of breastfeeding to her baby, and the potential dangers of bottle-feeding.

In many industrialized countries, including Great Britain, the US, Canada, France and Australia, experts advise HIV(type 1)-positive women not to breastfeed, because they consider the risk to their babies of getting HIV infection to be greater than the risk of not being breastfed.

However, HIV-1-positive women almost certainly *should* breastfeed if they live in areas of developing countries in which many babies die because of diarrhoea, other infectious diseases and malnutrition. In such places, not being breastfed means a child has nearly six times the risk of dying from these conditions.

- A South African researcher (2002) said, 'The overwhelming majority of babies born to HIV-infected women, and all babies born to uninfected women, will benefit from exclusive breastfeeding for about six months'.

In resource-poor settings in certain developing countries, 20 per cent of the babies of HIV-positive mothers are born with HIV – some have acquired it in the womb, others during delivery. However, if the mother receives one dose of an anti-retroviral drug (for example, nevirapine) in labour, and the baby is given one dose immediately after birth, the proportion of infected babies falls to 12 per cent. The infection is more likely to progress to AIDS (acquired immune deficiency syndrome) if they aren't breastfed, partly because breast milk contains several anti-HIV factors.

It's probably wise for an HIV-positive breastfeeding woman living in such circumstances to breastfeed exclusively.

It's also wise for her to:

- Look after her general health, for example, by eating a healthy diet, so the infection is less likely to progress.
- Make sure her partner uses a condom for sex, since, if he's HIV-positive too, sex without a condom could increase her body's viral load.
- Have skilled support with breastfeeding so she avoids sore nipples and mastitis as far as possible.
- Avoid feeding from a cracked nipple or a breast with an abscess.
- Have anti-retroviral drug treatment. Her baby needs this too.

However, when her baby is six months old, she should consider stopping breastfeeding if he is not yet infected. This is because the benefits of breastfeeding after six months may not outweigh the potential risk of him becoming infected.

Heat-treating expressed breast milk to 62.5°C (144.5°F) for half an hour, or simply boiling the milk, reduces its HIV load, but it's challenging for a mother always to have to express her milk, and giving expressed milk means she also has the bother of sterilizing a cup or spoon.

The virus is more likely to be present in the milk of a woman who becomes infected during the time she breastfeeds than if she became HIV-positive before or during pregnancy.

An HIV-positive woman living in a developed country is best off being treated with several anti-retroviral drugs in pregnancy and afterwards, and having a caesarean section. The overall risk of her baby being infected is then 'only' 1–2 per cent. It's better for her to bottle-feed, unless she is prepared to take the risk of her baby becoming infected by her milk.

Because so few babies catch HIV (type 2) from their mothers, there are as yet no specific recommendations.

Syphilis

Infection of the skin on the breasts means a baby shouldn't breastfeed, but he may be able to have expressed or pumped milk.

Leprosy

A mother with leprosy should breastfeed, as breastfeeding is valuable enough to outweigh any possible dangers of contact. However, she may be advised not to hold her baby at other times. Both mother and baby can have drug treatment.

OSTEOPOROSIS

Women with osteoporosis can breastfeed if they want to and their condition isn't too painful. They may, like other women, experience a temporary loss of minerals from their bones during pregnancy and breastfeeding. However, bone density lost while breastfeeding is recovered afterwards.

When you breastfeed, sit comfortably and in a well-supported position. If possible, ask someone else to pass your baby to you so you avoid lifting.

Research suggests that breastfeeding helps reduce the long-term risk of osteoporosis, and it's possible, though unproven, that this means it may also be beneficial in the long term for women who already have the condition.

HIGH PROLACTIN

A high level of the hormone prolactin can be treated with a drug called bromocriptine. This dries up breast milk, but women with high prolactin have traditionally been advised not to breastfeed anyway. This is firstly because breastfeeding raises their prolactin level further; secondly, because there seems to be a higher risk of a breast abscess; and thirdly, because a sizeable proportion have a pituitary tumour (prolactinoma) and it's feared that raising their prolactin further could make the tumour bigger – which, in turn, could lead to visual disturbances, including blindness.

- However, Swedish research (1986) which followed thirty-eight women with such a tumour concluded that it's safe to stop taking bromocriptine during pregnancy and while breastfeeding, provided a woman has had at least a year of treatment before pregnancy and has monthly prolactin tests and visual-field measurements so she can start taking bromocriptine again at the first suspicion of any increase in tumour size. Eight out of ten women in this survey breastfed successfully for up to two years.

AFTER A CAESAR

Many babies today are born by caesarean section (more than half in some US hospitals). There's no reason why you shouldn't breastfeed afterwards, but you'll need to be determined early on. You'll face two main challenges. First, your tummy will be tender. Second, you'll find it uncomfortable to feed in the normal sitting position with your baby on your lap, so you'll need to choose a position in which his weight isn't on your tummy and your abdominal muscles aren't strained by holding him to your breast.

Enlist the help of a nurse to position him next to you as you lie on one side in bed. When the time comes to change breasts, ring for the nurse to help you turn over and change the baby to your other side.

If you have a horizontal scar, you could also try sitting up, with your baby propped up on a pillow at your side, his head facing your breast, and his legs tucked under your arm on that side – so he isn't on your tummy. Alternatively, sit up straight (to avoid straining your abdomen), lie him on a pillow at your side with his legs across your thighs, and support his head either with another pillow or with your arm (itself supported by a pillow).

Unrestricted breastfeeds are just as important for you as for any other mother who wants to produce a good milk supply, so feed your baby frequently by day and night. It's just as easy to breastfeed as to express or pump your milk, and you're less likely to become engorged or get sore nipples if you feed like this from the beginning.

- A study in South Australia (2003) found that by the sixth day after birth, only one in five breastfed babies born by caesarean had regained their birthweight, compared with two in five breastfeds born vaginally. However, by then all were getting similar amounts of milk. So the slow start was unlikely to last long.

If you've had a general anaesthetic you may not be able to breastfeed immediately after delivery, but as soon as you are awake or well enough ask for your baby to be brought to you, even if he's asleep. Most caesareans are now performed under epidural anaesthesia, which means breastfeeding can get started sooner.

If your baby is in an incubator after delivery and the nurses can't bring him to you for feeds, express or pump your colostrum (and your milk when it comes in). The nurses can then give the breast-milk feeds by tube or cup until you can go to him. Don't be alarmed by the small amounts of colostrum you produce – remember there isn't much in the first day or so.

A caesarean, especially if unplanned, can undermine a mother's opinion of herself as a woman, but breastfeeding may help her think well of herself again. Breastfeeding also helps postoperative recovery, because it produces oxytocin, which assists the womb to return to its former size. A caesarean leaves some mothers feeling very tired for some time, so it's important to get enough rest. This doesn't mean that nights must be unbroken, with your baby given a bottle by the nursing staff, but that between feeds the day shouldn't be crammed full of activity on the ward or at home. Allow ample time to sleep or catnap. Painkillers may be necessary, especially in the first day or two, because the scar can be painful while healing, especially when coughing.

By the end of the first week you should feel very much better, though it will take many months before you're back to normal.

PRE-ECLAMPSIA

Severe pre-eclampsia (previously called pre-eclamptic toxaemia) can cause several problems with breastfeeding. For example, the baby may be preterm or small for dates and need to be nursed in an incubator. And the mother may still be at risk of having an eclamptic fit and therefore need treatment (including blood-pressure-lowering drugs, sedation and bed rest in a darkened room). The good news is that most mothers recover within twenty-four to forty-eight hours after delivery.

If such a woman can't put her baby to the breast, or if early feeds are unsuccessful and stressful, she may be advised to express or pump her milk. Some doctors consider the stress of this too risky for a woman who may have a fit, but expert nursing care can help make it as easy and stress-free as possible. The discomfort of having engorged, unemptied breasts would anyway be considerable. Also, a mother may be more anxious, unless heavily sedated, if her baby isn't breastfed.

It's vital to check that a baby (especially if ill or preterm) doesn't become sedated by drinking milk containing phenobarbitone from his mother's medication, since this would hamper his ability to feed. If your doctor is reluctant for your baby to drink your milk because of its high drug levels, you or the nurses can keep your milk supply going by expressing or pumping until your medication level is reduced.

If you are too ill to breastfeed, or for you or the nurses to pump or express your breasts, you can always get your milk supply back later when you are well again.

BREASTFEEDING AFTER BREAST SURGERY

Some women have had a breast lump removed before they ever got pregnant; a few need a breast lump biopsied (sampled via a needle) or removed while breastfeeding. Others have had plastic surgery to make breasts larger or smaller. So what about breastfeeding?

Biopsy or removal of a lump before breastfeeding

If you have to have a lump biopsied or removed, and there's any chance you might one day want to breastfeed, have a thorough discussion with your surgeon first. As little breast tissue as possible should be removed, and the incision should sever as few milk ducts as possible. If the lump isn't easy to feel, your surgeon may localise it first with dye or a wire.

If you've had a biopsy, or a lump removed, you won't know whether you can breastfeed until you try. However, if – even with the best advice and support – you can't feed from the side that had the procedure, simply let the milk in that breast dry up (by not feeding from it and by expressing only the tiniest of amounts to stop it hurting). You're highly likely to be able to make all the milk your baby needs from the other breast.

Biopsy or removal of a lump during breastfeeding

Make sure your surgeon knows you are breastfeeding and wish to continue. Breastfeed your baby as close in time to the start of the operation as possible, and ask the nurses to bring him to you afterwards. They will also help you breastfeed from the other breast as soon as possible. Feed from the operated side as soon as you can; you may find it helps to press very gently over the dressing while you feed.

Breast-reduction surgery

You may be able to breastfeed if you've had surgery to make your breasts smaller. Whether you can breastfeed fully depends on how much glandular tissue was removed, how many milk ducts were cut, whether the cut ends of the ducts have managed to join up with open ducts so milk can get to the nipple, and whether the milk glands with intact ducts can produce enough milk.

In one type of operation, the nipple and areola are cut away completely before being transplanted higher up. In the other, they are left attached to some breast tissue so some ducts remain intact.

The longer between surgery and pregnancy, the more successful breastfeeding is likely to be. The only way to know whether you can breastfeed successfully is to try. Even if you manage to give your baby only a little milk each day, it's worth it for both of you. If you have to give formula as well, you can give it while breastfeeding, by using a supplementer (page 302).

- An Australian survey (1994) of thirty women who had a baby after a breast reduction found that of the 93 per cent who wished to breastfeed, 73 per cent were doing so when they left hospital and 27 per cent three months later (though only one woman was exclusively breastfeeding).

If you contemplate this operation before you have children, and think you might ever want to breastfeed, be sure your surgeon knows so he can leave as many milk ducts intact as possible.

Breast-enlargement surgery

Many women breastfeed successfully after having breast implants. However, this surgery can cause problems with breastfeeding.

- A US study (1996) found that 64 per cent of breastfeeding women had insufficient milk after having implants, compared with fewer than 7 per cent of breastfeeders who didn't have them. An incision around the areola was more likely than an incision beneath the breast to be associated with a poor milk supply.

The scare in 1994 about whether breastfed babies of mothers with silicone implants might develop a stiff gullet because of drinking silicone-containing milk from leaking implants has died down. Tests on breast milk from mothers with implants have not detected any silicone.

DRUGS IN BREAST MILK

Virtually every drug a mother takes passes into her milk, though some get through in much higher concentrations than others. Most drugs have such low known risks that breastfeeding is considered safe. However, a few are potentially harmful, either because of known side effects which affect adults as well, or because they have a different action in a baby, become concentrated in milk or aren't broken down by a young baby's body. Some drugs can cause a sensitivity or allergy which may be dangerous with repeated doses.

Knowledge of how some drugs affect breastfed babies is far from complete because of the difficulty in doing trials in breastfeeding mothers. It is clearly unacceptable to give healthy women drugs to see what happens to their babies. And the numbers of breastfeeding women who need any but the most common of drugs is very small. There's also the very real difficulty of measuring drug levels in milk.

Ideally, a breastfeeding mother should not take any drugs, medical or recreational. However, this is obviously the counsel of perfection and sometimes a drug is essential, even life-saving. If it happens to be dangerous for her baby, she'll have to wean, even if only temporarily. If any one drug isn't safe for a breastfed baby, there's often an alternative that is.

If you need any drug while breastfeeding, first remind your doctor that you are breastfeeding so he or she can check the safety of the drug to your baby if necessary.

Babies born preterm or small for dates, or who have jaundice or a liver or kidney problem, a family history of allergy, or a deficiency of the enzyme G6PD may be particularly susceptible to the adverse effects of certain drugs.

Rather than list the many drugs known to be safe for the breastfed infant, here is a list of those that are known to be either unsafe or better avoided by a breastfeeding mother. Their possible side effects *in her baby* are mentioned too. If you are concerned about a drug that isn't listed, check with your doctor that it's safe to take while breastfeeding.

Anti-infective drugs

Antibiotics can cause diarrhoea but other adverse effects are usually uncommon – though see the individual drug.

Chloramphenicol – This can cause sleepiness and vomiting, and theoretically could harm the bone marrow and lead to aplastic anaemia and a low white cell count. It is best avoided.

Ciprofloxacin – This is best avoided because there is concern that high concentrations in milk could affect a baby's joints.

Clindamycin – The concentrations in milk can be several times those in the woman's blood. It is best avoided because of the risk of bloody diarrhoea due to bowel inflammation.

Co-trimoxazole – This is better not taken in the first two weeks because of the risk of jaundice and a deficiency of folate ('folic acid', an important B vitamin).

Dapsone – This is probably best avoided as haemolytic anaemia has been reported.

Metronidazole – Only traces appear in breast milk, but there is risk of decreased appetite, vomiting and diarrhoea and a theoretical risk of cancer. High doses are not advised for breastfeeding women. One study suggests that if it's necessary for trichomonas infection, the woman should first collect and store enough expressed or pumped milk to last for a day, then take a single 2 g dose, discard her milk for the next twenty-four hours, and meanwhile give her baby the stored milk.

Nalidixic acid – One baby whose mother was also taking amylobarbitone developed haemolytic anaemia. It has also caused raised intracranial pressure. Use with caution only if absolutely necessary, and observe the baby carefully.

Nitrofurantoin – The level in breast milk is not significant, but it isn't advised for mothers of preterm babies or those with G6PD deficiency (a rare enzyme deficiency).

Novobiocin – Not recommended because of the possibility of causing jaundice.

Penicillins – These appear in trace amounts in breast milk and could, theoretically, cause allergic sensitization in a susceptible baby. They can also encourage thrush.

Sulphonamides – These can worsen jaundice and cause a rash. Haemolytic anaemia has been reported in one G6PD-deficient baby. Cautious use and careful observation have been suggested if the baby is under one month old; however, other experts recommend avoiding these drugs completely.

Tetracyclines – Theoretically these can cause mottling of a baby's developing teeth, though absorption from the milk in a baby's gut is poor. They are probably best avoided.

Anti-cancer drugs

Breastfeeding usually has to be abandoned (though methotrexate and busulphan seem to present little hazard).

Anticoagulants

Bleeding episodes have occurred after surgery or trauma in babies of mothers on anti-clotting medication; bleeding is more likely if the baby is deficient in vitamin K. Warfarin and heparin are suitable, but other drugs should be used with caution. The baby should benefit from a supplement of vitamin K.

Antithyroid drugs

Some have the rare side effect of causing a potentially fatal blood disorder, so the baby's development and blood count should be monitored. Iodides (also found in some cough medicines) can suppress a baby's thyroid (which may need to be treated with thyroxine), so his thyroid hormones should be monitored. Iodides can also sensitize a baby's thyroid to other drugs (lithium, chlorpromazine and methylxanthines). Propylthiouracil concentrates less in milk than does carbimazole; however, carbimazole can be used in doses of up to 30 mg a day.

Central nervous system drugs

Alcohol – Amounts large enough to make you tipsy can inhibit the let-down reflex and intoxicate your baby, perhaps making him sleepy. Very large amounts on a regular basis could cause brain damage.

Amantadine – Contraindicated, as it can cause vomiting, urinary retention and rashes.

Antidepressants – These may make a baby sleepy. No long-term safety data are available. A baby takes a long time to break down fluoxetine, so an alternative may be preferable. Tricyclic antidepressants are excreted in milk but not metabolized by a young baby, which theoretically could result in accumulation. However, no side effects have been reported, and it would seem safe for the breastfeeding mother to take them provided the dose isn't too high and her baby continues to thrive. Imipramine is probably preferable to amitriptyline for short-term use.

Anti-convulsants – These are mostly found in lower concentrations in milk than in the mother's blood. Experts recommend continuing breastfeeding. See individual drugs.

Anti-psychotics – These are present in small amounts in milk, and many are either unsuitable when breastfeeding, or mean a doctor has to check the baby regularly to make sure the drug isn't causing an adverse reaction.

Barbiturates – These can make a baby drowsy and lethargic, encouraging poor feeding and weight loss. They may also react with other drugs; one case of cyanosis (blueness) due to methaemoglobinaemia occurred in a baby whose mother was also taking phenytoin.

Bromide – This usually produces drowsiness and may cause a rash.

Cannabis – This can accumulate in a baby's body. Babies of marijuana-smoking mothers have been reported to have delayed motor development at one year. Avoid this drug.

Carbamazepine – No side effects have been reported in babies whose mothers take this drug on its own. However, it's not advised if used in high doses or with other anti-epileptics, as significant levels can build up.

Chloral hydrate can cause drowsiness.

Chloroform has been reported to cause deep sleep.

Chlorpromazine could cause drowsiness, so may be better avoided.

Diazepam – There has been one report of lethargy and weight loss. Levels may build up in the baby's body and increase physiological jaundice. High doses should be used only with caution.

Dichloralphenazone causes slight drowsiness.

Doxepin – An alternative antidepressant is preferable because of the risk of sedation and breathing problems.

Ethosuximide – Significant levels can build up in a breastfed baby. Poor sucking and over-excitability have been reported.

Heroin can cause addiction in babies when taken by their mothers in pregnancy. Breastfeeding and very gradual weaning is one way of withdrawing the drug from such a baby. However, the American Academy of Pediatrics recommends that heroin-addicted mothers should not breastfeed.

Lithium – If a mother takes this drug she should watch her baby and report any unusual signs, such as lethargy, floppiness or blueness, to her doctor.

Morphine – Significant amounts may be excreted in the milk of addicts.

Phenytoin – Many mothers on this have breastfed their babies safely. However, it has been associated with vomiting, tremors and rashes, as well as an idiosyncratic reaction of blueness due to methaemoglobinaemia.

Primidone – The high levels in breast milk can make a baby sleepy.

Sulpiride – This can be associated with adverse affects in a breastfed baby and is not recommended.

Hormones

Diethylstilboestrol – If a 'dry-up' dose is given but you change your mind and later decide you want to breastfeed, you can work up your milk supply again.

The Pill – The combined (oestrogen plus progestogen) Pill can suppress both the volume of milk and the duration of lactation quite markedly. Two studies have shown a decrease in protein, fat and minerals in milk. Small amounts of the synthetic steroids in the Pill also appear in the milk. Isolated reports exist of breast enlargement in male babies, proliferation of the vaginal epithelium in females, and changes in bones, though these all occurred with oral contraceptives containing higher doses of hormones than are now used. One unconfirmed study showed a correlation between prior use of the Pill and breast milk jaundice.

Many experts recommend the progestogen-only Pill for breast-feeding women.

Progestogen contraceptive implants/progesterone vaginal contraceptive ring – Studies suggest these have no adverse effects. However, the World Health Organization suggests not starting them until six weeks after childbirth.

Miscellaneous drugs

Allopurinol and oxipurinol – These enter breast milk in high concentration, meaning a baby risks the same side effects as his mother.

5-aminosalicylic acid (mesalazine) – This is considered safe but can cause diarrhoea.

Anti-diabetes (hypoglycaemic) drugs – Monitor the baby for low blood sugar.

Aspirin – This is best avoided because of the very small risk of rashes, gastrointestinal side effects or, if a baby has a blood-clotting disorder, jaundice and bleeding into the brain. There is also a small risk of potentially fatal brain and liver damage (Reye's syndrome).

Atropine is said to diminish milk flow and cause constipation and retention of urine in the baby, though there is no good documentation.

Beta blockers – Atenolol can slow a baby's heartbeat. Propanolol is preferable. However, while only small amounts of propranolol appear in milk, there is a theoretical possibility of accumulation in the baby, where the enzyme systems responsible for its metabolism are immature, so close observation for heart slowing or low blood sugar is necessary.

Bismuth (formerly used in some nipple creams). This should not be used.

Bromocriptine suppresses lactation. Prolactin levels fall within a few hours.

Caffeine – See page 207.

Cocaine – This can concentrate in breast milk and accumulate in the baby, so breastfeeding isn't advisable.

Digoxin – Two recent reports conclude that even if a mother is on a high dose, the amounts secreted in her milk are small.

Dihydrotachysterol – Animal studies show this encourages bone mineral loss. Some authorities advise against breastfeeding.

Diuretics – These can decrease the milk supply.

Ecstasy and MDMA – Breastfeeding is not advised because of a lack of studies.

Ergometrine lowers prolactin levels. It has been suggested that multiple doses might suppress lactation. In some obstetric units ergometrine is now given after delivery only if the uterus fails to contract and expel the placenta naturally (which often takes half an hour or so) or if there is post-partum bleeding from the uterus.

Ergot alkaloids – In one study 90 per cent of breastfed babies whose mothers took these had diarrhoea, vomiting, a weak pulse and unstable blood pressure. These drugs can also lower prolactin and therefore suppress lactation.

Fluoride can cause mottling of teeth.

Ginseng – There has been one report of a breastfed boy of a woman taking large amounts of Siberian ginseng developing pubic hair, a hairy forehead and swollen nipples; he returned to normal when he stopped breastfeeding.

Gold salts can cause rashes and a low white cell count, and are best avoided.

Indomethacin – There is one report of convulsions, so it's probably best avoided.

Laxatives may cause diarrhoea.

Lead – Lead toxicity (including encephalitis) has occurred after the historical use of lead acetate ointment on nipples.

Mercury – Mothers exposed to high levels should not breastfeed.

Nicotine may reduce the milk supply and interfere with the let-down. Breastfeeding mothers who are smokers are more likely than non-smokers to give up breastfeeding early. There is one report of restlessness and circulatory disturbance in a baby. It may also cause stomach ache, nausea, vomiting and diarrhoea.

Phenylbutazone – Take only if there's no alternative and report any unusual signs to a doctor because of the possibility of a blood dyscrasia.

Reserpine – There's been one report of significant nasal stuffiness, slowing of the heart, and an increase in tracheo-bronchial secretions.

Sulphasalazine – There is one report of bloody diarrhoea.

Vitamin B_6 (pyridoxine) – One study showed a decrease in milk supply with doses of over 100 mg a day. Supplements are often taken for premenstrual syndrome or postnatal depression, but this is inadvisable while breastfeeding.

Vitamin D – A high dose could theoretically cause a problem.

Radioactive drugs

Experts differ in their advice and recommendations have changed over the years. The following is a safe summary.

67Gallium citrate, 75Se-methionine, Sodium 32P phosphate, Chromic 32P phosphate – Significant amounts of these radioactive substances are excreted in milk. Different experts advise that breastfeeding should be interrupted and milk discarded for between seventy-two hours and two weeks. Ask if the nuclear medicine department at your hospital will measure your milk's radioactivity so you can return to breastfeeding as soon as possible.

Iodine isotopes – Radio-iodine studies of the thyroid should not be done in breastfeeding women. Hyperthyroidism and thyroiditis can reliably be diagnosed using pertechnetate (technetium 99m) imaging in combination with clinical criteria and plasma hormone levels.

99Tcm-pertechnate (technetium 99m) – Discard breast milk for twelve hours.

99Tcm-MAA – Discard breast milk for six hours.

99Tcm-DTPA, 99Tcm-EDTA, 99Tcm-MDP, 99Tcm-erythrocytes, 51Cr-EDTA and 111In-leucocytes – There's no need to stop breastfeeding, but some experts seek to reassure mothers alarmed by radioactivity to discard milk produced in the four hours after a test.

If you're advised to have any radioactive isotope investigation or treatment, discuss with your doctor whether there's an alternative – either not using an isotope at all, or using one which comes through into milk in small amounts.

If the interruption is to be short, plan ahead and store expressed or pumped milk in the fridge or freezer to be given to the baby during that time. While breastfeeding is interrupted, keep your milk supply going by expressing or pumping frequently and discarding the milk.

ENVIRONMENTAL CONTAMINANTS

Organochlorine pesticides (such as DDT, hexachlorobenzene, chlordane, dieldrin and heptachlor epoxide) are restricted in some countries and banned in others. These chemicals are fat-soluble and enter breast milk. Their concentration is highest in milk from mothers living in contaminated areas or eating contaminated produce. This makes their breastfed babies a special risk group. However, there's a lack of information on any side effects. And organochlorine levels in breast milk are declining in the UK. The World Health Organization continues to monitor the situation and to recommend tight controls over their use and the use of alternative, environmentally friendly measures.

Despite the need for vigilance, experts say that the advantages of breastfeeding far outweigh any risks for all except an extremely small minority of exposed babies.

Chlordane – This insecticide and its derivatives can enter breast milk, and the acceptable daily intake (ADI) is easily exceeded in contaminated areas. Its effects on breastfed babies are unknown, but chlordane and its derivatives persist in the body for at least five years. The intake for breastfed babies in the UK (1991) does not exceed the ADI.

DDT – Although DDT is present in breast milk in contaminated areas – and from mothers who smoke or have ever smoked (because DDT is used on some tobacco crops), no ill effects have been observed.

Dieldrin – The acceptable daily intake from breast milk is very easily exceeded in contaminated areas where some people consume up to twenty-two times the ADI! Also, Dutch research (1992) showed that the more often a woman ate meat and dairy produce, the higher were her milk levels of dieldrin.

Dioxins and furans – These are released by burning plastic made from PVC and wood treated with preservatives and are among the most toxic poisons known. They enter breast milk in industrially contaminated areas and it's been suggested that severe contamination of milk could lead to a bleeding disorder (late haemorrhagic disease of the newborn) due to vitamin K deficiency in young breastfeds.

Heptachlor – The acceptable daily intake (ADI) from breast milk is exceeded in every exposed baby, according to one study. Some intakes are up to seven times the ADI. Long-term exposure in animals can damage nerves, kidneys and immunity. The intake of breastfed babies in the UK (1991) does not exceed the ADI.

Hexachlorobenzene – Many infant deaths occurred in Turkey after mothers ate wheat treated with this fungicide. It is one of the most persistent organophosphates and the acceptable daily intake (ADI) from breast milk is easily exceeded in contaminated areas. Some intakes from the milk of exposed mothers contain up to forty-eight times the ADI.

PCBs (polychlorinated biphenyls) – The industrial use of PCBs is now banned in some countries and restricted to closed electrical systems in the European Union. The disposal of PCB-containing articles (such as transformers, capacitators and painted items) remains a problem. However, PCBs aren't thought to harm breast-fed babies and the levels in breast milk have only rarely (after unusual exposure) exceeded safe limits.

Thousands of drugs are available over the counter in the Western world. While most are perfectly safe in normal doses, talk to your doctor or pharmacist if you aren't sure what to do.

RESTARTING YOUR MILK SUPPLY (RELACTATION)

You may want to restart your milk supply days, weeks, months or even years after stopping feeding.

If your baby has been on formula for several weeks and your milk supply has dried up, start it up again by putting him to the breast frequently. He may be frustrated at first by feeding at an empty breast, partly because the shape of the nipple isn't such a strong stimulus to sucking as the shape of a rubber teat. You can try two things. Either let him have some formula from a bottle to satisfy his initial hunger, then let him feed from you. Or give him formula from a cup or spoon, so avoiding the stimulus of the rubber teat, then let him feed from you. Once you start to produce some milk, try to get your let-down working before putting your baby to the breast. You may also find a supplementer helpful (page 302).

After each feed, express or pump your breasts to encourage your milk supply to build up. Remember that the more often your baby breastfeeds, the more quickly your milk will reappear. After about two weeks you'll probably be producing enough milk to be able to do without formula.

The keynote to success is confidence. The experience of women all over the world is that their breasts are capable of producing milk again even after several years of being dry, *as long as they have enough stimulation.*

BREASTFEEDING AN ADOPTED BABY

Many women have fully breastfed adopted babies. Once your breasts have been prepared for lactation by a pregnancy, they always retain their ability to produce milk. If they've produced milk for any length of time, they'll be even more able to do so years later. This is why grandmothers in many parts of the world sometimes breastfeed their grandchildren.

All women can stimulate their milk production and build up their milk supply over time by putting their baby to the breast frequently, or by expressing or pumping their breasts. You can do this even if you've never had a baby – in which case it's called 'induced lactation' – though you'll have to persevere, and supplement your milk with other food. And you'll need a cooperative baby.

A woman who breastfeeds her own baby has had months of pregnancy for her breasts to prepare for breastfeeding. So you must expect to take a long time to prepare your breasts too. Start building up your milk supply at least six weeks before your baby arrives, by expressing or pumping at frequent intervals.

When the baby arrives, you'll probably need to give formula as well. However, some mothers have fed their adopted babies with breast milk from the baby's mother, from a breast milk bank or from a breastfeeding friend until their own milk became plentiful enough.

A supplementer (page 302) is a useful piece of equipment for relactating mothers. The original one was developed by a man for his wife who successfully built up her milk supply to feed their adopted baby.

How long will it take to build up your milk supply? It has been done within two weeks by mothers who weaned their own baby as long as six years before. It usually takes much longer. The pleasure it gives can far outweigh the difficulty involved, though be prepared for it to take some time.

In the next chapter we'll look at breastfeeding the older baby.

THIRTEEN

Feeding the older baby

Two practical issues for breastfeeding women are when to give their babies something other than breast milk and when to stop breastfeeding. First, though, let's clear up some confusion over the basic terminology.

The word 'weaning' comes from an old English word for 'accustoming'. Many people use it to mean weaning from the breast – gradually stopping breastfeeding as a baby gets used to other foods. However, it can also mean accustoming a baby to other foods while still breastfeeding.

When, how and why you start giving other foods, and when, how and why you stop breastfeeding, are up to you and your baby. However, a wealth of experience from other mothers, plus many years of scientific research, provide some useful guidelines.

INTRODUCING OTHER FOODS

The day you give your baby something other than your milk is an important milestone. Some babies take to it enthusiastically; others are less eager, especially at first.

When should you start solids?

Weaning foods are traditionally called 'solids', however runny they are.

The World Health Organization (WHO) recommended in 2001 that babies should have no foods or drink other than breast milk for their first six months. This means you shouldn't give formula either. In 2003, the UK Department of Health also recommended exclusive breastfeeding for six months, meaning no formula milk, other drinks, or solids until then.

Before these recommendations, quite a few mothers were giving solids before four months. For example, in a large survey in the UK in 2000,

- by six weeks 3 per cent of babies were on solids; by three months the figure had risen to 24 per cent; by four months, 85 per cent. By six months, 98 per cent were on solids; by nine months, 100 per cent.

However, it's better to wait until your baby is six months old before you start offering solids. Six months seems a natural time, because many babies allowed to decide for themselves when they want to start solids (by picking up pieces of food) don't begin until around then. This is also the time when many get their first tooth.

Before the WHO recommendation, quite a few mothers were giving formula before six months too. For example, in a large survey in the UK in 2000,

- 45 per cent of breastfed babies aged four to five months were receiving formula as well.

When's the latest to start?

Most babies benefit from starting solids at no later than eight or nine months old. A few, though, are satisfied and well nourished on breast milk alone for longer. (Indeed, studies in Africa and in Australia suggest that exclusive breastfeeding is adequate for some babies for as long as fifteen months.)

How to start solids

Many mothers start by spoon-feeding, or even, the first few times, by offering a little taste from their (washed) finger. Others wait until their baby picks up food for himself. If your baby likes it, give a little more.

When giving your baby anything other than root vegetables for the first time, don't give it again for four days, so you can see whether he develops any symptoms (such as diarrhoea, a runny nose or a rash) that could mean he's sensitive to it. This also gives him the chance to get used to each new taste.

After the first two or three weeks, you can give two or more foods in the same meal. However, some babies (like some adults) prefer foods to be kept separate.

Be sensitive to your baby's appetite and let him guide how much you give.

Spoon-feeding

Give your baby the breast first, then offer food in a spoon that has a fairly flat bowl. Put the laden spoon into his mouth, then gently withdraw it against his upper gum and lip so some of the food stays in his mouth. He may try to suck in some of the food from the spoon. End by giving another drink of milk from your breast. Choose a food that's soft enough to swallow easily. Babies start chewing at around six months, and as they become more used to it you can give them gradually more lumpy foods. However, the average baby doesn't become efficient at chewing for another month or so.

Finger foods

Some inquisitive six-month-olds like to investigate by grasping food from their mother's hand or plate. This is fine as long as it's suitable and not too hot. Good 'finger foods' to pick up and suck on, chew or bite include any raw fruit, such as a large piece of peeled apple, a rusk of baked wholemeal bread, or anything hard that won't be likely to break into pieces and choke him. He'll probably like the taste and will eat some of it by gradually dissolving it in his mouth.

Many babies love the new sensations involved in eating solids. They smack their lips and look for more at once. Others are taken by surprise, but a screwed-up face or a look of amazement doesn't necessarily mean your baby doesn't like the food, just that it's unfamiliar. Wait a moment, so he doesn't feel pressured, then try again. A lot of what goes in his mouth will probably come out again, but simply scoop this up gently from his chin with the spoon and try again.

WHAT TO GIVE

This is an up-to-date guide on what's suitable.

From four months at the very earliest – ideally not before six:

- Vegetables – avocado, broccoli, carrots or other root vegetables, cauliflower, courgette, squash.
- Grains without gluten – rice, corn (such as polenta), millet and other starchy carbohydrate foods, such as tapioca, sago.
- Fruit – apple, apricot, banana, pear.

From five months at the very earliest – ideally not before six:

- Chicken, turkey.

From six months:

- Dairy food – full-fat cows' milk, cheese, yoghurt.
- Other meats.
- Peas.
- Gluten-containing grain (wheat, barley, rye, oats) foods – for example, bread, baked bread rusks, breakfast cereal, flour-based sauce.

From eight months, add:

- Beans, tofu, lentils (if windiness at night stops your baby sleeping, avoid these at supper).

From nine months, add:

- Eggs – cooked well so the yolks are more digestible; raw or lightly

cooked eggs are unsuitable for under-ones because of the risk of salmonella infection.
- Fish.

From one year, add:
- Nuts and seeds – but don't give whole or chopped nuts, or whole seeds, to a child under five years old, as there's a small risk of inhalation.

You may want to purée a food for a baby who can't yet chew. Do this by mashing, pushing it through a sieve or mouli or whizzing it in an electric blender. Meat is one of the most difficult foods to chew, so finely chop it, or blend or mince it, until your baby is around ten months, when it may be all right simply cut up small.

To thin a savoury purée and make it easier to eat, add a little of one of these:

- Expressed breast milk (its familiar sweet flavour makes a new food more attractive).
- Water in which you've cooked vegetables.
- Water.
- Vegetable or chicken stock (previously frozen in an ice-cube tray and used cube by cube.

To make a sweet purée easier for your baby to eat, add a little of one of these:

- Expressed breast milk.
- Water in which you've cooked fruit.
- Water.

A healthy diet

At first your baby will still get nearly all his nourishment from your milk. This means you needn't worry about balancing his diet until he's eating more solids, and breast milk plays a less important role.

Go easy on added sugar, and avoid it for under-ones where possible. Sugar can encourage tooth decay and provides 'empty' calories, meaning it doesn't contribute worthwhile or irreplaceable nutrients. The intrinsic sugars in fruit, vegetables and milk often taste pleasantly sweet anyway. The occasional food containing added sugar won't hurt older babies. But it's wise not to give sweetened snacks or drinks between meals or at bedtime, unless you clean your baby's teeth and gums afterwards.

Avoid added salt as it can be dangerous for a baby if given in excess. Don't give your baby breakfast cereals containing added bran, as this could prevent iron, calcium and zinc being properly absorbed. It's also very filling, which could spoil his appetite.

Under-ones should not have unpasteurized honey, as there's a tiny risk of food poisoning from botulinum toxin.

Home-made or shop-made?

Many mothers like to give home-made food most of the time, often giving their baby whatever they are going to eat, perhaps mashed or sieved first. This is cheaper than commercial baby foods, and lets your baby get used to family food. If you cook food especially for your baby, it's convenient to freeze portions in ice-cube trays, so that you have something for when the family meals isn't suitable.

But up to 95 per cent of mothers in industrialized countries give their babies some commercially prepared foods, perhaps mainly when it's particularly convenient, for example, when out with their baby.

DRINKS

What drinks can your baby have? Under six months it's best to give only breast milk. However, as your baby grows older, you can start introducing other drinks. Remember, though, that giving more than the occasional drink could diminish your milk supply, so it isn't wise if you intend breastfeeding for a year or more.

Let's look at the various options.

Water

Your baby will do very well if you give him only water.

Fruit juice

For a change, try the juice of an orange, diluted with water or on its own. This is best given at mealtimes, as its vitamin C encourages iron absorption from other foods. Apple juice is a popular drink too.

Fruit juice is best not given between meals, or at bedtime, as its acid and sugar encourage tooth decay unless you clean your baby's teeth and gums afterwards. Fruit drinks contain added sugar or artificial sweeteners and are best avoided.

Fruit squashes or diluted syrups

Orange squash or blackcurrant syrup diluted with water are popular. However, syrups and most squashes contain a lot of sugar and, because they are sugary and slightly acidic, encourage tooth decay unless you clean your baby's teeth and gums afterwards. While some contain vitamin C, not all do and many contain no natural fruit juice at all.

Herbal baby drinks

These are popular, but even if they contain only a little sugar, they encourage tooth decay if given between meals or at bedtime – especially if given from a bottle. Such decay can occur even before the very first tooth shows through the gums. Dentists say fruit-containing herbal drinks are the worst culprits for damaging teeth. So clean your baby's teeth and gums afterwards.

Cows' milk

Does a baby need cows' milk during or after weaning? The answer is, it depends.

In developing countries, babies have traditionally been weaned on to a diet that doesn't include cows' milk. However, they tend to get the benefit of breast milk for far longer than infants in developed countries.

In many developed countries in which the traditional diet includes cows' milk and other dairy foods, women are used to incorporating milk into their family's diet. Indeed, most expect to give their babies cows' milk and might find it difficult, without extra information or help, to know how to ensure their baby gets a balanced diet, with enough fat and calcium particularly, without it.

Whether you give cows' milk depends partly on your baby's age, because if you stop breastfeeding before six months (the minimum recommended), you'll probably substitute your breast milk with cows' milk formula. You can carry on giving formula until your baby is a year old, or give 'follow-on' milk from six months to a year. Alternatively, give your baby full-cream cows' milk after six months if you find he can easily digest it.

Cows' milk is a good source of calcium and fat. Growing babies need more fat in their diet than do older children and adults, so giving your older baby some milk each day in addition to your family food readily fills this need. However, semi-skimmed milk is unsuitable for children under two years old, and skimmed milk is unsuitable for children under five years old.

HOW LONG TO GO ON BREASTFEEDING

In 2001 the World Health Organization recommended exclusive breastfeeding (meaning no other foods or drinks) for the first six months, and continued breastfeeding for up to two years or beyond. This recommendation is based on an enormous amount of research into babies' and mothers' health. In all, more than seventy countries worldwide now recommend exclusive breastfeeding for six months, and continued breastfeeding for a year or more beyond. These include the US, UK, Costa Rica, Brazil, Australia, Egypt, Kenya, India, Iran, Hong Kong, Mongolia, France and Bosnia.

For example, in 2000, the US Surgeon General recommended breastfeeding exclusively for the first six months, and continuing to breastfeed throughout the first year. Note that a Texan anthropologist who studied weaning times in different mammals thought it appropriate to breastfeed human babies for a minimum of two and a half years.

In 2003 the UK passed a resolution encouraging exclusive breastfeeding for six months and continued breastfeeding up to two years or beyond.

In 2003 Australia's National Health and Medical Research Council recommended exclusive breastfeeding for six months and continued breastfeeding up to one year or beyond.

In 2004 Health Canada was working on a draft resolution recommending exclusive breastfeeding for six months and continued breastfeeding up to two years or beyond.

Yet even if they advise women to breastfeed exclusively for six months and to carry on afterwards, many countries have a long way to go to meet WHO recommendations.

Here's the proportion of all mothers who are breastfeeding at six months in a selection of countries:

- UK (2000) – 21 per cent.
- US (2003) – 32 per cent.
- Australia (2001) – 48 per cent.
- Norway (2003) – 80 per cent.

Note, though, that the above figures aren't for exclusive breastfeeding.

- In the UK (2000) – probably only about 10 per cent of mothers breastfeed for six months without giving any formula.

Figures for 1995–2004 from UNICEF show the proportion of women who breastfed exclusively for at least three months:

- Middle East/North Africa – 9 per cent.
- Sub-Saharan Africa – 34 per cent.
- Latin America/Caribbean – 37 per cent.
- South Asia – 46 per cent.
- East Asia/Pacific – 57 per cent.

There's serious intention in many countries to improve on the figures.

For example, in 2004, the US Department of Health and Human Services' Office on Women's Health launched a campaign to increase the proportion of mothers starting to breastfeed to 75 per cent by 2010 (up from 70 per cent), and of those breastfeeding at six months to 50 per cent (up from 32 per cent). Particular help is needed for those who are least likely to carry on breastfeeding, for example, African Americans and women in low-income homes.

Australia has set itself high goals, with 2003 guidelines by the National Health and Medical Research Council recommending as important objectives that 90 per cent of babies should start off breastfed and 80 per cent should still be breastfed at six months.

- In Australia (2001) 23 per cent of babies were being breastfed at one year old and 1 per cent by two years.

Breastfeeding after six months

There are three major advantages to breastfeeding after six months:

1. Your baby goes on receiving protection against infection. This advantage continues to eight months in developed countries and for much longer in developing countries.
2. You and your baby probably enjoy feed times.
3. You may reduce your risk of pre-menopausal breast cancer and of ovarian cancer, rheumatoid arthritis and osteoporosis in later life.

How long will your milk supply last?

It'll last as long as you want, if breast milk is the major source of your baby's fluid intake. However, as soon as you give him meaningful amounts of other drinks, with only one or two breast-feeds a day, it will slowly dry up (though having said that, some women continue with only one feed a day for many months).

It isn't unusual for women who breastfeed into the second year to produce a pint (over half a litre) of milk a day. Wet nurses used to feed one baby after the other for years, and many mothers the world over feed their children or even their grandchildren for several years. The Western idea that milk automatically dries up after a few months is totally wrong.

Breastfeeding the older child

You can breastfeed your baby into his second year if you want, or until he is two, three or older. Breastfeeding an older child is more important for psychological comfort and pleasure than for nutritional reasons, since other foods almost always supply sufficient nourishment by then.

An older child may feed primarily to get off to sleep, or during the night for comfort. Or there may be little pattern to his feeds: he may come for a drink when he feels like cuddling and being close to his mother, perhaps when he's upset or tired.

You may notice a difficult patch between four and six months when you wonder whether you want to go on. You may be feeling much livelier in yourself and want to do more in the outside world. Your baby probably wants more attention and is more aware. He may want more to eat, and unless you give yourself time to increase your milk supply, you may feel you haven't got enough milk. Or you may have become disenchanted with breast-feeding, perhaps even feeling it's gone on for long enough.

If you've had enough, give up gradually. It's better to stop breastfeeding and continue developing a loving relationship with your baby than to resent feeding him.

If you continue breastfeeding as your baby passes his first birthday, your main challenge will probably be coping with criticism from friends, neighbours and relatives. Many will be surprised you are going on long after other mothers have stopped. This can be off-putting, but if you and your baby want to continue, it's up to you. To spare their amazement or your embarrassment, you may prefer to feed your older baby alone. It's scarcely surprising that a society that sometimes finds it hard to deal with the sight of a young baby being breastfed finds it even more difficult to cope with seeing an older one at the breast. If your child tugs your clothing, or asks for a feed when you are out visiting, go into another room to feed him if you prefer.

How long you go on is your personal choice. But however long it is, you'll know you've done your best for him, and it'll probably have given you a lot of pleasure too.

Breastfeeding during a period

Breastfeeding during a period won't harm you or your baby, though some women find their babies rather fractious around this time. This may be because they have premenstrual tension which their babies sense. Some babies have slight diarrhoea for a couple of days; others seem to dislike the taste of the milk (see page 32).

Changes in milk volume may occur during a period because of altered blood flow in the breasts.

Breastfeeding in pregnancy

You can breastfeed throughout your next pregnancy if you want, though some women find their breasts are more tender than usual.

Your milk may decrease, probably because pregnancy hormones affect milk production, but a month or so before your next baby is due it will automatically increase again.

Breastfeeding an older child as well as a baby

Carry on feeding your toddler when your new baby arrives if you want, but let your newborn have first call on your milk. Breastfeeding two children of different ages is called tandem nursing.

Researchers aren't yet sure whether mature milk made by pregnant breastfeeding women becomes enriched, when their next baby is born, by the extra antibodies, protein, zinc and other minerals, vitamins A, E, B_6 and B_{12} and live cells normally found in colostrum. However, it seems highly unlikely that a newborn baby would be at any disadvantage.

STOPPING BREASTFEEDING

Some women take a unilateral decision about when to stop; some take their cue from their baby, thus making a joint decision; others let their baby be the one to decide. Whoever decides, many women experience mixed feelings of loss and pleasure at moving on.

Baby-led weaning from the breast

'Baby-led' means letting your baby decide when he wants to stop. Some babies lose interest in the breast relatively soon, others want to go on much longer, and some don't want to give up at all.

Sudden baby-led weaning

Sometimes a happily and fully breastfed baby may suddenly refuse to feed. There may be an obvious reason, such as his nose being blocked by a cold, or teething, or an unpleasant experience (such as a loud noise) while at the breast. At other times there's no apparent cause. Nourish him by giving your expressed or pumped milk in a cup for the time being, but offer the breast before and after each cup feed. He may just be having a temporary nursing strike.

The easiest way

If you want – or have – to stop breastfeeding, it's easier to do it gradually. If you try to stop quickly, you may have a fractious baby and painful, engorged breasts. There's no place for drying-up pills.

1. Give up first the feed at which you have least milk. Most women find this is in the later afternoon or early evening. Give your baby something else to drink. If you have to wean early, remember that young babies benefit from sucking, so a bottle may be better than a cup.
2. After a week or so, give up another feed. Carry on cutting out one more feed every week or so until you are feeding only once a day. You may find it's most comfortable to give up the earliest morning feed last, as you'll probably have most milk then. But many mothers prefer to give up the final feed of the day last, as their babies enjoy this the most and sleep well afterwards.

Weaning is best done unhurried and unworried. Don't wean in an emergency if you can avoid it. Your baby will find it hard to understand why he is suddenly denied the breast and might be upset for some time.

If he asks for a feed by nuzzling against your breast several days after you've stopped feeding him, and you let him suck, he'll soon realize there's little, if any, milk there – though he may want to have a go anyway.

If you find yourself wishing you hadn't stopped so soon, you can take steps to increase your milk supply.

FOOD SUPPLEMENTS

Fluoride

If you live in an area with low fluoride levels in the drinking water, your doctor or dentist may recommend fluoride supplements in the form of tablets or drops. Adequate levels of fluoride can cut tooth decay by half, but too much can mottle the teeth.

Children's vitamin drops

Most children don't need extra vitamins. However, in some countries, such as the UK, vitamins A, C and D are recommended for all children from six months to at least two years, and preferably five, to protect those who would otherwise go short. Some breastfed babies need extra vitamins because of illness, because their mothers aren't eating a healthy diet or because neither they nor their mothers spend enough time outside in bright daylight each day. Ask your doctor or other professional adviser about your baby's needs.

The majority of breastfeeding women neither take vitamin supplements themselves nor give their babies supplements, so they need to protect themselves and their babies by eating a healthy diet, and by spending some time outside each day with their babies to benefit from daylight on their skin (obviously without burning) – which is the best way of ensuring they get enough vitamin D.

Clearly the way to breastfeed and wean your older baby is to be led by him, by sensible guidelines and by common sense. The next chapter explores how sex and breastfeeding influence each other.

FOURTEEN

Breastfeeding and sex

The juxtaposition of the words 'breastfeeding' and 'sex' still raises eyebrows, even in cultures in which it's hardly possible to open a newspaper or magazine or view a television programme without being confronted by a sexual message of some sort.

MOTHER, LOVER . . . OR BOTH?

A surprising number of women harbour the belief that a woman should shut off her sexual side when she becomes a mother. Some women come to the end of their first pregnancy feeling somewhat ambivalent about breastfeeding from the sexual point of view. Until now they've seen their breasts mainly as sexual objects that gave pleasure to themselves and their man. Now another function is asserting itself, and confusion reigns. Some men, too, have difficulty in seeing their partner as both 'Mother' and 'Lover' and some, unwittingly, to be fair, force her to make a choice. As a result, breastfeeding can suffer.

THE PLEASURES OF BREASTFEEDING

Part of the confusion is that breastfeeding can be a highly pleasurable experience for a woman, and for some even sexually arousing. In fact, some women find feeding their baby one of the more sensual experiences they've ever had. Indeed, breastfeeding, just like intercourse, must have been enjoyable throughout history, or the human race would have died out.

But a few women feel uncomfortable, even guilty or ashamed, about any perceived link between sexuality and breastfeeding. They may be particularly concerned if they feel aroused when breastfeeding a boy, or notice he occasionally has an erection while feeding. How, a woman's unconscious may wonder, could she possibly cause such a response in her own son? Incest is a major taboo, and this sort of incident puts some women off breastfeeding, though it's not the sort of thing people usually talk about with their friends, let alone mention to researchers!

MEN'S AND WOMEN'S VIEWS OF SEX, SEXUALITY AND BREASTFEEDING

Men, by and large, think of sex mainly in terms of their desire for penetrative intercourse, with themselves and, perhaps, their partner having an orgasm. However, most women think differently. Sex to them is closely bound up with many other factors, such as their wish to find a lifetime partner who will look after them and father their children, the need for contraception, and the possibility of one day getting pregnant, becoming a mother and, perhaps, breastfeeding. In other words, women tend to find intercourse more meaningful and fateful because it's they who carry and nurture babies. It is also part of a much larger 'sexual' and emotional picture than it is for a man.

While to most men breastfeeding is simply a superior way of feeding a baby, to many women it's an extension of their initial commitment to getting pregnant with a particular man – a commitment that in some mystical, let alone practical, sense, they ideally want to last a lifetime.

Another reason for the difference in perceptions of sex is that any one man can, in theory, impregnate many women in a lifetime; he produces semen every day of his life, and once he's ejaculated he simply makes more. On the other hand, a woman produces only one mature egg a month; once she has conceived she can't become pregnant again for many months, and when her ovaries' stock of immature eggs is eventually used up she has her menopause. So eggs are clearly more valuable to a woman than sperm to a man. How a woman 'invests' these eggs is therefore likely to be highly significant.

In traditional cultures many millions of women are pregnant or lactating for most of their reproductive lives, and breastfeeding is still by far the most important form of contraception. The average Western woman, though, doesn't want to be ruled by her cycles, and doesn't have babies every two or three years. On the contrary, she spends much of her reproductive life avoiding pregnancy. Such a woman increasingly wants very few babies, and prefers to look flat-bellied, slim, even masculine in body style. However, she may still want to experience the whole range of female sexuality, including pregnancy, birth and breastfeeding. Not surprisingly, these diverse desires are sometimes difficult for her to reconcile, let alone for society as a whole. Men too can have problems with these conflicting concepts.

WHAT BREASTS REPRESENT

Breasts are the erotic focus for millions of men in many countries. However, many cultures around the world don't eroticize breasts, and it's noticeable that women in such cultures breastfeed for long periods.

Could it be that 'breast-erotic' societies have become so deprived over the last century of the experience of being comforted and nourished at the breast – and so habituated to seeing images of the eroticized and 'unmotherly' breast – that their men seek to replace their unmet infantile needs and primitive drives in other ways, albeit later in life? Such ways could, perhaps, include compulsive behaviours such as promiscuous sex and various methods of oral gratification, including overeating, smoking and drinking.

Alternatively, could society's eroticization of the breast make women less likely to want to breastfeed and men less likely to support them? With both men and women putting such emphasis on breasts as sex objects it's hardly surprising that erotic overtones can militate against breastfeeding before a woman even gets pregnant. Studies have shown that some women won't even consider breastfeeding because they believe it will ruin their figure and render them sexually unattractive.

BREASTFEEDING AND SEX

There's a certain similarity between sexual arousal and lactation, because they both make a woman's breasts larger and more sensitive, and because many women feel protective or motherly after intercourse and when breastfeeding. This is no accident because the level in a woman's blood of the powerful sex hormone oxytocin increases during both these events. More than half of all women get a lot of pleasure from their breasts when masturbating or making love; some, indeed, say they can get an orgasm from breast-play alone. And breast stimulation from breastfeeding can make some women at least partially sexually aroused. All this is hardly surprising, given that the nipples and genitals are interconnected by nervous pathways in the brain.

The degree of sexual arousal caused by breastfeeding is very variable. Some women notice nothing; some report feeling 'nice'; others have increased vaginal moisture; and a few feel they could climax. Some women feel euphoric or contented after a feed in a similar way to after an orgasm. Some such women find that these experiences enhance their feelings towards their man, and so feel emotionally and sexually closer to him. Indeed, some studies show that breastfeeders return to having sex earlier after childbirth than other women. However, whether lactating women in general tend to feel more sexy than bottle-feeders isn't at all clear from research. Some feel more sexy, others less so. And any one woman may feel different from one baby to another, or during any one lactation.

- One interesting study (2002) reported in *New Scientist* suggests that women who spend time with breastfeeding mothers experience greater sexual desire. This is thought to be partly because these mothers produce pheromones (hormone-like substances in their sweat and other skin secretions) whose 'invisible' scent affects nearby women at an unconscious level. It's possible that pheromones act as a signalling system to inform a woman that it's safe for her to reproduce.

OFF SEX AFTER CHILDBIRTH?

Recently delivered women are traditionally advised to wait for several weeks before having intercourse again, though they can cuddle before that, the man can masturbate himself, or be masturbated, any time, and the woman too may enjoy breast and clitoral stimulation without vaginal penetration.

However, when they get the all-clear from their doctor, some women find their sex drive is dampened by other factors, while some simply don't feel sexy. There are several possible reasons.

Fatigue

One of the most likely reasons is that they are overwhelmed or exhausted after recently giving birth. Undoubtedly the tiredness experienced by many mothers of young babies who are waking at night, whether breastfed or not, often puts them off sex simply because they are too exhausted even to think about it! Indeed, tiredness is possibly the biggest antidote to sexual desire at this stage of a couple's life together. If your baby wakes often, consider having him by your bed so you can easily feed him without having to wake properly. Or you could have him in your bed. You can make love with your baby alongside you if you wish.

Stretched or stitched vagina

The second most likely reason is that their vagina, including its opening in the vulva, is still recovering from being stretched while giving birth, or healing after being torn or cut and stitched. Time and patience will eventually prevail, but it may help to insert just one finger (your own or your partner's) into your vagina the first few times you make love, then, as it becomes reaccustomed to having something inside, to insert two, then three fingers, then eventually the penis. Use a lubricant if necessary.

Tender breasts

Your breasts may sometimes be so full and tense that they are tender to the touch. A way round this is to encourage your partner to suck your nipples as you start making love; there's no need to worry about him stealing milk from the baby – there'll be plenty there. Alternatively, you could express a little milk yourself. Just taking some pressure off your breasts will eliminate any tenderness; it may also help you get aroused!

Leaking milk

You may feel embarrassed about leaking that occurs as you become aroused or have a climax, or concerned about the milk soiling your bedclothes. Some men, too, are put off by leaking. You can reduce the chance that you'll leak by taking off a little milk before you make love, as above. Some women feed their baby before lovemaking, for this very reason.

Too much responsibility

For a few women the experience of having total responsibility for a baby and all the other pressures of motherhood (for first-timers especially) is too much, and they lose interest in sex because they feel so anxious and overwhelmed.

Not ovulating

Another possible reason for feeling less sexy in the early months after childbirth is that exclusive unrestricted breastfeeding suppresses ovulation, and for many women their peak of sexual interest is around the time they ovulate.

Shocked by childbirth

Some women are so shocked by the experience of giving birth that they avoid sex because they don't want any chance of another pregnancy.

No need for the previous intimacy they had with their man

Some women find the relationship with their new baby, and the sensations they experience when breastfeeding, so powerful and fulfilling that they no longer need the sensual and erotic experiences they used to have with their man. Such a woman turns her sexuality inward to focus on the mother–baby relationship. Her partner can, understandably, feel excluded, though whether he is upset or not depends on his background and his personality. To some extent a woman's intense interest in her newborn baby is normal; it is also relatively temporary. Prevent or deal with any problems this causes in your relationship with your partner by being open and frank with each other.

Shows up their lack of intimacy with their man

Some women say the level of intimacy and delight they share with their baby, and the way they feel wanted, special and needed by their baby, stand in stark contrast to the poverty of emotional intimacy and pleasure they share with their man. Indeed, a few women stay with their man only because of the rewards they get from their relationship with their baby.

However, relying for your emotional sustenance on your relationship with your baby is at best short-sighted, at worst even abusive. Young children rely on parents to meet their needs, but parents shouldn't rely on their children to meet theirs – this is the wrong way round.

If an unsatisfactory relationship with your partner is an issue for you, consider seeing a counsellor or therapist for help in making your relationship more rewarding to you both.

Want to avoid intimacy with their man

A few women unconsciously use their commitment to breastfeeding and mothering as a way of avoiding sexual or emotional intimacy with their partner.

Transferring their affection to their baby is what certain women, unconsciously, or even consciously, have wanted all along. After all, not every relationship is a good one.

Need a 'comfort blanket'

The first year of their child's life is one of the most common times for a man to have an affair or the couple to break up. A woman betrayed in this way may focus intensely on breastfeeding or mothering as a way of diverting her attention, consoling herself, boosting her self-esteem and obtaining some degree of emotional intimacy.

FOCUSING ON YOUR MAN

If your partner encourages you in breastfeeding, you are more likely to do it successfully. Some men, though, resent their baby intruding into their sexual and emotional life, and want to get back to the status quo as soon as possible. Their spoken or unspoken messages make their partner less likely to breastfeed for as long as she wants. If this happens to you, find verbal and non-verbal ways of letting your man know he is still central to your life, that you love him and that he is very important to you. Obviously you'd like him to be a tower of strength as you adjust to being the parent of a newborn baby. But this particular challenge is happening to both of you at the same time, and at an unconscious level it may well be making this grown man feel like a needy, frightened or angry little boy. Psychologists call new parenthood the 'third childhood', because its various challenges can evoke emotional issues that we didn't resolve in infancy (our 'first childhood') or adolescence (our 'second childhood').

A loving couple can usually resolve this by addressing the situation honestly and explaining how they both feel about parenthood, breastfeeding and sex – or the lack of it. But remember that you may – perhaps only temporarily – need support and encouragement from someone other than him, just as he may need support and encouragement from someone other than you!

A problem can occur if a man who's psychologically thrown by the experience of new fatherhood, and his partner's concentration on her baby, continues to feel rejected and abandoned.

It's possible that some of these feelings go back to his own experiences of being mothered in babyhood. Part of an infant's emotional development is to think of important experiences or things as either all good or all bad. For example, the breast that isn't there when a baby boy is desperately hungry becomes a 'bad' or even 'punishing' breast belonging to a 'bad' mother. As he grows, provided he has good enough mothering, he resolves this stage of 'splitting' important experiences or things into good and evil, and comes to see the breast – and his mother – as both good and bad, not either/or. However, if he doesn't completely resolve this stage, then any important stressor in future, such as new parenthood, can bring up his original infantile tendency to see things as all good or all bad. Although this operates at an unconscious level, it can have far-reaching effects on his conscious attitudes and behaviour. And this time his partner bears the brunt!

Your man has a responsibility in all this, and it will help if he tries to become more aware of his feelings, and practises sharing them with you – or with a trusted friend – rather than acting them out in unhelpful and inappropriate ways, such as storming off to the pub, criticizing your lack of interest in him, or even having an affair in an effort to find the love he fears he's lost.

When discussing all this, make a pact to express your feelings using 'I' language, rather than 'you' language. For example, say, 'I feel such and such . . .', rather than, 'You make me feel such and such . . .'. This is more honest and less threatening.

FOCUSING ON YOU

Some women think their lactating breasts, with their initially increased size, look particularly sexy, and enjoy showing them off to their man. Others, though, are shy about their breasts, some even in front of their man. And some find that their large, full, possibly tender and leaky breasts make them feel anything but sexy and attractive. If you feel that your larger breasts make you more womanly and 'female', your whole perception of breastfeeding will be different, and its chances of success better, than if you dislike the way they look and the way they make you feel.

Breastfeeding is most likely to be successful if a woman likes her breasts, enjoys them being played with and touched by herself and her man, and sees them as a vital part of her femaleness and femininity. One US study some years ago found that women who had sexual hang-ups were much less likely to breastfeed successfully. Other studies looking at women's reasons for failing to feed as they intended have discovered that in a substantial minority this was because they found the whole thing 'distasteful' or 'immodest'. Such women see their breasts as private, and the notion of having to expose them other than for washing or medical examination completely unacceptable.

Indeed, a few women are revolted at even the thought of a baby sucking their breasts. They say it's too animalistic . . . too primitive . . . not what they want at all. The roots of such feelings are often very deep. Just as the experience of new fatherhood may make a man think at an unconscious level of the breast (and breastfeeding . . . and his partner as the symbolic mother) as bad, so may this happen to her.

Whether you feel like a mum or a sexual playmate in bed, you may be happy for your partner to play with your breasts as he did before. He may also want to suck your nipples and taste or drink your milk, which is fine if it's OK with you.

Once you start making love again after childbirth you'll probably notice a few changes. Some women say their nipples don't erect and their breasts don't swell during sexual excitement like they used to. This is most likely when their breasts are full of milk, so try taking off a little. And try changing the positions in which you make love if swollen breasts get in the way of your old favourites.

The foundations for successful breastfeeding are influenced by a woman's early experiences with men. If she's learned to value and enjoy her breasts in her sexual relationships, she'll be more receptive to breastfeeding.

It may help to focus on your breasts when pregnant. For example, you can stimulate your nipples when masturbating and you may like your man to play with them and suck them when lovemaking.

Once you have your baby, involve your partner in your enjoyment of breastfeeding, if he wants. And aim to keep up some aspects of your 'lover' image, so you don't give your partner messages that you've gone off him in favour of mothering. However, it may take time before you begin to feel sexy again, so be gentle and patient with yourself meanwhile.

Remember that, as in most areas of life, honest communication between new parents is at the heart of a successful relationship between them. It also encourages enjoyable and effective parenting, and successful breastfeeding. Imagine going mountaineering with people you didn't like, or had problems getting on with. Or more to the point – who didn't like climbing. The adventure would be unenjoyable at best and could even fail as a result. It's the same with breastfeeding.

Many couples make breastfeeding a time of personal growth, and succeed in nourishing not only their *baby* but also their emotional and sexual relationship.

> Many couples find breastfeeding enriches their sexual insights and broadens their relationship. In the next chapter we'll look at the subject of work and breastfeeding.

FIFTEEN

Work and breastfeeding

Women are an important part of the workforce in many countries, and young women are often brought up to think of themselves as important economic units. For some, raising children has to fit in with maintaining their standard of living and with their career plans. It's difficult to know how many mothers with young children work, because so many of those who do so work part-time or at home, and their activity is unrecorded by government agencies. Such statistics as are available show that only a small minority of mothers with young babies work outside the home; only a few women give up breastfeeding to go back to work; and full-time workers tend not to breastfeed for as long as those who work part-time.

Here are a few figures:

- In a US survey (2003) 69 per cent of full-time working women started breastfeeding (compared with 70 per cent of all women), but only around 25 per cent were still breastfeeding at six months (compared with 33 per cent of all women).
- In a large UK survey (2000), 53 per cent of the small group of mothers who didn't give up work were still breastfeeding at six months. This compared with 37 per cent of those who returned to work by four or five months and 38 per cent of those who returned by eight to nine months.
- A large survey in Great Britain (1990) found that only 8 per cent of mothers with babies aged between six and ten weeks returned to work.
- In the same British study (1990), 14 per cent of breastfeeding mothers with two- to three-month-old babies, 23 per cent with three- to four-

month-old babies and 15 per cent with four- to nine-month-old babies, stopped breastfeeding so they could work. The corresponding figures in 1980 were 6, 2 and 6 per cent.

- A large US survey (1987) found that at six months, about one in four mothers who'd chosen to breastfeed and were not employed were still breastfeeding. This compared with only one in ten who'd chosen to breastfeed and were employed.

Breastfeeding women either carry on as long as they want and go back to work at a time to suit themselves, or find ways of continuing to breastfeed when they return to work. But full breastfeeding is compatible with full-time work outside the home only with considerable effort and determination.

SUPPORT AT HOME

It's particularly vital for a breastfeeding woman who works to get all the support she needs to help her look after her baby and herself, maintain a home and enjoy her relationship with her partner, family and friends. Your partner may be the obvious person to help out at home, but if he's too busy with his own work, or you don't have a live-in partner, then, whoever your assistants are, you need to be completely clear and specific about what needs to be done. Management skills aren't only for managers at work. They're very important for working mothers at home too. Assess the situation every week or so early on, so you can work out more effective ways of using your joint resources if necessary.

SUPPORT AT WORK

Facilities and support for women to breastfeed at work are very important if women are to breastfeed exclusively for six months and carry on for a year or more.

- In Chile (1999), researchers found that 53 per cent of working mothers who were given support with breastfeeding continued with exclusive breastfeeding until six months, compared with only 6 per cent of working mothers not given special support.

The International Labour Organization recommends that nursing mothers should have a break of at least half an hour twice in the working day. Many countries recognize these breaks. They mean a breastfeeding woman can feed before work, express or feed once during a morning nursing break at work, once in her lunch break at work, and once in an afternoon nursing break at work. She can then breastfeed as much as necessary at home during the evening and at night.

In France, Egypt, Argentina and China, for example, breastfeeding mothers can take two thirty-minute breaks in the working day. In Italy, a full-time worker can have two one-hour 'rest' periods; if she likes she can take these together at the end of the day so she can go home earlier. In Portugal, breastfeeding mothers can take two hour-long breaks. In Spain, breastfeeding mothers can take a single one-hour break, or two half-hour breaks. In Russia, breastfeeding mothers are allowed a half-hour break at least every three hours. And in Turkey and Austria, breastfeeding mothers can take two forty-five-minute breaks a day.

In many countries employers must, by law, provide a room for breastfeeding. In France, for example, establishments employing more than one hundred women must provide nurseries. In Denmark, if an employer has twenty-five or more women on the payroll, there must be a breastfeeding room.

Sweden has generous provision for paid parental leave, gives all babies access to a crèche and has legislation entitling women to paid breastfeeding breaks in the workplace. However, few women use breastfeeding breaks at work as they have time to stay at home as long as they want before returning to work anyway. In parts of Africa, relatives sometimes bring the baby to the working mother so she can feed him, or mothers take their babies to work and have them by their side.

In contrast, in the UK very few organizations have nurseries, so it's usually impossible to take a breastfed baby to work. However, new guidance to employers from the Equal Opportunities Commission in the UK should help breastfeeding mothers. This states that if an employee is breastfeeding when she returns from maternity leave, she needs time during the day to express milk or feed her baby. The employer should give her rest periods, access to a comfortable private room in which she can express or feed, and access to a fridge where she can store her milk. If there is a workplace nursery, and she uses it for her baby, she should have rest periods and a private room in which she can breastfeed. Also, there should be no health and safety risk that could affect her health or that of her baby. Lawsuits concerning cases that don't meet these recommendations are already being tried.

As for the US, the Department of Health and Human Services released a policy document in 2000 asking employers to institute programmes to facilitate breastfeeding or breast milk expression. It included a list of recommended practices for corporations to consider when developing mother-friendly policies. However, it didn't make specific recommendations about legislation that would support a mother's plan to breastfeed.

Although it's a challenge to combine breastfeeding and paid employment, it can be done. First, though, why do some women want or have to combine the two?

PROS AND CONS OF WORKING AND OF STAYING AT HOME

Women's expectations have changed a great deal over the last three generations, and as a result both they and society as a whole are still trying to adjust. The issues involved when deciding whether to return to work outside the home, or to stay at home, are many and complex.

Money

Many couples find the cost of living so high that the man's income (if he has a job) simply isn't enough to run a home. However, it may be worth challenging this assumption. Think what you'd actually have to go without if you didn't work, then weigh up the advantages of being able to be with your baby and breastfeed more easily. Some women, on reflection, prefer to cut back financially and enjoy staying home with their child. If both a woman's and her partner's salary are needed to pay the mortgage, this could mean moving to a cheaper home, or arranging with the mortgage company to take a prolonged break in interest repayment – a 'mortgage holiday'.

Don't forget to consider the hidden costs of working when making your decision, including such things as clothes, travel and meals out. Equally, make sure you're clear about your long-term financial plans if you put work on hold for a while. For example, find out the position over your pension.

Quite a few women say they need to work for the money, when other reasons are really more important to them, though possibly not at a conscious level. In effect they shroud these reasons with economic excuses which may seem or sound more acceptable.

Maternity allowances and job protection vary from one country to another, but their generosity or otherwise can make a big difference to a woman deciding about breastfeeding. One reason why so many women breastfeed in Norway, for example, is that they are entitled to ten months' maternity leave on full pay, or 12 months on 78 per cent pay. In the US, by contrast, the Family and Medical Leave Act offers only twelve weeks of unpaid parental leave. The UK offers twenty-six weeks' maternity leave, during which you may, depending on your employment history, be paid by your employer or receive a maternity allowance; you can take a further twenty-six weeks' leave, but this is unpaid. And France offers only sixteen weeks of maternity benefits at 84 per cent of the minimum daily wage for the first and second child (twenty-four weeks for subsequent children).

Career

Some women don't want to lose their place on the career ladder. While it's true this can be important, it's equally true that many women return to what turns out to be a rewarding, even illustrious, career after a long break to mother their children. There are no absolutes, and the employment tide is turning in women's favour, with fewer jobs for life for anyone nowadays.

You could consider having a break while you breastfeed for as long as you want to, and then, if you want to or have to work, starting again in a completely different way, perhaps even working from home. If you work for a large organization it may be worth discussing with your employer whether there's any way you could take a career break and return to work when your child is older. Job-sharing is another option that works well for some breastfeeding mothers.

Self-image

Some women are disturbed by the thought of becoming a full-time mother. They want to maintain their status by returning to work, thereby retaining their image of themselves as independent, working, financially productive women. Indeed, increasing numbers of women measure their self-worth by their ability to earn.

However, having some time away from work doesn't necessarily extinguish the part of a woman that thrives in the world of work, it simply puts it on hold until such time as she chooses to return. Many women see motherhood, being with their baby and breastfeeding as ways of *adding* to their self-esteem, their understanding of who they are, and their maturity – not detracting from it.

Company and stimulation

Some full-time mothers of young children are lonely and crave adult company. Others are bored and miss the buzz of their previous job. Many adults today have most of their need for company and stimulation met at work. However, most women who stay at home find ways of meeting people and making friends in their community – indeed, they may have more opportunities than before to do so. There are also special groups to which mothers of young children are invited, for example, in the UK, National Childbirth Trust post-natal groups.

Others, though, feel very isolated by being at home with only a young baby for company. With today's small family units, some women are alone with their young children much of the time. Not surprisingly, some don't enjoy their experience and seek a way out. Some even admit to taking a job to have a break from the baby or to 'keep sane'.

Things are different in many parts of the world. For example, in rural parts of certain African countries, a mother and her baby aren't parted at all for the first fifteen months. Researchers who studied a sample of such mothers to see if they became irritated by being with their children so closely for so long found no ill effects in the mothers or their babies. However, such women are generally surrounded by other people and never lack company or practical and emotional support.

Company and stimulation for the baby

It's a popular myth that babies benefit from attending a nursery while their mothers work because they need exposure to other adults and to children for optimal social development. There's no evidence this is so unless a mother is very depressed or unable to interact for some other reason. Young babies benefit most from sensitive and responsive one-to-one attention, and the opportunity for two-way interaction, when they need it most. A nursery is very unlikely to be able to provide staffing levels that would enable someone to give your baby the same amount of attention and opportunity for interaction as you can at home. If you spend time playing with, talking to and listening to your baby, and you get out and meet people so you get *your* needs met, there's no reason why he should miss out at all and every reason why he should gain a lot. This said, your baby will almost certainly benefit from the stimulation of having other people around while he is with you.

COMBINING WORK AND BREASTFEEDING

If you intend to work, the easiest solution is to work at home if you can. All kinds of home-based jobs, from making things, word-processing and writing, to telephone-selling, could enable you to breastfeed and fit in your work to suit you and your baby.

The next easiest option is to work part-time and locally. Working locally cuts down on commuting time and means you can pop home easily and quickly in an emergency. With local part-time work your baby may need feeding only once while you're away. If you leave him with a minder, you can put expressed breast milk in the fridge to be given from a cup.

Working part-time a long way from home, or full-time anywhere, means being away from your baby a lot longer. You can express or pump enough milk to leave for him while you're away, but this requires considerable effort, time and determination. While it's good because he'll have breast milk while you're at work, and you'll keep your milk supply going, it also means both you and he will miss out on the pleasure of breastfeeding. And, of course, he has no chance to be at the breast when he wants to be particularly close to you for reassurance or comfort.

A few women manage to leave enough milk for their baby while they're out at work just by expressing after the early morning feed, when their breasts are usually fuller than at any other time of day. However, most need to express milk after each feed at home. And many find they can't leave enough milk for their baby unless they also express at work, and take this milk home for their baby to have next day. This can become very time-consuming.

Expressing milk

Aim to express at least every three hours while you and your baby are apart – more often if necessary, for example, if your baby is very young – and express after feeds at home too. You'll probably get only a very small volume of milk when you express after a feed, but if you add several small volumes together they soon mount up. You'll quickly learn what's best for you.

Make sure your minder knows how to shake and warm your milk and, unless you're sure you've left enough, tell her what to give your baby if he were still to be hungry after having the milk you've left for him. Boiled, cooled water will fill his tummy until you get home. But if he ever does need water while you're out, take steps to increase your milk supply so you'll be able to leave more breast milk in future. Formula should be a very last resort.

Reasons for expressing at work

1. So you can add it later to the milk you express at home and thereby leave enough for your baby the next day.
2. So your breasts don't become too full. If they do, you risk not only discomfort but also a blocked duct or breast infection, and a gradual reduction in your milk supply. You can always throw away the milk your baby doesn't need.
3. So you can make more milk. Expressing boosts prolactin, which encourages your breasts to produce more milk. However, it doesn't stimulate the breasts quite as well as your baby does, so to make up for this you may have to express more often or use a pump as well.

Expressing is rather tedious, takes longer than feeding a baby and calls for privacy and somewhere comfortable to sit. However, one very good reason for doing it is the satisfaction of knowing your baby can still have your milk.

If you do it at work, express into a previously sterilized plastic container, cover it, and keep it cold (it can be warmed later for a feed). If you can't put your milk in a fridge at work, put the sterilized container in a wide-necked vacuum flask containing some ice you put in before you left for work in the morning. Such a flask will also be useful for taking the milk home. Failing a flask, take a small cooler containing a frozen ice pack to work with you; put the ice pack in the freezer compartment of a fridge at work, so it's ready for you to put back in the cooler before you take your little container of expressed milk home.

If you don't want to express at work, this doesn't necessarily mean you can't breastfeed. You can feed your baby before you go to work in the morning and as soon as you get back, as well as in the evening and at night. However, when deciding whether to go back to work, bear in mind that getting up at night and working full-time can be very tiring. Also, some babies so like to be with their mothers that they get in the habit of waking very frequently at night, as if to make up for lost time during the day. For your sake you should make night-time feeds as boring as possible! So keep the light dimmed or off and keep quiet. You can make a fuss of your baby in the morning!

When at home in the evenings or at weekends (or at other times if you work shifts), feed your baby on an unrestricted basis. This, combined with continued regular expression at work, should keep your milk supply going so you can carry on breastfeeding for as long as you and your baby want.

- The large British study (1990) mentioned earlier in this chapter found that by the time breastfed babies of working mothers were nine months, 6 per cent went to work with their mothers (and could be breastfed there), 4 per cent received expressed breast milk while their mothers were at work, 39 per cent had other milk (such as formula), and the rest got by without milk while their mothers were at work (presumably these last babies received solids and other drinks – such as water or fruit juice).

Should you get him used to the bottle?

Many women wonder whether they should accustom their baby to a bottle before they return to work. In the first few months, before breastfeeding is properly established, it's better not to. Simply carry on breastfeeding until the day you go back to work. When your baby is hungry he'll almost certainly take your expressed breast milk from a cup given by the minder (though he may understandably refuse a cup if *you* offer it). If the baby isn't interested at first, the minder should persevere and all will eventually be well. In the early months a cup is better than a bottle because some babies given a bottle soon learn to prefer it to the breast, then make a fuss when it comes to having a breastfeed. Giving expressed breast milk from a spoon is another option. If you want your baby to have your milk from a bottle when he's older than four months or so, this should be no problem from the point of view of him continuing to breastfeed when you're there.

Looking after yourself

If you're a working breastfeeding mother, the odds are you'll be tired, especially if you have older children as well. This makes it even more essential to look after yourself.

Enjoying your baby

Some working mothers encourage their babies to stay awake in the evenings so they can spend more time with them. Others say night feeds become precious times when they and their baby can take a delight in each other's company. Whatever you decide to do, remember you'll probably have only one or two babies in a lifetime and they'll only be really tiny and dependent on you for a short time. Make the most of this time together and you'll both benefit hugely.

Do everything you can to stay home with your baby for the first six months at the very least. If you go back to work you can carry on breastfeeding – but don't forget to take care of yourself. The next – and last – chapter is mainly for fathers.

SIXTEEN

Mainly for fathers

The role of fathers has altered a great deal over the last three decades since the first edition of this book was published, and looks set for even more change. In the late 1970s most people expected a young child's parents to be married and living together, with the man the main breadwinner and the child's biological father.

While this is still so for many young children today, it has become less so, and things are on the move. When a man is resident, he may not be the biological father of the child. In the US, more than one in three children lives apart from their biological father. In the UK, nearly one in five firstborn babies begins life without their biological father living with them. And similar trends are happening in some other westernized countries too. Even when the man in the home is the biological parent, his lifestyle is likely to be considerably different from that of a father of similar age thirty years ago.

Fathering today tends to fall into one of two types. In the first, the man is employed and works to keep his job and support his family. Many such men find the modern workplace insecure and stressful. In the second, the father is either out of work, or employed on a temporary basis, and therefore feeling financially insecure much of the time. He may even feel panicky over whether his family has security of tenure in their home. Both groups of fathers may therefore find themselves either overstretched or otherwise stressed, if for different reasons, and if so they may have little time or energy for their family.

It's a paradox that social welfare systems are not always beneficial to family life, but many countries are now rethinking their arrangements. Some of the changes that have been made, such as the option for paternal leave after a child is born, can benefit breastfeeding. However, an overstretched or otherwise stressed man may not welcome a request from his partner for him to take time off work so he can support her by looking after domestic arrangements after the birth. He may also fear that his colleagues and employers will interpret his absence as a sign that he lacks commitment to his job.

In addition, if his partner has been contributing significantly to the family income, or is the major breadwinner, he may prefer her to go back to work as quickly as possible to take the pressure off him. If he imagines that work and breastfeeding don't mix, he may encourage her to bottle-feed.

Some men don't much care about breastfeeding anyway, because they simply don't know about its many advantages. Once they learn, they can see how important their contribution to supporting it can be.

WHY YOU ARE SO IMPORTANT TO BREASTFEEDING

The father of a breastfed baby is a very important person and can play several very helpful roles. Just as when a baby gorilla is born the father lifts the baby to the mother's breast so she can suckle it, so you too can offer your partner help with breastfeeding!

For example, a few hospitals even today still give breastfed babies water, glucose water or formula unnecessarily, especially at night. If this isn't what your partner wants (which it almost certainly isn't if she's aiming to breastfeed successfully), you can help prevent it happening. Remind the staff that you and your partner want your baby to be totally breastfed and don't be fobbed off by someone trying to persuade you it doesn't matter if he has the occasional bottle. It may well matter if you want breastfeeding to have the best chance of success.

Stay with your partner after the birth if she wants you there. She's just been through one of the most important events in her life and may need your company and support. She may also feel emotionally and physically keyed up, or exhausted, and anything you can do to help, support and encourage her could help get breastfeeding off to a good start.

In the US some women are asked immediately after childbirth whether they want to breastfeed, and if the answer is 'no' they are given an injection to dry up their milk. This happens in some other countries too. However, if a woman hasn't yet made her final decision, she'll probably be in no fit state to decide in the few minutes after giving birth. Some women who decide at this time to bottle-feed wish later that they'd had more time to think. In the UK dry-up drugs are given only rarely, but if your partner is offered them, ask if she really needs them, or whether, if she's going to bottle-feed, she could instead let her milk dry up of its own accord. If she's had dry-up drugs, then changes her mind, she should be reassured that she will be able to get her milk back, though restarting her milk supply will take time, effort and determination.

Some women feel low in the first week after childbirth, and it's then that they may need most help with breastfeeding. One experienced breastfeeding counsellor says she thinks that successful lactation depends on a woman's helpers, not her ability to produce milk. You could be one of your partner's most valuable helpers.

However useful you are when your partner is in hospital, you can help even more when she gets home. Take a couple of weeks off work if you can, so you can be there for her and look after any other children. You'll be particularly important as a provider, protector and general helper over the next few weeks and you'll play an even more valuable part in family life than usual. Most of us only ever have two children, so it's well worth making the effort to give her the support and help she needs at this crucial time. Many women hope, or expect, the home to run as it did before they had the baby, and many men feel much the same. But if your partner is to breastfeed successfully, and you can't take time off work, you'll almost certainly need to help in the home, unless you have close family who can step in, or you can afford paid help.

She'll need emotional back-up too, because breastfeeding is a deeply emotional business. So use empathic listening whenever possible. This involves putting your own concerns aside while you focus entirely on her; trying to understand how she's feeling so you can identify her main emotions; and, finally and most important, letting her know what you sense is going on for her emotionally. Most of us like to know that someone understands where we're at. An additional benefit of listening well is that it could help fend off post-natal depression, because this is particularly likely in women who feel emotionally alone in their new role. Research has shown that mammals of many species (including humans) produce less milk, or even stop producing it, if disturbed or stressed while breastfeeding. Serenity fosters successful breastfeeding, and having you to listen to how she's feeling will allow her to let off steam and enjoy her baby. Having her feelings heard makes her realize that you care, and that she isn't alone.

The majority of women are highly emotional after having a baby, partly because of the physical and emotional upheaval of childbirth and becoming a mother and partly because their hormones are keying them up to breastfeed and respond to their baby. But they may also react to the world around them in a way that's atypical for them. Even the most able and well-balanced professional woman may cry for no apparent reason. And this may be because she's happy, not sad. This can be a challenge for her partner to understand.

It's wise to be especially sensitive, and careful what you say. As her partner you'll play a vital role in the success or otherwise of breastfeeding. A casual or thoughtless remark can destroy a woman's confidence and make her feel inadequate.

If you have other children you'll need to look after them, or organize others to, so your partner can get all the rest she needs. You can also act as a buffer between her and the outside world. Relatives, friends and neighbours may be keen to see her and the new baby, but make sure they come in small doses. Many's the time a recently delivered mother becomes so exhausted from regaling friends with the saga of her delivery – and wanting to please everybody – that she simply hasn't the energy to relate to her new baby or get feeding off to a good start.

Encouragement is another thing you can provide. Studies show that a woman whose partner doesn't want her to breastfeed rarely manages to do so. Even if he's merely neutral, the chances of successful feeding are greatly reduced. One American breastfeeding counsellor who guaranteed success wouldn't accept a woman as a client unless her man approved of breastfeeding. It's best if your attitude is positive from the beginning, as your partner may find breastfeeding particularly challenging in the first few days while she's learning how to do it. She'll need plenty of loving encouragement and support and the odds are that she will especially value it coming from you.

SOME COMMON CONCERNS

Two things that concern men most about breastfeeding (or at least the things they most often talk about, which isn't necessarily the same) are whether their partner will (*a*) go off sex and (*b*) lose her figure. There's more about sex and breastfeeding in chapter 14 but let's look at the figure question here.

Whether breastfeeding experts like it or not, virtually every man thinks of breasts first and foremost as sex objects. Of course, breasts are for feeding babies too, as most men reluctantly agree, but during the years of a couple's life together, which could be many decades, the erotic role of the breasts is much more important most of the time. This makes it foolish to ignore any fears a man may have about his partner having droopy breasts after breastfeeding.

But let's consider what actually happens. All breasts enlarge in pregnancy, regardless of how a woman intends to feed her baby. If she breastfeeds, her breasts stay bigger for longer than if she bottle-feeds. This can be a real bonus, of course, for the man who likes large breasts! Indeed, some men are greatly turned on by their breastfeeding partner's relatively large breasts and more erectile nipples. Research into breastfeeding and breast size is scanty. One study reported that women who breastfed for two weeks or more thought their breasts became slightly droopier; they also said their pleasure from breastfeeding far outweighed this slight change. Wearing a well-fitting bra by night and day during the later months of pregnancy, and while breastfeeding, supports the heavier-than-usual breasts and prevents the skin becoming overstretched, which helps maintain their original shape. Many women find their breasts are relatively soft after they stop breastfeeding. This is because the milk glands and ducts can shrink quite abruptly after stopping. However, as the weeks and months pass, and body fat becomes redistributed, and the breasts' contours gradually fill out again.

But whatever happens, does it matter anyway? The fashion for perfect breasts isn't just a little crazy it's also wholly unrealistic, because most men don't marry girls from the centrefold of *Playboy* in the first place. Breasts quite normally change with age and if pregnancy or breastfeeding hastens this change at all, it's only a very little. Any man who sees his partner as a pair of walking breasts has other problems in his relationship that probably need attention.

YOU AND YOUR BABY

Many fathers like the idea of their partner breastfeeding, partly because it's such an intrinsically feminine thing to do, but it can leave them feeling there is little they can do for their baby. Indeed, some men like the idea of bottle-feeding because they can then give their baby the occasional feed. And at a time in history when increasing numbers of young men feel useless, helpless and even hopeless, feeding their baby is something they feel they can do to contribute. This certainly isn't a good reason for persuading his partner not to breastfeed, though, because there are innumerable things a father can do with his breastfed baby, including cuddling, playing and bathing – all of which are much more fun than bottle-feeding!

Some new fathers feel shut out of the excitement of the first few days. The mother is closely involved with her newborn, and he may feel she and the baby are hogging the limelight and excluding him. However, although a new father isn't centre stage, this can be a wonderful time for him and potentially for his self-development too. He can be proud of bringing a new life into the world. He also has the opportunity to practise being selfless and to learn how to back up his partner, service her, if you like, while she finds her feet looking after and breastfeeding their child. For many fathers of a newborn baby this 'mothering' role is a completely new experience.

While this comes easily to some men, others find it a challenge. They may have been used to being looked after by their partner, just as their mother looked after them before that, and can't easily change roles.

Talking all this through may help a man accept and enjoy his new role, and discussing it with other men can be useful too.

Caring for his breastfeeding partner can add a whole new dimension to a man's relationship – one in which he matures from being a big boy to a real man who gives as much, or more, than he receives. This can be a quantum leap in a couple's life together.

BENEFITS OF BREASTFEEDING TO YOU

Having a breastfed baby and a breastfeeding partner can provide you with benefits you might not have considered.

- You won't have to get up at night to take your turn preparing bottle-feeds – and that's no mean advantage for a working man.
- You can't run out of milk powder at awkward times, and it's one less thing to buy! Even allowing for the cost of the little extra food your partner may need, several studies agree that breastfeeding is less expensive than bottle-feeding.
- Having a breastfeeding baby means there's less baby equipment to carry when you go out anywhere. This makes travelling, going on holiday and going out a lot easier.
- Finally, there's the pleasure you'll get seeing your partner enjoying the feelings of femininity, fulfilment and intimacy so many women experience with breastfeeding, and knowing you are contributing by being there to back her up. In this sense, breastfeeding is a joint effort, with you as the most important member of the fan club!

LOOKING AFTER YOURSELF

With all the fuss, commotion and excitement over your new baby, it's easy to forget yourself and your needs. Both you and your partner have to get used to the physical and emotional needs of the new member of your family, and this isn't always easy. You are a very important person and you'll enjoy this time more and have more to offer if your well of energy, health and well-being is full.

Here's a checklist that might help, and of course you can add things to it yourself:

- Are you getting enough sleep? If you're waking a lot at night when your baby wakes and your partner breastfeeds, you may find yourself dropping off during the day. Perhaps you could learn to catnap for half an hour or so at work after lunch, sleep in another room for part of the night or have forty winks in the early evening or when you've helped get any other children to bed.

- Are you getting enough good food? Ensure that you eat healthily so as to keep up your stamina while you are being such a source of support and strength to your partner.
- Are you looking after yourself outside the home? As a new father you'll benefit from being on top form. Keep up your own interests and hobbies, even if you have to put a few things on ice in the very early weeks. There's no need for a man to give up all his interests and become a second mother to the baby. As with so many things in life, balance is everything.
- What about exercise? Time is often short at this stage in life, but if you work those muscles and get your circulation going you'll enjoy higher levels of 'feel good' endorphins and keep yourself in trim for your new role.
- Is there someone around for *you*? Your partner may be too absorbed while she's getting used to the new baby and, if it's her first child, to motherhood, yet you too may need someone to help you adjust to your new role. Many men, given the chance, benefit from talking about their feelings on becoming a father, with all the changes and responsibilities of their new lifestyle. Few men find it easy to 'let it all hang out', but a friendly ear, a shared joke and the sense of relief you get from being honest with a friend or relative about the highs and low of your new lifestyle can be a godsend. Getting out with friends can also help keep everything in perspective.

PASS ON THE MESSAGE

As the dad of a breastfed baby, and partner of a breastfeeding woman, you are in a position to do some very valuable work. It involves letting some of the men and boys in your local community know about the benefits of breastfeeding and the value of being a supportive father. So, if your circumstances permit, consider asking local antenatal teachers or schoolteachers if they'd like you, your partner and the baby to attend a class to talk about your role, your feelings and the importance of breastfeeding.

Most boys today never see a baby being breastfed and never get the chance to talk about being a father. If their own father has left the family, they may never be exposed to a man who's a positive role model for fathering either. So your contribution, however small it may seem, could have enormous and lasting significance. If you have any 'ins' to a school, talk to whoever teaches biology or personal and social development. You may at first feel you are making yourself potentially vulnerable to criticism as you go public as a 'breastfeeding dad', but experience suggests you'll be very warmly received both by boys at school and by fathers-to-be at antenatal classes.

Helping your partner breastfeed can give both of you pleasure and your baby the best possible start. Over a lifetime as a father you'll lavish huge amounts of time, money and energy on your child. That journey starts here, so don't underestimate the importance of the time, support, empathy and affection you give your partner. You are helping lay the foundations for your new family – and you can make a huge difference.

SEVENTEEN

A word for helpers

Helpers include relatives, friends, neighbours, voluntary breastfeeding counsellors, midwives, doctors and, in the UK, health visitors.

WHAT MAKES A HELPER MORE EFFECTIVE?

1 **Practical skills** learned from the experiences of successful breastfeeding women, from good teachers and, possibly but not necessarily, from their own experiences of breastfeeding.

2 **Up-to-date and reliable information** about the benefits and practicalities of successful breastfeeding. If as a professional or voluntary helper you aren't offered in-service training, ask for it or arrange it yourself. However much you know, you can deepen your knowledge and broaden your understanding at any time – if you give yourself the chance.

3 **Empathy** – recognizing (through words, body language and other unspoken messages) what a woman feels about breastfeeding and being a mother; check this out with her, and you'll help her learn and grow.

4 **Humility** – accepting that no one knows everything about breastfeeding.

5 **The desire to go on learning** – particularly for voluntary counsellors and professional helpers.

6 Enthusiasm about breastfeeding.

7 Acceptance that each mother–baby pair is unique and the needs, behaviour and experience of each woman and baby are special.

8 Encouragement – A few words of encouragement can give a breastfeeding woman confidence that may last a lifetime. I vividly remember sitting in King's College Hospital giving my first daughter one of her earliest feeds. A midwife (Staff Nurse Benjamin) came and stood for a while, smiling with approval, as she watched. She said 'Mrs Stanway, you're a wonderful mother.' The warmth, generosity and encouragement of her comment as I was starting out as a mother have stayed with me ever since. If a woman has a breastfeeding problem, then identifying what she is doing well – and telling her – may help her persevere and find a solution by generating inner feelings of warmth, self-esteem and belief she can succeed.

9 Awareness of their own feelings about breastfeeding – so that difficult and unresolved issues don't unwittingly adversely colour the advice. If these were unchecked, a helper could act out his or her emotional state by encouraging bottle-feeding. For 'sticking a bottle between baby and mother' would destroy the triggers that make these painful emotions surface (see below). We've already looked at a mother's and a father's feelings about breastfeeding; these can also apply to any helper who is a parent.

10 Satisfaction of their needs for nourishment and love – Without this, it's difficult, if not impossible, to be a good breastfeeding helper, as unmet neediness is likely to get in the way. Watching breastfeeding is a situation almost above all others that can trigger an awareness of having had insufficient love or nourishment oneself. If you realize you are very needy, ask someone you trust either to help or to recommend where you can get help in coming to terms with your feelings and getting your needs met.

ESPECIALLY FOR HEALTH PROFESSIONALS

Several things are particularly significant for health professionals. Let's see how you can make the time you spend with pregnant and breastfeeding women into a time of golden opportunity for them and for you.

1 **Be positive and enthusiastic** – Being enthusiastic is important – *not putting pressure on women to breastfeed, bullying them or putting them off with an evangelistic attitude,* but being positive about its benefits. Many studies confirm that an enthusiastic health professional can encourage women not only to start but also to continue. A woman who wants to breastfeed will also be much more prepared to overcome any problems if she knows you are interested.

Don't forget that people mainly take in ideas visually, so having pictures of breastfeeding mothers in your clinic or consulting room will help you get your message across.

2 **Be encouraging** – Polish up your encouragement skills and learn to give well-focused, specific encouragement, describing exactly what a woman can be pleased about. This is especially important for a woman who is starting to breastfeed or having problems. There'll be something you can encourage in every situation – even simply the woman's readiness to seek help.

3 **Don't imagine you'll make women feel guilty** – Many health professionals are reluctant to tell women about the benefits of breastfeeding for fear of making those who don't (or can't) breastfeed feel guilty or inferior. This fear is best recognized and then put to one side.

It's only fair to respect each woman's right to make an informed decision, but she can do this only if she has information. If she then decides not to breastfeed, that's her choice as an adult able to weigh the pros and cons as she sees them. Hopefully she'll weigh them carefully and have confidence in what she believes is right for her and her baby. Just as if she were buying a car, she'll then stand or fall by her decision. It is *her* responsibility to decide and it is within her gift to live with the consequences.

Most women who choose to bottle-feed do so because they actively *don't want to breastfeed*. A woman may feel pleasure and/or regret, or indeed any other emotions resulting from her choice. Whether she feels guilty or not depends on whether she has come to terms with her reasons for bottle-feeding or feels bad or ambivalent about it. Professionals don't have the power to *make* women feel guilty, nor should they predict that women will experience guilt rather than other emotion. Women aren't little girls who need a parent-figure to take responsibility for their emotions. The effort to protect women from some potential guilt they might feel is misguided at best and arrogant at worst. And it's a way in which some professionals unwittingly seek to infantilize pregnant and newly delivered mothers at the very time they should be encouraging and supporting them. Your responsibility as a health professional is to give pregnant women accurate, up-to-date and unbiased information about the benefits of breastfeeding.

The argument about the guilt (or disappointment) of the woman who *can't* breastfeed is another matter. First, most of those who 'fail' to breastfeed might have succeeded with better support, encouragement, information and advice. Only a very few women physically can't breastfeed. Also, virtually every woman who wishes to breastfeed can give her baby some breast milk and you can reassure her that a little is better than none.

Some bottle-feeding women know they are putting their needs first. Their emotions and concerns about their choice are far better acknowledged and discussed than hidden away and allowed to seep out as guilt.

It's important to consider whether the guilt you imagine a woman might feel could have more to do with you than with her. Do you think she *should* feel guilty? In other words, do you think she is 'bad' or 'naughty' because she doesn't breastfeed? If so, this may suggest your whole life is too full of 'shoulds' and 'oughts' (both for others and for yourself) and you'd be happier and serve your patients better if you relaxed a bit. It isn't appropriate for someone who works with pregnant women and new mothers to apportion blame. And could it also be that your fear that a woman will feel inadequate if she can't breastfeed is really a projection of your own fear of being an inadequate helper (see below)?

Women who want to breastfeed but find they can't may have all sorts of feelings, including anger and sadness, about the loss of the experience of breastfeeding. Our task is to support them in their mourning and help them grow both in their mothering skills and as human beings, empowered and enriched by dealing with their feelings and learning from their experience of 'failure'. Many women who want to breastfeed *do* see bottle-feeding as a failure, and learning to deal with failure is an extremely important task in anyone's personal development.

4 **Become more self-aware** – An important part of being a better listener is becoming more aware of our own emotions. We're unlikely to be able to help women deal with feelings which we've suppressed ourselves. And once we're aware of our feelings, we can put them to one side so they don't interfere with our work.

If we know in our heart that our advice tends to sabotage breastfeeding, we need to examine our emotions carefully. Talking about, watching and helping with breastfeeding may trigger painful emotions (in our mind or body) which unwittingly distort our advice about breastfeeding. Such emotions may stem from difficult and unresolved situations in our childhood or in our past or current life. They may also reflect our feelings about our own mothers and the mothering we had, and about the love and emotional nourishment we have or, indeed, do not have, today.

As an exercise, look at your feelings about breastfeeding by asking yourself these soul-searching questions, because just recognizing and naming them can be a great help:

a Do I know what I'm doing and am I a 'good enough' helper?
b Do I at some level dislike breastfeeding?
c Will I lose face if I'm not seen to be authoritative?
d Will this baby starve?
e Will it be my fault if the baby starves?
f Can I bear it if this woman feels guilty because of what I tell her?
g Will this woman dislike me if I tell her what she needs to do to breastfeed successfully?
h What will my colleagues think if this woman doesn't breastfeed, or doesn't succeed in breastfeeding?
i Can I bear giving up control to this mother and her baby?
j Am I being unkind if I don't suggest that this woman with breastfeeding problems bottle-feeds instead?
k Can I cope with the implicit sexuality of breastfeeding?
l Do I want to watch this demanding baby who never seems to stop feeding?
m Why haven't I got a baby I can love and who will love me?
n Does my advice echo my personal experiences of breastfeeding?
o Am I comfortable seeing this baby cared for so lovingly when no one seems to care for me and I don't feel I received the love and nourishment I needed from my mother?

If any of these questions rings bells for you, ask yourself how it makes you feel. For example, questions *a*, *b* and *c* make some people feel afraid; *g* makes some feel helpless; *k* makes some feel jealous and unloved; *g*, *k*, *l* and *n* make some feel angry; *l* and *n* make some feel a sense of desperate longing and neediness; and *k*, *l* and *m* make some feel envious.

If these emotions aren't familiar, either they don't apply to you or they may be suppressed in your unconscious mind.

Suppressed emotions usually stem from unresolved experiences in infancy and childhood. We aren't consciously aware of them because we've erected defences to stop them hurting us. But anything – particularly the deeply significant act of breastfeeding – that disturbs these defences can stir up our suppressed emotions and allow them out. This can cause problems – or, better, challenges.

One relevant challenge might be knowing that you often give poor breastfeeding advice (see below) even though this isn't what you consciously want to do. (Others might include compulsive behaviour – such as overeating, promiscuous sex, dependence on alcohol and drugs, or overwork – or depression or anxiety.)

So ask yourself whether rather too many of the women you advise choose to bottle-feed or give up breastfeeding earlier than they would have wished. If this is the case, could your advice be based on a need to avoid the painful feelings resulting from your 'yes' answers to the questions above? Are your difficult feelings, recognized or unrecognized, making you give irrational or inconsistent breastfeeding advice? By *not* giving sound information, advice and encouragement about breastfeeding, could you really be attempting to meet your own emotional neediness?

> — In other words, are you unconsciously seeking to separate a breastfeeding mother and baby by putting a bottle between them so as to prevent your own painful feelings?

Or are you even, unwittingly and symbolically, seeking to punish your own mother for being 'bad', under the guise of punishing all the mothers you meet by sabotaging their breastfeeding?

This may seem fanciful but it's astonishing how many health professionals who choose baby and child care as a career have old wounds from their own past that so obviously need healing. Or perhaps it isn't!

If you are aware of any problems in this area, and if you work on them, you can use the insights you gain to improve the quality of your life in many ways. Many health professionals need to spend more time caring for themselves, listening to their inner voice and finding ways of getting their emotional needs met if they are to care for others more effectively. Otherwise, their own neediness could interfere with them being effective breastfeeding helpers.

When we're unaware of our own needs and feelings, it's all too easy to seek to 'rescue' people from their predicaments in life. We do this instead of helping ourselves, since we see our own problems only in others. However, being aware of our emotional pain and seeking to resolve it can transform us into a 'wounded healer' who is more effective as a helper.

A wounded healer is someone who has been emotionally wounded but has taken steps to recognize painful feelings and deal with them effectively. The result is that he or she learns and matures emotionally.

The need for helpers to be aware of their own emotional woundedness (and all of us are wounded to some degree) is rarely more important than in the fields of midwifery, obstetrics, paediatrics, mother-and-child care, and breastfeeding. This is because these areas are, by definition, so primal and, as we've seen, so resonant with our own past experiences. As health professionals in these areas, we owe it to mothers, fathers and babies to be among the most aware of all health professionals.

5 Share your feelings – If you'd like to come to terms with any painful emotions triggered by helping women breastfeed, a wish to change may not be enough. You may need to discuss your feelings with a trusted friend or colleague. If you have the opportunity of discussing feelings about breastfeeding in a small group at work, it may be a more effective use of your time if you can work with a trained facilitator. Staff who make an awareness of feelings (both their own and those of others) a part of their professional skills can be a powerful source of expertise. A few helpers find they benefit even more from one-to-one work with a counsellor.

6 Polish your empathic listening skills – It's particularly important for all health professionals – not just those dealing with pregnant and breastfeeding women – to keep their listening skills well polished. Good listening skills enable you to help a woman recognize and understand how she feels about breastfeeding. Talking to you about her emotions may clarify things considerably for her. If she has difficult or negative feelings, recognizing and discussing them may enable her to come to terms with them and perhaps decide to breastfeed even though she'd planned not to.

7 Practise what you preach – It's all very well *talking* about breastfeeding, but it's another doing it! If *you* have a baby, remember that how you care for and feed him will have an important modelling role for everyone who knows you are a health professional. If *you* breastfeed, they'll think it really must be good. If you don't, or you do it only half-heartedly, they'll find it hard to believe you think much of it.

Unfortunately, health professionals are often hard on themselves – and on their babies. Some of them work so hard that they have to carve out time to be with their babies, breastfeed them and enjoy them.

- A study in the US (1985) reported that health care workers (doctors, nurses and technicians) returned to work earlier than other employed mothers. And doctors whose babies were cared for in hospital crèches were often late for their babies' feeds.

8 Remember you too need encouragement and support – You are a valuable person and a skilled professional caring for mothers and babies at a vitally important time in their lives. If you can find ways of polishing your self-esteem and your pleasure – in yourself, the way you live your life and the way you do your job – you'll help more effectively.

You might like to discuss the importance of well-focused encouragement with a group of colleagues and agree to find ways of encouraging each other.

9 Affirm yourself – Make time to recognize the good work you're doing and give yourself a pat on the back. It's surprising what a difference this can make.

10 Look after yourself – Take extra special care to look after yourself as you learn to recognize and adjust to your feelings about helping mothers breastfeed.

Treat yourself as a valuable person who deserves an enjoyably healthy diet, regular exercise, time spent outside each day and ample opportunity for rest, relaxation, entertainment and laughter. You well deserve it!

Appendix

RECOMMENDED READING LIST

When reading anything aimed at helping you feed, bring up or look after your child, remember that the information is there for you to assess and use if it seems right for you and your family. No author can get everything right and certainly no author can address him or herself to each individual reader. It's up to you to decide on what seems most suitable, discuss it with friends, family, professional advisers and counsellors, and then to act on a mixture of this information plus a good helping of common sense.

Mothercare New Guide to Pregnancy and Babycare, ed. Penny Stanway (London: Conran Octopus).
The Politics of Breastfeeding, Gabrielle Palmer (London: Pandora).
Breastfeeding: A Guide for the Medical Profession, Ruth A. Lawrence (London: Mosby).
Breastfeeding: A Guide for Midwives, Dora Henschel with Sally Inch (Hale: Books for Midwives).

From La Leche League (*see pages 419 and 420*)

The Womanly Art of Breastfeeding, La Leche League International (New York: New American Library).
Nursing Your Baby, Karen Prior (NY: Pocket Books).
The Manual of Natural Family Planning, Anna M. Flynn and Melissa Brooks (London: Thorsons).
Three in a Bed, Deborah Jackson (London: Bloomsbury).

LLL also sells a wide variety of leaflets, including:

Increasing Your Milk
Positioning and Attaching Your Baby at the Breast
When You Breastfeed Your Baby: The First Weeks
Crying – Why and What to Do
Breastfeeding and Sexuality
The Breastfeeding Father
Does Breastfeeding Take Too Much Time?
Breastfeeding Your Premature Baby
Breastfeeding a Baby with Down Syndrome

From NCT Maternity Sales (*see page 420*)

Bestfeeding: Getting Breastfeeding Right for You, Mary Renfrew, Chloe Fisher and Suzanne Arms (Berkeley, California: Celestial Arts).

Successful Breastfeeding, Royal College of Midwives (Edinburgh: Churchill Livingstone) a detailed guide for those supporting breastfeeding mothers.

NCT Maternity Sales also sells a variety of leaflets on various aspects of breastfeeding.

BREAST PUMPS

Electric pumps

Ameda Egnell Ltd, Unit 1, Belvedere Trading Estate, Taunton, Somerset TA1 1BH, UK, 00 44 (0)1823 336362, www.ameda.demon.co.uk

Egnell Elite Breast Pump – Mainly made for hospitals, this is also available from medical supply houses and on hire from many National Childbirth Trust branches (call 0870 444 8707 from the UK for your nearest one). It works by suction together with stimulation of the nipple and areola against the side of the flange.

It is quiet and efficient and has variable suction with a resting phase, and two sizes of funnel (for different shaped breasts). It has two cups so you can pump both breasts at once and the extra stimulation this provides encourages let-downs and halves the pumping time compared with pumping one breast at a time. In the UK you can rent the pump you used in hospital, or have one delivered to your home the next working day; rental costs £44 for thirty days and £25 for each subsequent thirty days.

Ameda Lactaline Personal-Dual Breastpump – This lets you pump both breasts at once. It's available from the company's website and from the National Childbirth Trust (Maternity Sales – see page 420) and costs £79.95.

Medela UK, Huntsman Drive, Northbank Industrial Park, Irlam, Manchester M44 5EG, UK, 00 44 (0)161 776 0400, www.medela. co.uk

US readers can find out more at www.medela.com; distributors in other countries are listed at www.medela.ch

The ***Symphony*** is a new model that offers '2-phase expression', meaning it mimics a baby's sucking and milking rhythm so as to encourage a faster let-down, increased milk flow and decreased pumping time. It pumps both breasts at the same time. It costs £995 plus VAT, but you can rent one from a hospital that acts as an agent for £35 a month plus a one-off payment of £21 for the starter pack (containing a bottle, tubes, etc. – to enable you to use the pump); or you can rent directly from the company for £35 a month plus £42 for the starter pack.

The ***Lactina*** is their older model. It costs £445 plus VAT and can pump both breasts at the same time if you like. You can rent it from a hospital that acts as an agent for £19 a month plus a one-off payment of £14 for the single-breast starter pack, or £21 for the double; or you can rent it directly from the company for £19 a month plus £35 for a single-breast starter pack, or £42 for a double.

The ***Mini Electric Breast Pump*** can be battery operated or plugged into a mains socket; it costs £42.95 and in the UK is also available from Boots and from Maternity Sales (see page 420).

Intavent Orthofix, Burney Court, Cordwallis Park, Maidenhead, Berkshire SL6 7BZ, UK, 00 44 (0)1628 594500; offers three electric pumps:

The ***Axicare CM12*** has a variable suction strength, adjustable to three levels, and its sucking rhythm can be preset or controlled by a fingertip and its suction strength is adjustable. It comes complete with a carrying case, and costs £480 plus VAT. The collection kit is an extra £16.75 plus VAT.

The ***Axicare CM10*** is a fully automatic pump with an automatic sucking rhythm but an adjustable suction strength. It comes with a carrying case, and costs £480 plus VAT. The collection kit (pack of five) is an extra £36.60 plus VAT.

The **Axicare CM8** is a semi-automatic pump providing constant suction whose strength and duration can be controlled to create the most comfortable sucking rhythm. It comes with a carrying case, and costs £340 plus VAT. The collection kit (pack of five) is an extra £36.50 plus VAT.

Hand pumps

Avent Isis pumps – This is an easy-to-use piston-action pump with a squeeze handle and a collecting funnel designed to mimic the action of the baby so as to stimulate let-downs and milk production. It is available from Cannon Avent Ltd, Glemsford, Colchester, Suffolk, UK, 00 44 (0)178 726 7000, www.aventbaby.com, and from some pharmacies and babycare outlets; it costs about £25.

Ameda One-Handed Breastpump – This piston-action pump is available from Ameda Egnell (see above) for £19.95.

Ameda Lact-h Hand Operated Breastpump – This costs £14.95.

Medela Harmony – The action of this pump mimics a baby's sucking and nursing rhythm; it's available in the UK from Medela UK (see above) or NCT Maternity Sales (see page 420) for £32.95. US readers can find out more at www.medela.com; distributors in other countries are listed at www.medela.ch

FREEZER BAGS

Freezer storage bags for expressed breast milk are available from NCT Maternity Sales (see page 420) and some chemists and baby shops.

FEEDING CUPS

Feeding cups suitable for preterm and older breastfed babies are available from NCT Maternity Sales (see page 420).

The Baby Beak – A small plastic cup with a big spout, suitable for feeding breast milk to young babies who can't yet take enough (or any) milk from the breast. Call the Baby Beak Company on 00 44 (0)1592 771962; one baby beak costs 25 pence plus the cost of a first-class stamp.

NURSING BRAS

NCT Maternity Sales (see page 000) has an excellent range of nursing bras, both drop cup and zip cup, in a variety of sizes (up to 46HH).

Blooming Marvellous has a good range of attractive nursing bras with matching knickers; call 0870 751 8977 from the UK for a catalogue, or visit www.bloomingmarvellous.co.uk

BREAST PADS

Washable pads

Ameda breast pads – Machine-washable 100% cotton pads from Ameda Egnell (see page 412) and from NCT Maternity Sales (see page 420).

Lansinoh Washable Nursing Pads from many independent pharmacies in the UK; more information at www.lansinoh.co.uk

Cone-shaped pads

Boots own cone-shaped pads available in the UK from Boots.

Lansinoh contoured, non-slip breast pads – from most local independent pharmacies in the UK; more information at www.lansinoh.co.uk

NIPPLE CREAM

Lansinoh cream – A pesticide-free lanolin cream for sore nipples; available in the UK from many independent pharmacies; more information from www.lansinoh.co.uk

HYDROGEL DRESSINGS

VioGel Breastfeeding Discs – Call 00 44 (0)1825 733566 or visit www.viohealthcare.com

AVENT NIPLETTES

These are made by Cannon Avent Ltd, Glemsford, Colchester, Suffolk, UK, 00 44 (0)178 726 7000, and are available from pharmacists, though you may have to ask for a special order; alternatively, visit www.aventbaby.com and order over the Internet. One costs £19.99; two, £29.99.

BREASTFEEDING SUPPLEMENTERS

Medela Supplemental Nursing System – Made in Switzerland, this is available in the UK from Medela UK by calling 00 44 (0)161 776 0400 and costs around £20. Distributors in other countries are listed at www.medela.ch

Lact-Aid Nursing Trainer System is the original supplementer; more information from www.lact-aid.com

MILK BANK NEWSLETTER

Milk Banking: News and Views, a newletter, is available from Gillian Weaver, Human Milk Bank, Queen Charlotte's and Chelsea Hospital, Goldhawk Road, London W6 0XG, UK.

The UK Drugs in Lactation Advisory Service, for health professionals, is available from the Trent Medicines Information Service, Leicester Royal Infirmary, Leicester, www.ukmicentral.nhs.uk.

BREASTFEEDING INFORMATION ON THE INTERNET

Anyone whose work involves helping women to breastfeed is welcome to seek or exchange information about breastfeeding and lactation via email on the Internet. If you'd like to do this, email LISTSERV@library1.UNMED.edu and write in the message box: Subscribe LACTNET, your first name, your last name (but use no punctuation).

BREASTFEEDING EDUCATION PACKS FOR SCHOOLS

Breastfeeding Matters packs for different ages are available from the Norwich Joint Breastfeeding Initiative. Prices and mail order details from the NJBI, Lawson Road Health Centre, Lawson Road, Norwich NR3 4LE, UK.

OPEN-SIDED CRIB AND COT

These are made by Huggababy – call 00 44 (0)1874 711 629, or visit www.huggababy.co.uk; they are sturdy and attractive and designed to be placed next to the parental bed for easy night-time breastfeeding. With the crib or cot alongside your bed, its open side next to you, you simply slip your baby across into your bed when he needs a feed and slip him back when he's finished.

The Bedside Crib has one side that drops completely and multiple height options, allowing the cot mattress to be exactly level with your bed; it costs £99 (including UK delivery but not including a mattress).

The Global Bedside Cot has a drop side that lifts and slides up and over so it's completely out of the way. This can be converted into a four-sided cot, or a bed without sides, and costs £145 (including UK delivery).

FERTILITY PREDICTION

Fertile Focus 'Lick and Look' ovulation detector – If relying on breastfeeding and the symptothermal method for contraception, this microscope-like gadget the size of a lipstick can help by revealing the fern-like pattern in your dried saliva that's present only during fertile days (from three or four days before ovulation to two to three days after). It costs £21.23 from Med-Direct International, at www.fertilitytest.co.uk

First Response Ovulation Prediction Kit – This can be a useful guide for breastfeeding women using the symptothermal method of contraception. Available from pharmacies, it can be useful when periods have returned to predict when ovulation is likely to return. This is because, when used towards the middle of the cycle, it indicates whether you are likely to ovulate by measuring hormone levels in urine. If ovulation is on its way, you can use additional contraception during the fertile days five days before and the day after ovulation.

If your periods haven't yet returned, it's too expensive to use each day but can be useful as an additional guide if you've observed changes in bodily signs (e.g. vaginal mucus) which indicate that ovulation is near.

Fertility Awareness Kit – This costs £19.99 and contains an explanatory video, thermometer and charts. Details from the Family Planning Association (0845 122 8600 in the UK).

ORGANIZATIONS IN THE UK

La Leche League of Great Britain (LLL GB) – BM 3424, London WC1N 3XX, UK; call 0845 120 2918 in the UK, or visit www.laleche.org.uk

La Leche League has many leaders and groups, and also provides a wide range of information, including books and many leaflets and details of products including baby slings.

Also, *for the blind or visually handicapped*, many publications in Braille, on cassette-tape or reel-to-reel. Ask for LLLI's special publications list.

For a price list, send a stamped self-addressed business-size envelope. For information in languages other than English, ask for the translation list (No. 508).

National Childbirth Trust (NCT) – Alexandra House, Oldham Terrace, London W3 6NH, UK; call 0870 444 8708 in the UK with breastfeeding queries or visit www.nctpregnancyandbabycare.com.

The NCT's Breastfeeding Promotion Group has many counsellors and a wide range of information including books and leaflets. Its Experience Register lists women who have breastfed in special situations and are willing to discuss these with other parents.

NCT Maternity Sales (call 0870 112 1120 in the UK or visit www.nctms.co.uk) offers a wide range of nursing bras, underwear, nightwear and various baby-care products.

The Association of Breastfeeding Mothers – This organization has local groups and counsellors who offer information and support; call 00 44 (0)20 7813 1481 or visit www.abm.me.uk

SOME OF THE MANY OTHER ORGANIZATIONS

Australian Breastfeeding Association – (formerly Nursing Mothers Association of Australia), 1818–1822 Malvern Road, East Malvern, Victoria 3145, Australia; call 0061 3 98850855, or visit www.breastfeeding.asn.au

La Leche League International, – 1400 N. Meacham Road, Schaumburg, IL 60173–4808, call (001) 847 519 7730, or visit www.lalecheleague.org

International Lactation Consultant Association – 1500 Sunday Drive, Suite 102, Raleigh, North Carolina, 27607, USA; call (001) 919 861 5577, or visit www.ilca.org

Any prices mentioned are correct at the time of going to print.

Index

PETER HOBSON

The Cradle of Thought

Exploring the Origins of Thinking

PAN BOOKS

In this widely acclaimed book, Professor Peter Hobson suggests that it is the quality of a baby's exchange with its parents and carers during the first eighteen months of life that lays the foundations for emotional engagement and entry into the realm of communication and culture.

'Hobson presents in clear terms a theory about thinking that has implications for the origins of language, for what it means to be human and – the aspect most likely to disturb the general public he wants to reach – for parenting'
THES

'This is a superb book . . . providing a theory of human development that has social contact at its core. *The Cradle of Thought* is both beautifully written and scientifically provocative'
Professor Paul Bloom, Yale University

CLAIRE GILLMAN

The Best of Boys

Helping your sons through their teenage years

PAN BOOKS

'Raising sons can be wonderfully rewarding, but it can be challenging. As a parent, you can benefit from sharing ideas and take comfort in knowing that others are undergoing similar experiences.'

Growing up is never easy, but for boys today the pressures seem to be increasing. With depression and suicide rates among male adolescents on the up, giving them the right support and guidance is vital. This book offers parents all the information they need on the enormous changes boys go through from eleven to eighteen. Practical, informative and reassuring, it draws on advice from experts, a wide range of other parents and from teenage boys themselves.

With the message that we should celebrate teenage boys, this down-to-earth, positive book is essential reading for all parents of sons.

OTHER PAN BOOKS

AVAILABLE FROM PAN MACMILLAN

PETER HOBSON		
THE CRADLE OF THOUGHT	0 330 48828 7	£7.99
CLAIRE GILLMAN		
THE BEST OF BOYS	0 330 41149 7	£8.99
LYNNE ROBINSON & HOWARD NAPPER		
INTELLIGENT EXERCISE WITH PILATES & YOGA	0 330 49389 2	£12.99